Foundations of Health Professions Education Research

Foundations of Health Professions Education Research

Principles, Perspectives and Practices

Edited by

Charlotte E. Rees
The University of Newcastle, Callaghan, New South Wales, Australia

Lynn V. Monrouxe
The University of Sydney, Camperdown, New South Wales, Australia

Bridget C. O'Brien
University of California San Francisco, San Francisco, California, USA

Lisi J. Gordon
The University of Dundee, Dundee, Scotland, UK

Claire Palermo
Monash University, Clayton, Victoria, Australia

WILEY Blackwell

Registered Offices
John Wiley & Sons, Inc., 111 River Street, Hoboken, NJ 07030, USA
John Wiley & Sons Ltd, The Atrium, Southern Gate, Chichester, West Sussex, PO19 8SQ, UK

For details of our global editorial offices, customer services, and more information about Wiley products visit us at www.wiley.com.

Wiley also publishes its books in a variety of electronic formats and by print-on-demand. Some content that appears in standard print versions of this book may not be available in other formats.

A catalogue record for this book is available from the Library of Congress

Paperback ISBN: 9781119839484; ePub ISBN: 9781119839507; ePDF ISBN: 9781119839491

Cover Design: Wiley
Cover Image: Courtesy of Lynn Monrouxe

Set in 10.5/13pt STIXTwoText by Integra Software Services Pvt. Ltd, Pondicherry, India
Printed and bound by CPI Group (UK) Ltd, Croydon, CR0 4YY

C9781119839484_270723

We dedicate this book to our current and past research students, research assistants and fellows, as well as the early and mid-career researchers we have collaborated with, supervised, and mentored. We have truly learnt so much about research (and ourselves as researchers) from working with you and your projects. It has been a privilege to share the research journey with you.

Contents

Foreword: Foundations?

This book is about foundations; the foundations of a field that many scholars have built up over the years to the point that a volume reassessing and outlining those foundations has become necessary. But what does it mean for something to have foundations? I ask you to pause and reflect before diving deeper into this book as thinking about the significances and meanings of foundations will help make your exploration of this volume all the more rewarding.

The term 'foundation' can refer to whatever a structure, whether physical, social, or cultural, has been built upon. Foundations may be deliberately constructed as a basis for what follows, or they may simply be what was there before. There is a temporality to this sense of foundation. Foundations precede, they imply something historical, something archaeological, something focused on the contexts that gave rise to something else and within which those later things need to be understood. The foundations of health professions education research (HPER) from this perspective imply therefore that there was a 'before' on which HPER was built. And yet, although the history of health professions education (HPE) can be linked to the founding of schools and programmes, and to system-wide reforms, HPER did not start at one point in time; it coalesced out of many threads and actions over an extended period of time. In terms of education, we might think back to the influence of Hippocrates or Galen, William Harvey or Thomas Sydenham, or to the traditions of medical training developed at Padua or Edinburgh, all of which have contributed to the foundations of HPE.

Foundations in this sense are akin to the tributaries of a great river. Some are long and deep like sociology, psychology, economics, and organisational science, while others are more obscure such as the epidemiological philosophies of science, or the emergent practices of action research and design research implied in the work of innovators and inventors. These foundations are often philosophies of science, scientific disciplines, or paradigms, each with their own histories and narratives, which beyond historical curiosity, may have limited relevance to HPER today. Who today worries much about the contested threads of 'continental' philosophy and how Kant and later Nietzsche shaped the thinking of Husserl, whose work in turn shaped phenomenology and much of the hermeneutic aspects of the qualitative sciences that HPE researchers employ? The foundations of HPER are primarily the foundations of the social sciences in general, albeit infused with beliefs and values from medicine and from the basic sciences.

Foundations can also refer to the deliberate creation of something new, such as the founding of a school or university, or the functions of a foundry where things of substance are forged and cast. In this case, although historicity is implied, the focus is more on the intent and the acts of the founders. Indeed, this is the sense invoked whenever the emphasis is on the foundational person or people, or on their intentions, vision, hopes, or values. This is often a normative perspective that considers how things should have been according to some definitive source, and how reality has diverged from this founding vision ever since.

Foundations can also refer to that which underlies something in the present moment. From this perspective, foundations focus instead on the here and now and surveying and appraising the reasons for the current form and function of things; warts and all. This usually means unravelling the peculiar entanglements of different elements, traditions, structures, and practices that may never have been designed to interact. Foundations from this point of view can therefore be understood as a palimpsest of earlier things inscribing those that follow them. Examining foundations in this light can tell us much about the morphogenesis of contemporary HPE and HPER. For instance, in HPER we can think of the idiosyncrasies of professional identity formation with its jumble of service, vocation, agency, hierarchy, status, and other principles. Some of this foundational thinking comes from ancient tradition, some from current social realities. Some comes from guild-like collectivism, some from entrepreneurial competitiveness. As another example, we might consider Norman's generational model [1], starting with a coalescence of scholars from very different backgrounds moving in and out of the, as yet undefined, spaces of HPER. These pioneers were followed by those who trained in other disciplines but pursued careers in HPER and established it as a distinct field, and they were followed in turn by scholars who trained in HPER, who knew little else, and who thought of it as a discipline as much as a field [1]. Each generation reinvented (and will reinvent) the foundations they encountered such that foundations become a standing wave defined both by tradition and the changing perspectives of the scholars in the field over time. For instance, that the historical figures I mentioned earlier were all men reflects a male-dominated past that is not reflected in the present or (I hope) in the future of our field.

Finally, foundations can mean covering over things or erasing them altogether. Indeed, although concealment and elision are not what one may first consider in thinking about foundations, they are important concerns. Foundations may simply just cover over what preceded, forming another stratum of change and development, such as the widespread adoption of Internet technologies over the past three decades. Foundations may also deliberately erase what went before, creating a *terra nullius* on which something new and better might be built. This sense of foundations is reflected in the episodic paradigm changes in scientific fields and disciplines that are often as much about what is rejected as they are about what replaces such ejecta. For example, some examples of historical people and places I gave earlier were drawn from Western and Anglophone perspectives, but what about others? The elision of non-Western traditions' influence on the foundations of Western medicine and healthcare is a long-standing concern, reflected, for instance, in the extent to which Hippocrates and Galen are celebrated while the influence of Ibn Sina, Ibn Rushd, and Confucius (among many others) is rarely acknowledged.

Whether we focus on the unintended or deliberately shaped bases on which other things were built, or on the simple facts and consequences of precedence, or on acts of founding, or even on the underlying assumptions and idiosyncrasies of origins and their consequences, a consideration of foundations may tell us many things. Exploring foundations can help us to remember that science is not itself an objective or natural phenomenon; it was created by many people, working both together and in parallel, as well as cumulatively over time. Not one of them laid the foundations for science alone; they all contributed to them. We do not stand only on the shoulders of giants; we stand on the shoulders of everyone who has preceded us – giants and lesser mortals alike.

Although we talk about foundations as single entities, the foundations of HPER are made of many parts, as this book outlines. Chapter 1 argues the foundational purposes of HPER are both *'to generate new knowledge and to improve education'*. Chapter 2 explores theoretical and philosophical foundations of HPER with a particular focus on the purposes and bases of scientific disciplines in the context of HPER. Chapter 3 outlines the ethical and moral foundations of HPER. Chapter 4 considers different methodological foundations and their meaning in designing and appraising quality in HPER. These foundations are then expanded on in exploring different approaches to HPER with their differing foundational ideas. Chapter 5 illustrates scientific foundations, Chapter 6 outlines realist foundations, Chapter 7 outlines interpretivist foundations, Chapter 8 explores critical foundations, and finally, Chapter 9 outlines pragmatic approaches and their associated foundations. The book closes by describing the foundations of participation in HPER communities and discourses, with Chapter 10 outlining the foundations of expressing and communicating HPER in putting studies together, Chapter 11 describing the foundations of disseminating HPER once a study has been completed, and Chapter 12 outlining the foundations of translating HPER into practice and the potential impacts thereof.

There are clearly many dimensions to the foundations of a field like HPER. However, when we speak of foundations, we imply coherence and contiguity among their constituent parts. As much as this book outlines where this contiguity can or might be found, like any area of human activity, there are also gaps and conflicts. Indeed, if HPER had been deliberately designed, it would not resemble the HPER we have today, which has evolved organically and haphazardly over time. A study of foundations can tell us how we got to where we are. To that end, we might employ concepts of morphogenesis or poststructuralist discourse analyses. A study of foundations can also tell us why it is we do what we do when we know it is not ideal. From this perspective, we might draw on bounded rationality theory to consider the symbolic orders within which we practice [2]. A study of foundations can get us to reappraise and deepen our understanding and commitment to what we do in terms of moral agency and paradigm (ideology). A study of foundations can help us to be more selective and critical of why we do what we do; many scholars change track mid-career once they develop deeper understandings of the foundations of their chosen field or paradigm. A study of foundations can also help us to better appraise the evidence base we draw on, all of which is inevitably made up of past events and historical thinking.

This book may, in your hands, do some, many, or all of these things. It may also take you to other places or lead you to question the foundations of why this book was written, how it was written, and what influence it might have. These are all good things. I encourage you to think about why it is you are reading this, and what it is you seek or hope to find in this book or through it. You should also think about the various worlds of HPER in which you live or that you hope to explore, not just in terms of how they are right now but where they came from and where they are going. To do that you must attend to foundations.

In closing, let me return to the idea of foundations as an investment in the future, as a way of protecting and nurturing that which is good (as in Isaac Asimov's Foundation novels). Laying down a solid foundation is not just to react to the present but to protect against and to embrace whatever the future may bring. To that end, foundations are a form of stewardship, and they are a form of defence against attack and decay. They are also the basis of hope and continuity from which better things might be built. Either way, foundations are an investment in the future, and they are the investments one makes in those who will follow. Your foundations are your ancestors, but you put down foundations for those who will follow you. Your successors will stand on your shoulders, as you have stood on the shoulders of those who came before you. The foundations of science serve us, and they are us.

Rachel H. Ellaway
University of Calgary, Alberta, Canada

REFERENCES

1. Norman G. Fifty years of medical education research: waves of migration. *Med Educ.* 2011;45(8):785–791.

2. Gigerenzer G. What is bounded rationality? In Viale R, ed. *Routledge Handbook of Bounded Rationality*. London and New York: Routledge; 2021:55–70.

About the Editors

Charlotte E. Rees BSc (Hons), GradCertTerEd (Mgt), MEd, PhD, PFHEA, FRCP (Edin)
Charlotte is Head of School, School of Health Sciences, The University of Newcastle, New South Wales, and Adjunct Professor, Monash Centre for Scholarship in Health Education (MCSHE), Faculty of Medicine, Nursing & Health Sciences, Monash University, Victoria, Australia. With over 20 years' postdoctoral experience in health professions education and research, Charlotte has expertise in workplace learning, healthcare professionalism, identities, and transitions. She employs realist and interpretivist approaches including longitudinal qualitative research, narrative enquiry, and realist evaluation methods.
@charlreessidhu

Lynn V. Monrouxe BSc (Hons), PGDip, PhD, FAcadMEd
Lynn is Professor and Academic Lead for Healthcare Professions Education Research, and Convenor of Waranara (Healthcare Professions Education Research Network), The University of Sydney, New South Wales, Australia. After completing her PhD in cognitive linguistics using experimental methods, she has 20 years' experience in health professions education and research. With expertise in professional identities, healthcare professionalism, and workplace learning, she employs realist, interpretivist, and pragmatic approaches including qualitative and quantitative methodologies. She is especially interested in interactional analyses (narrative, conversation, and discourse) using audio and video data.
@lynnmonrouxe

Bridget C. O'Brien BSc, MSc, PhD
Bridget is Professor of Medicine and Education Scientist, Center for Faculty Educators, University of California. San Francisco, San Francisco, USA. She has more than 15 years' postdoctoral experience as a researcher and educator in health professions. Bridget's research focuses largely on understanding and improving workplace learning among health professionals using interpretivist and pragmatic approaches that employ a variety of qualitative and mixed methodologies. She has also studied various aspects of publishing including authorship and peer review.
@bobrien_15

Lisi J. Gordon BSc, MSc, PhD, FHEA
Lisi is Senior Lecturer in the Centre for Medical Education, School of Medicine, University of Dundee, Scotland, UK. Lisi has 10 years' experience as a physiotherapist, and 20 years as an educator including 10 years' doctoral and postdoctoral experience in health professions education research. Her expertise focuses on transitions, leadership, diversity and inclusion, and identities. She employs interpretivist and critical approaches including longitudinal qualitative research, narrative enquiry, diary-based, and visual methods.
@lisigordon

Claire Palermo BSc, MNutDiet, MPH, GradCertHthProfEd, PhD, PFHEA, Fellow DA

Claire is Associate Dean (Teaching and Learning), Faculty of Medicine, Nursing & Health Sciences, Monash University, Victoria, Australia. With 10 years' experience as a dietitian and 15 years each as a teacher and education researcher, Claire has expertise in competency-based education and assessment, and workforce development employing critical and pragmatic approaches (using qualitative methodologies especially).

@ClairePalermo

Author Contributions

This book represents the culmination of editors' individual and collective efforts over many years; including years of conducting health professions education research (HPER), supervising others' HPER, and teaching research philosophies, methodologies, and methods through workshops, short courses, and award-bearing courses like Masters and Doctorates in Health Professions Education.

Charlotte led the development of this book proposal in January 2020; based on work done in 2017 with Claire at Monash University to develop a five-day intensive course introducing learners to HPER. This initial book proposal was substantially improved through discussions with, and suggestions from, Lynn, Bridget, Lisi, and Claire, who helped shape the final book proposal submitted to, and accepted by, Wiley Blackwell.

At the start of this book-writing project, we agreed that this would be an edited textbook, but that Chapters 2–12 would be written and edited by at least one editor (often two), including one to three external contributors as co-authors, mostly early career researchers (ECRs). This was especially important to us because we wanted the book to be developed *with* and *for* those relatively new to HPER. And the more senior you get, the harder it is to put yourself in the shoes of an ECR. Indeed, our external contributors have been priceless in reminding us what is understandable, and what is not, throughout the process of writing this book.

In terms of the editors, we decided on editor order based on contribution (rather than alphabetical), but with Claire's position as last author akin to senior author given the Monash-based genesis of the book. Charlotte led the overall book project, managing regular editorial meetings, progress, and timelines, and liaising with the publisher. She led the writing of five chapters (Chapters 1, 2, 5, 6, and 12), edited Chapters 3 and 13, and gave extensive feedback on the remaining chapters. She, along with Lynn, also edited the whole book. Lynn led the writing of three chapters (Chapters 3, 7, and 13), edited three others (Chapters 1, 6, and 12), gave feedback on additional chapters, took the book photographs, and worked with Anique on the book cover. Bridget led the writing of two chapters (Chapters 4 and 9), contributed to the writing and editing of one chapter (Chapter 11), edited another chapter (Chapter 3), gave extensive feedback on other chapters, and section-edited Part I of the book. Together with Charlotte and Lynn, Bridget managed our half-yearly webinars with external contributors. Lisi led the writing of Chapter 11, contributed to the writing and editing of another three chapters (Chapters 2, 7, and 8), and section-edited Part III of the book. Finally, Claire led the writing of two chapters (Chapters 8 and 10), edited another three chapters (Chapters 4, 5, and 9), gave extensive feedback on other chapters, and section-edited the largest part of the book (Part II). Claire also managed our book's data repository and contributor email communications. All editors were involved in pulling together the Book Glossary, with involvement of all chapter authors. From an editorial perspective, we largely stuck to guidelines about writing style, tone, and level, as well as chapter formatting, in order to maintain consistency across the chapters and parts, thereby benefiting learners reading the whole book in chronological order. However, you will note some differences between chapters due to variations in writing style and chapter content: some chapters are more philosophical/theoretical; others are more practical.

All nineteen contributors to Chapters 2–12, provided illustrative cases for their selected chapters (thirty cases in total across the book representing diverse topics, approaches, methodologies/methods/theories, study participants, healthcare professions, and countries/regions). All contributors also commented on and/or edited their chapter, plus all bar one provided peer-review feedback for another chapter. Additionally, some contributors were more involved in the writing process, for example, about half wrote the first draft of a chapter section. Six of our chapter contributors (all early career researchers from Monash University) also peer-reviewed one of the three book parts: Part I (Dr Van Nguyen and Dr Mahbub Sarkar), Part II (Dr Jonathan Foo and Dr Olivia King) and Part III (Dr Louise Allen and Dr Ella Ottrey). They also worked together to co-author the Afterword for our book. Furthermore, as mentioned above, Dr Anique Atherley worked tirelessly on book cover designs. We include brief biographies for our contributors here (in alphabetical order):

Louise Allen BNutDiet (Hons), GradCertEdDes, PhD

Louise is Lecturer, Monash Centre for Professional Development and Monash Online Education, Monash University, Australia. She is a dietitian by background and an early career researcher having completed her PhD in 2020. Her PhD used a pragmatic approach to explore the broad impacts of continuing professional development in the health professions. She completed a Fulbright Postdoctoral Scholarship 2022/2023 furthering her research in continuing professional development and her qualitative research skills.
@Louise_Allen3

Lulu Alwazzan MD, MMEd, PhD

Lulu is Assistant Professor of Medical Education and Head of the Assessment and Examination Unit, College of Medicine, Imam Mohammad Ibn Saud Islamic University, Saudi Arabia. With a medical degree and postgraduate medical education training, she is currently the chairperson of the Department of Medical Education. Having received her Medical Education PhD in 2019, her scholarly work examines leadership/leadership development and professional development using qualitative methods.
@Alwazzan_L

Anique Atherley MBBS, MPH, PGCUTL, PhD

Anique is Assistant Professor, Academy for Teaching and Learning, Ross University School of Medicine, Barbados. She is an early career researcher who received her PhD in Medical Education in 2021 through dual candidature with Maastricht University, Netherlands and Western Sydney University, Australia. Anique has been working in medical education research since 2012 and has interests in transitions, academic and research coaching, and using qualitative social network analysis, longitudinal qualitative research, and review methodology.
@aniqueatherley

Maria A. Blanco EdM, EdD

Maria is Associate Dean for Faculty Development and Associate Professor, Department of Psychiatry, School of Medicine, Tufts University, USA. In 2002, she earned her Masters in Education at Harvard Graduate School of Education, followed by a Doctor of Education in 2007. Maria has been an educator and researcher in health professions for more than 24 years. Her scholarly work covers various topics (e.g., mentoring, faculty development, diversity, equity, and inclusion) and involves qualitative and mixed methodologies.
@MariaABlanco1

Gabrielle Brand BN, MN (Research), PhD
Gabrielle is Associate Professor, Monash Nursing & Midwifery, Monash University, Australia. After gaining her PhD in 2013, Gabrielle focuses on narrative medicine, health humanities, and creative and critical pedagogy including co-design. She leads a health humanities research programme called *Depth of Field*, drawing on healthcare consumers' voice (narrative) and art (narrative artefacts and visual methodologies) to co-design strengths-based, consumer-driven health professions workforce education resources.
@GabbyBrand6

Megan E.L. Brown MBBS(H), PGCHPE, PGCRT, PhD, FHEA
Megan is Senior Lecturer in Medical Education and Programme Lead for the Postgraduate Certificate in Medical Education, University of Buckingham, UK. She is also Teaching Fellow in Medical Education Research, Imperial College London, UK. With a medical background, she is now a full-time medical educator and researcher since her PhD completion in 2022. Her research interests include the philosophy of medical education, longitudinal learning, and professional identity, and using creative approaches to qualitative research.
@Megan_EL_Brown

Jeffrey J.H. Cheung HBSc, MSc, PhD
Jeffrey is Assistant Professor, Department of Medical Education, University of Illinois College of Medicine at Chicago, USA. He received his PhD in 2019 from The University of Toronto, Canada where he also completed his research fellowship at The Wilson Centre. Drawing on scientific approaches, his research primarily applies theories from cognitive psychology to clarify how educators can design learning experiences that better prepare learners for clinical practice, and how to assess learners' capacity to be flexible with their knowledge/skills.
@CheungJJH

Anna T. Cianciolo BA, MA, PhD
Anna is Associate Professor of Medical Education, Southern Illinois University School of Medicine, USA and Editor-in-Chief of *Teaching and Learning in Medicine*. She 'emigrated' to medical education in 2011 after 10 years conducting performance-based training research/development for the US Army (PhD, 2001). Her research interests include small-group collaborative and peer-assisted learning, clinical teaching, learning and assessment, clinical reasoning, and scholarly professional development. She draws on diverse approaches/methodologies to investigate practical problems.
@cianciolo_anna

Paul E.S. Crampton BSc (Hons), MSc, PhD, SFHEA, FAcadMEd
Paul is lead for the Health Professions Education Unit (HPEU), Lecturer in Medical Education, and Programme Director for the MSc in Health Professions Education at Hull York Medical School, University of York, UK. Paul has been working in medical education since 2008 and gained his PhD in 2015. He has expertise in subjects such as interprofessional learning, professionalism, quality assurance, longitudinal placements, workplace learning, fitness to practice, and continuing professional development, drawing on diverse methodologies.
@pes_crampton

Jonathan Foo BPhysiotherapy (Hons), PhD
Jon is a Physiotherapist and Lecturer, Department of Physiotherapy, Faculty of Medicine, Nursing & Health Sciences, Monash University, Australia. He is an early career researcher (PhD 2021) with a passion for optimising resource allocation – promoting

research, education, and healthcare that makes best use of available resources. His quantitative work has primarily focused on the application of economic theory and methodologies, including within the context of health professions education research. @JonFromAus

Ghufran Jassim BSc (Hons), MD (Hons), HPEC Diploma, MSc, PhD, ABMS, ICGP, Advance HE Fellowship Cert
Ghufran is Associate Professor and Head of Department of Family Medicine, Royal College of Surgeons in Ireland (RCSI), Bahrain. With a medical background, she received her PhD in 2014, and has recently completed the RCSI health education profession diploma programme and fellowship in advanced higher education. Her research interests include women's health and medical education and her expertise is primarily with bioethics research including quantitative, qualitative, and review methodologies.
@Ghufranprof

Olivia A. King BPod (Hons), Grad Cert Diabetes Education, PhD
Olivia is Manager, Research Capability Building, Western Alliance and Adjunct Research Associate, Monash University, Australia. She is an early career researcher (PhD 2018) and is passionate about developing research capability in rural and regional health workforces. Her research interests include health professions education, allied health workforce, and sociology of the professions. Her expertise is primarily with qualitative methodologies.
@Oliviaaking

Van N.B. Nguyen BN, MN, PhD
Van is Lecturer, Monash Nursing & Midwifery, Monash University, Australia. For her PhD (conferred 2017), Van developed and validated the Clinical Nurse Educator Skill Acquisition Assessment (CNESAA) tool and is passionate about using this to explore factors contributing to nurse educators' clinical teaching confidence. As an early career researcher, Van is interested in health professions education and workforce capacity building research, as well as expanding her expertise in diverse research methodologies.
@VanNBNguyen

Ella Ottrey BNutrDietet, BNut (Hons), PhD
Ella is Senior Research Fellow, Monash Centre for Scholarship in Health Education, Monash University, Australia. She has 10 years' experience as a dietitian and three years' postdoctoral experience in health professions education research, having completed her PhD in 2019. Ella has research expertise and interest in preparedness for practice, transitions into practice, and healthcare workforce development using interpretivist approaches.
@ellaottrey

Nicole Redvers BSc, ND, MPH
Nicole is a member of the Deninu K'ue First Nation in Denendeh (Northwest Territories, Canada) and has worked with Indigenous patients, scholars, and communities around the globe across her career. She is Associate Professor, Schulich School of Medicine and Dentistry, University of Western Ontario, Canada. She is actively involved at regional, national, and international levels promoting the inclusion of Indigenous perspectives in both human and planetary health research and practice.
@DrNicoleRedvers

Eliot L. Rees MBChB, PGCert, MA, FHEA
Eliot is Lecturer in Medical Education, Keele University and National Institute for Health Research (NIHR) Academic Clinical Fellow in General Practice, University College London, UK. Eliot has been working in medical education research since 2012 and is submitting his PhD thesis in 2023. He has research expertise in selection, widening access, peer teaching, and primary care medical education using diverse approaches including quantitative, qualitative, and review methodologies.
@ELRees1

Mahbub Sarkar BEd (Hons), MEd, PhD, SFHEA
Mahbub is Senior Lecturer of Educational Research, Faculty of Medicine, Nursing & Health Sciences, Monash University, Australia. Having gained his PhD in STEM Education in 2012, he made the transition to health professions education research in 2018. He has over 15 years' experience researching educational issues from early years to undergraduate levels. His current research interests include developing employability capital for healthcare students and improving professional learning for university educators. He primarily employs qualitative and mixed methods approaches.
@MahbubS

Ahsan Sethi BDS, MPH, MMEd, PhD, FDTFEd, FAIMER Fellow, FHEA
Ahsan is Associate Professor and Programme Coordinator for the MSc in Health Professions Education, Qatar University, Qatar. He is also faculty at institutions internationally (e.g., University of Dundee, UK; Khyber Medical University, Pakistan). He completed his PhD in Medical Education (2016) at the University of Dundee. With over 12 years' experience as a dentist, educator, and researcher, his research focuses on curriculum, assessment/accreditation, blended learning, and professional development. He largely draws on pragmatic approaches employing mixed methods.
@drahsansethi

Marieke van der Schaaf PhD
Marieke is Professor of Research and Development of Health Professions Education. She is Director of the Utrecht Center for Research and Development of Health Professions Education, University Medical Center Utrecht and of the Life Sciences Education Research PhD programme, Graduate School of Life Sciences, Utrecht University, Netherlands. She earned her PhD in 2005 and has interests in health professionals' expertise development, feedback, and educational innovations. She uses a pluralism of approaches and methods (e.g., mixed-methods).
@MariekevdSchaaf

Acknowledgements

It takes a community to pull together an edited textbook, so we have numerous people and organisations (plus the odd pet) to thank here; without whom the book would have been challenging at best, impossible at worst.

First, we would like to thank our contributors (most of whom are early career researchers) for your wonderful inputs into Chapters 2–12 – for your writing, editing, and peer-reviewing. Across these chapters, we share over thirty diverse case studies based on our contributors' (and our own) research. These case studies are diverse in terms of the health professions education (HPE) topics covered (e.g., teaching, learning, assessment, simulation, professionalism, professional identities, faculty development, transitions, well-being), the research approaches taken (i.e., scientific, realist, interpretivist, critical, and pragmatic) and methodologies/methods/theories employed, the study participants included (learners, educators, patients), the health professions researched (medicine, nursing, allied health), and countries/regions included (Asia-Pacific, Australia, Canada, Europe, Middle East, UK, USA). We would also like to thank the co-authors of the papers featured in the case studies (noting that our interpretations of these cases are ours alone and may not represent those of our co-authors). Returning to our contributors, we would especially like to thank seven who went beyond the call of duty in either helping us design the book cover (Dr Anique Atherley, Ross University School of Medicine, Barbados) or peer-review entire book sections (as well as chapters) and writing our book's afterword. All from Monash University, we thank (in alphabetical order): Dr Louise Allen, Dr Jonathan Foo, Dr Olivia King, Dr Van Nguyen, Dr Ella Ottrey, and Dr Mahbub Sarkar. Extra thanks go to Ella for her detailed proofreading of the whole book. We are also hugely appreciative to Professor Rachel Ellaway, University of Calgary, for writing the book's thought-provoking foreword – thanks Rachel for taking the time and for sharing your wisdom so generously. Lastly, in terms of our contributors, we would like to thank Associate Professor Narelle Warren, Monash University, for her peer review of the ethics chapter.

Second, we would like to thank our institutions for providing us with resources (e.g., time, IT, library) to develop, write, and edit this book: The University of Newcastle (Charlotte), Murdoch University (Charlotte), The University of Sydney (Lynn), University of California San Francisco (Bridget), University of Dundee (Lisi), and Monash University (Claire). We also thank our colleagues at these institutions for giving us the space to write, as well as allowing us to bounce our ideas off them. And we especially thank our colleagues in the Monash Centre for Scholarship in Health Education (Dr Olivia King, Dr Van Nguyen, and Dr Mahbub Sarkar), who helped two of us (Charlotte and Claire) co-create a five-day intensive course on health professions education research in 2017 on which this book proposal was based. We would also like to thank our research students, assistants, and fellows across our careers for putting our ideas on the spot – encouraging us to continuously think about and question research, how it ought to be done and why, and what that means for who we think we are (and ought to be) as researchers.

Third, we would like to thank the supportive and encouraging Wiley Blackwell team for commissioning the book, giving us feedback on the proposal, chapters, and book, and for helping us navigate (often COVID-related) challenges along the way.

Thanks especially to James Watson (Commissioning Editor), Jenny Seward (Managing Editor), and Ella Elliot (Editorial Assistant).

Finally, we would like to thank our wonderful families and friends for their support and encouragement, and for reducing their expectations of our time and attention during two years of busy thinking, writing, and editing (often at unsociable hours). More specifically, our personal thanks go to:

Charlotte: Thanks to my chapter contributors (Lulu, Jeff, Paul, Jon, Olivia, and Van) – I have enjoyed learning with you and from you in the write-up of our chapters. Thanks as ever go to my enormously patient family – Sid and Kitty – who put up with considerable periods of inattention when I get into the zone of reading and writing. I love you both. And thanks to my Miniature Schnauzer Herbert whose twice-daily walks have kept me sane – during COVID and this book-writing project. Many of my best ideas happen on our shared walks and he is also good for cuddles. Finally, thanks to Lynn, Bridget, Lisi, and Claire; all of whom I have worked with previously but never all together before. You are formidable women – individually and collectively. Thanks for your insights, suggestions, advice, support, good humour, and your unwavering patience whenever I got my knickers in a knot about our book progress and timelines.

Lynn: First and foremost, I would like to thank you, Charlotte: for your strength in leadership for the team across the many months of work (intellectually and emotionally). It is never easy working with a team of strong-minded academics, and at times I am sure it felt like you were herding cats. But here we are, on time, within the word limit and more knowledgeable for it. I would also like to thank my other co-editors, and sometimes co-authors: Bridget, Claire, and Lisi. Always supportive, always communicative, always a pleasure to work with. Thanks too for my early-career co-authors: Ella, Megan, Olivia, Paul, and Van. Learning with you, and about your work, is a delight. For inspiring work on the book illustrations, I would like to thank Anique. Thanks also to my Waranara colleagues for stimulating conversations (and occasional references) to help my thinking. Finally, there is Foohey (my Greyhound), sitting beside me, always reminding me that five o'clock *walkies* are more important than writing (in his world, at least!).

Bridget: When I joined the team of editors and authors on this book, I broke my promise to decline any more book projects. I am so glad I did. Working with an international team of editors (Charlotte, Claire, Lisi, and Lynn) and co-authors (Anique, Anna, Eliot, Ghufran, Louise, and Marieke) has been an incredibly rewarding and enriching experience. It makes me truly excited for the future of health professions education research and I am grateful for the opportunity. I also wish to thank my partner Damian, my pup Maddie (who occasionally shares her perspective during our meetings), and my colleague and mentor at UCSF, Patricia O'Sullivan, who now knows almost as much about pragmatic approaches as I do. Finally, I thank the editors for converting my American English to British – 'z's' are starting to look foreign to me and 'u's' are popping up all over the place!

Lisi: I would like to start by thanking co-editors Charlotte, Bridget, Claire, and Lynn for inviting me to share this adventure – you are all such brilliant academics, I still feel a bit star struck! Thanks to my co-writers (Anique, Anna, Ella, Gabrielle, Lulu, Megan, and Nicole); I have learned so much from you all. There are so many colleagues who have supported my academic career; I thank you all. I want to especially mention Professors Charlotte Rees, Divya Jindal-Snape, and Martina Sliwa, whose encouragement and belief in me (even when I wobble) has led me to do things I did not think I could. Finally, my husband, Iain, my 'little' boys Dougie and Fergus (both of whom grew past six foot during the writing of this book), and my friends: the

'Bookless Club' ladies (Amy, Anna, Fiona, Heather, and Susie). Your love and laughter are the touchstones that have kept me grounded.

Claire: I would especially like to thank Charlotte for having the idea for this book and making it happen. Thanks also go to my chapter co-authors (Jeff, Jon, Eliot, Gabby, Nicole, Maria, and Mahbub). I would like to thank Wayne Hodgson and Michelle Leech for their continued belief in me and for encouraging me to take on the challenge of working at the Monash Centre for Scholarship in Health Education. A very special thanks to Charlotte who significantly advanced my 10 years' postdoctoral experience as a health professions education researcher and developed my capabilities so much further. The time you invested in me, and your honest and timely feedback has developed me in more ways than you probably realise. Thanks to Carl, my husband, for being my biggest fan. To the rest of the editorial team, thank you for having me along this journey with you and for all your hard work and critique.

CHAPTER 1

Introducing Foundations of Health Professions Education Research

Charlotte E. Rees[1,2] and Lynn V. Monrouxe[3]

[1] The University of Newcastle, Callaghan, New South Wales, Australia
[2] Monash University, Clayton, Victoria, Australia
[3] The University of Sydney, Camperdown, New South Wales, Australia

Health professions education research (HPER) matters: it involves the creation and sharing of new knowledge about healthcare students and professionals' education and development. HPER considers a plethora of topics from student admission to healthcare professionals' (HCPs') retirement; with the aim of not only developing HCPs for their own benefit, but also for the benefit of others and organisations. Research priorities across HPER internationally, therefore, point towards diverse topics (e.g., preparedness for practice, transitions, assessment/feedback, workplace learning, educational methods) for the improvement of student learning and well-being, graduate employability, evidence-based education, organisational cultures, as well as addressing current challenges with education, policy, and political agendas [1–13]. Ultimately, HPER is about making better practitioners to improve patient health, safety, and well-being.

Based on the collective research supervision, teaching, and mentoring experiences of our interdisciplinary and international editorial team, we know that the number of individuals wanting to conduct HPER for the first time is increasing, and that existing HPE researchers want and need to improve the quality and impact of their HPER. Furthermore, our experience is backed up by evidence of: 'a solid increase of publications, numbers of specialized journals, professional associations, national and international conferences, academies for medical educators, masters and doctoral courses, and the establishment of many units of HPE scholarship' [14 p. 510]. Therefore, foundational guides such as this book serve to help novice and more experienced HPE researchers alike to build their understanding of the *principles, perspectives*, and *practices* of HPER. Using the latest evidence-based theoretical and methodological thinking, illustrated through our numerous case studies (including from early-career researchers), this down to earth guide will help build your capabilities in HPER; improving the quality and impact of your research.

In this introduction chapter, we clarify what we mean when we say *research* in section 1.1, and outline two key purposes of HPER in section 1.2. In section 1.3, we discuss past and future trends in HPER methods. In section 1.4, we discuss why you should read this book and how. Finally, in section 1.5, we outline what the book comprises. We hope this book will facilitate a smooth navigation of your HPER journey – helping you to choose your preferred route, as well as manage any inevitable detours (or potholes) along the way.

1.1 HEALTH PROFESSIONS EDUCATION RESEARCH (HPER)

Research is: 'a process of investigation leading to new insights, effectively shared' [15 p. 60]. But not all educational investigations offering insights are *research* [16]. It is therefore important that you understand what HPER is and what it is not. Educational research typically applies, tests, and/or builds theory (see Chapter 2). Educational research also involves systematic, rigorous, and peer-reviewed methodologies and methods with careful sampling, data collection, and analysis (see Chapters 5–9). We can contrast this with teaching evaluation activities that you might engage in for the purpose of developing your own practice. While an important activity, such work typically involves quick, non-systematic educational evaluations employing non-validated scales [17, 18]. We can also contrast education research with other published work such as commentaries, practical tips for educators, and education innovation dissemination [16]. The primary focus of educational research is the discovery of generalisable knowledge to benefit other researchers, with any resulting applications at the national and even international levels. This contrasts with teaching evaluations that focus on applying findings to your own local practice: making judgements about specific programmes within specific contexts [18–20]. This is not to say that HPER simply focuses on building new knowledge and theory for other researchers. HPER is a highly applied field continuously looking to make improvements to educational practice and policy (see Chapter 12).

1.2 WHAT ARE THE PURPOSES OF HPER?

Two key purposes of HPER can be seen as sitting at opposite ends of the same continuum: (1) to generate new knowledge; and (2) to improve education [19]. At the knowledge generation end of the continuum, research focuses on producing findings for other research producers (i.e., researchers). Consequently, research problems are defined by researchers (often due to gaps in knowledge). The focus here is on creating knowledge and theory, with other researchers evaluating research quality through peer review (see Chapter 4) [19, 21]. At the other end of the continuum, research centres on producing findings for research users (e.g., practitioners, policymakers, students) with research problems being typically defined by practitioners (often due to current problems with education). The focus here is on solving such educational problems through research, with users evaluating research quality through its uptake and use (see Chapter 12) [19, 21]. It is therefore important at the outset of your HPER that you understand the purpose(s) for conducting your project and where you sit on the continuum: is your primary purpose to generate new knowledge, is it to improve education, or is it to do both? Indeed, most HPE researchers nowadays (and we include ourselves in this camp) try to marry theory and practice in our HPER by making novel contributions to educational knowledge and/or theory *and* making a difference to education through improving educational practice and/or policy. It is not unusual for educational scholars to occupy multiple different roles: for example, as teachers, assessors, curriculum developers, educational leaders, educational policymakers, and educational researchers. Each of these roles we occupy might place us in various and changing positions on this producer–user continuum. It is therefore not uncommon that your position might shift on this continuum depending on context (e.g., different projects), the role you occupy (e.g., teacher in this project, leader in another project), or different time periods.

1.3 WHAT ARE THE TRENDS IN HPER METHODS?

In the UK and USA, the emergence of HPER occurred throughout the early- to mid-twentieth century triggered by multiple factors, not least policy-driven, including the: Atherlone, Goldmark, Wood, and Brown (UK/US nursing) [22], Flexner and Gies (US medicine and dentistry) [23], and Nuffield (UK pharmacy) reports [24]. Other contributing factors comprised the growing importance of scientific research, increased funding, journals, and publications for educational research, and calls for research accountability [25–31]. This has led the field to both retrospectively and prospectively consider trends in HPER topics and related approaches to develop strategic, forward-thinking HPER. And while research has tended to focus mainly on the *whats* of HPER (e.g., past topics under study and future needs), there is a select body of work that comments on trends in research approaches. Thus, commentaries and studies across a range of HPE disciplines, employing a variety of methods (e.g., bibliometrics, content analysis, critical discourse analysis, narrative review, scoping review, social network analysis, text network analysis), have examined HPER internationally across a time period of over fifty years (1963–2022) [29, 31–44]. Within this work, two key trends have been identified.

Firstly, there appears to be a distinct shift from primarily empirical research conducted within a positivist framework (see Chapter 5), towards the inclusion and acceptance of a wider range of research approaches (see Chapters 6–9) [26, 34, 37, 42, 43]. Indeed, due to the influence of clinically or experimentally trained researchers, it has been commonplace to: 'methodological[ly] transplant' [34 p. 14] gold-standard research approaches from those clinical fields to educational research [45]. So, the early years of HPER were dominated by randomised control trials (RCTs) and experimental methodologies (see Chapter 5). Over this lengthy time period, HPER has been influenced by psychology, thereby focusing on individuals (i.e., learners or teachers) [31]. Indeed, a great deal of early research has employed scientific approaches (see Chapter 5) focusing on programme effectiveness (i.e., justification studies) [46], rather than studies exploring what works, how, and why (i.e., description or clarification studies) [31, 44, 46–48]. Although this culture continues in some geographical and disciplinary domains [32, 38, 44], over the years, researchers from a wider range of disciplines have joined the field. And this has triggered the discipline's developing interest in wide-ranging topics: 'there is now a stronger emphasis than ever before on the need for multifaceted approaches to the diverse issues' [42 p. 31]. Indeed, it is clear to many of us with long-standing editorial and peer-reviewer roles that the last decade has seen a considerable rise in qualitative HPER, as well as non-experimental quantitative research [30, 49]. Furthermore, recent work (spanning 2000–2020) has identified the key role played by sociology in examining socialisation, professions, social control, knowledge production, and stratification, alongside examining the field of HPER itself [36]. Clearly, this trajectory of HPER approaches reflects a broader shift whereby: 'educational researchers have moved into ... systems, classrooms, and workplaces and have found a complex and multifaceted world that they feel is not well described by traditional research techniques' [50 p. 35]. This shift has moved educational researchers to consider a wide range of research approaches enabling a greater understanding of the complexity of HPE systems. For example, promotion of realist approaches to evaluate complex interventions in areas such as simulation-based education (see Chapter 6) [35].

Secondly, responding to calls for greater evidence in HPE and the explosion of new HPER, there has been a growth in articles using a range of knowledge syntheses approaches (e.g., literature reviews, bibliometric reviews) [31, 33, 39, 40, 51, 52]. For example, in the largest study of its kind in HPER, Maggio et al. [39] conducted a biblio-metric analysis to characterise the frequency, types, and patterns of knowledge synthe-sis publications in medical education across twenty years (1999–2019). From the 963 studies identified, they found a 2620% increase over that period in knowledge synthe-sis articles, compared to an overall increase of 204% for non-knowledge synthesis arti-cles. Systematic and critical reviews were present at the beginning of the period, with realist and scoping reviews being published from 2010 and 2011 respectively.

1.4   WHY SHOULD YOU READ THIS BOOK AND HOW?

As mentioned above, this book serves to help you build your understanding of the fundamentals (i.e., *principles, perspectives*, and *practices*) of HPER. We have pitched this book at readers who are novice HPE researchers, as well as more experienced HPE researchers who want to better understand the fundamentals of less-familiar approaches. So, if you are studying postgraduate qualifications (e.g., Masters, PhD) in HPE, or if you are an experienced biomedical or clinical researcher wanting to con-duct educational research for the first time, this book is for you. This book is also for you if you are an experienced HPE researcher with responsibilities for supervising students or teaching HPER methodology/method courses. Indeed, the original idea for this book was inspired by one of our own courses (based at the Monash Centre for Scholarship in Health Education, Monash University) and triggered by our desire to develop a foundational guide to recommend to our own students in degree-awarding programmes (e.g., Masters, PhD) and non-degree short courses (e.g., continuing pro-fessional development). Therefore, we set out to ensure that this book is broad in its scope, focusing on HPER (not just medical education research) with global relevance. With a multidisciplinary, international authorship team, the book draws on litera-ture and case studies from diverse countries (including Western and non-Western cultures) and healthcare professions (including dentistry, dietetics, medicine, nurs-ing, pharmacy, physiotherapy, and others).

We believe that this book is unique compared to other texts currently available. Firstly, our book focuses on the key foundations of HPER, so privileges *principles, perspectives*, and *practices* rather than providing a how-to methods textbook (we rec-ommend that novice readers read our book as a prelude to how-to methods texts). The uniqueness of our approach, in terms of the scope of our book, means that you can use this as a guide as you design, develop, conduct, and publish your research. Furthermore, we have written this book for, and most importantly with, early-career HPE researchers across the globe, to ensure that each chapter is maximally appropri-ate and relevant to our primary audience. Additionally, aligned with others' sugges-tions of broadening the scope of HPER to give more attention to interactional and organisational levels, and perspectives from sociology, economics and so on [31], we include some novel chapters not yet appearing in other texts (e.g., realist approaches, critical approaches, pragmatic approaches, research impact). Each chapter aims to facilitate your learning. While Chapters 1 and 13 do so by providing you with the necessary introductory material and discussing synergistic elements across the chapters, bringing together key recurring themes, the remaining chapters offer examples and exercises to stretch your mind. And while we cover significant foundational ground, we encourage you to make links and connections between that theory and your own and others' HPER throughout.

Thus, Chapters 2–12 start with learning outcomes, and contain several case studies from our own research (including examples of Masters and PhD research), bringing concepts to life. These chapters also include 'pause and reflect' activities, 'stop and do' activities, and recommended reading. We therefore anticipate you engaging actively with each Chapter's learning processes. Chapters can be read as stand-alone depending on what best suits your needs during your learning journey; however, we have written the book to be read chronologically with Part I (*Principles*) foundational to Part II (*Perspectives*), and Part II foundational to Part III (*Practices*). All chapters include links to earlier and later chapters to help you make connections between them, and to guide your decision-making around which chapter to read next should you not adopt a chronological reading approach.

1.5   OVERVIEW OF THE BOOK

Our book is organised in three parts, with Part I (Chapters 2–4) providing a synopsis of HPER *principles*, Part II (Chapters 5–9) giving an overview of key *perspectives* to HPER, and Part III (Chapters 10–12) presenting cross-cutting *practices* in HPER. Thus, our opening chapter in Part I, Chapter 2, will help you better understand what theory is, the different purposes of theory, and the challenges in applying theory in HPER. It will facilitate your appraisal of the different ways theory can be employed in HPER and reflect critically on theories relevant to your own research. Chapter 3 will help you understand why it is necessary to consider ethics in HPER, analyse key theoretical ethical perspectives in HPER, and summarise the practical elements of doing ethical research (including the role of institutional review boards, research ethics committees, and codes of conduct). It will also enable you to review key issues around research integrity in HPER. Chapter 4 will support your understanding of quality and why it matters in HPER, alongside specific aspects of quality relating to different research approaches. It will also help you distinguish between critical appraisal tools and reporting guidelines, explain the strengths and weaknesses of different quality tools, and employ tools to appraise the quality of HPER.

Part II provides you with similarly structured overviews of five different approaches to researching HPE: scientific (Chapter 5), realist (Chapter 6), interpretivist (Chapter 7), critical (Chapter 8), and pragmatic approaches (Chapter 9). Each chapter will help you understand the philosophical underpinnings (ontology, epistemology, and axiology) of the chosen approaches, summarise common methodologies, and identify key principles of methods (i.e., sampling, data collection and analysis) within each approach. Part II chapters will also help you understand the main indicators of quality within each approach, and evaluate their strengths and challenges, as well as reflecting on the applicability of the different approaches to your own HPER.

Part III begins with Chapter 10, designed to broaden your understanding of the different purposes of HPER proposals, appraise the key components of high-quality proposals and discuss appropriate writing styles for HPER proposals. It will also help you explore common errors made in HPER proposals and enable you to critique them. Chapter 11 should expand your understanding of the importance of disseminating HPER, outline different forms of dissemination, and summarise guidance for disseminating your HPER. It also includes tips for developing high-quality outputs and for managing the often emotion-laden processes of disseminating your HPER. Chapter 12 will help you summarise different understandings of research impact, explain the philosophical underpinnings of different impact approaches and critique research impact pathways in HPER. It will also help you evaluate the key enablers and barriers of HPER impact, outline different ways of assessing HPER impact, and help you develop strategies to plan for, and enhance, impact from your own HPER. We present our conclusion in Chapter 13. Here, we summarise Parts I-III of the book, explicating cross-cutting matters (relating to research, relationships, and the self) and the future of HPER. Together, we hope that the chapters in this book, rather like graduate studies as the quotation below shows, will be a developmental force as your journey progresses in HPER:

> Part of graduate studies in any discipline is developing the language and methods that would make you recognizable to others in the field as 'one of them' … learning an accepted body of knowledge and a methodological tool kit for making sense of this knowledge and/or contributing to knowledge generation. [53 p. 1128–1129]

REFERENCES

1. Ajjawi R, Barton KL, Dennis AA, et al. Developing a national dental education research strategy: priorities, barriers and enablers. *BMJ Open*. 2017;7(3):e013129.

2. Dennis AA, Cleland JA, Johnston P, et al. Exploring stakeholders' views of medical education research priorities: a national survey. *Med Educ*. 2014;48(11):1078–1091.

3. Palermo C, King O, Brock T, et al. Setting priorities for health education research: a mixed methods study. *Med Teach*. 2019;41(9):1029–1038.

4. Sleep J, Bullock I, Grayson K. Establishing priorities for research in education within one college of nursing and midwifery. *Nurse Educ Today*. 1995;15(6):439–445.

5. Thompson CJ. Research priorities for nursing education: application to clinical nurse specialist education. *Clin Nurse Spec*. 2017;31(5):285–288.

6. Yau S-Y, Babovič M, Liu GR-J, et al. Differing viewpoints around healthcare professions' education research priorities: a Q-methodology approach. *Adv Health Sci Educ*. 2021;26(3):975–999.

7. Cash RE, Leggio WJ, Powell JR, et al. Emergency medical services education research priorities during COVID-19: a modified Delphi study. *J Am Coll Emerg Physicians Open*. 2021;2(4):e12543.

8. Fincher R-ME, White CB, Huang G, et al. Toward hypothesis-driven medical education research: task force report from the Millennium Conference 2007 on educational research. *Acad Med*. 2010;85(5):821–828.

9. Stefanidis D, Cochran A, Sevdalis N, et al. Research priorities for multi-institutional collaborative research in surgical education. *Am J Surg*. 2015;209(1):52–58.

10. Tootoonchi M, Yamani N, Changiz T, et al. Research priorities in medical education: a national study. *J Res Med Sci*. 2012;17(1):83–91.

11. Van Schalkwyk SC, Kiguli-Malwadde E, Budak JZ, et al. Identifying research priorities for health professions education research in sub-Saharan Africa using a modified Delphi method. *BMC Med Educ*. 2020;20(1):443.

12. Wilkinson TJ, Weller JM, McKimm J, et al. Programmatic research in medical education: a national collaboration. *NZ Med J.* 2010;123(1318):24–33.

13. Hodges BD, Albert M, Arweiler D, et al. The future of medical education: a Canadian environmental scan. *Med Educ.* 2011;45(1):95–106.

14. ten Cate O. Health professions education scholarship: the emergence, current status, and future of a discipline in its own right. *FASEB BioAdvances.* 2021;3(7):510–522.

15. Research Excellence Framework. Draft guidance on submissions. UK: REF; 2018. https://www.ref.ac.uk/media/1016/draft-guidance-on-submissions-ref-2018_1.pdf (accessed 26 Aug 2022).

16. Anderson MB. When I say ... really good stuff. *Med Educ.* 2020;54(11):979–980.

17. Hooper B, Gupta J, Bilics A, et al. Balancing efficacy and effectiveness with philosophy, history, and theory-building in occupational therapy education research. *Open J Occup Ther.* 2018;6(1):11.

18. Sandars J, Brown J, Walsh K. Research or evaluation – does the difference matter? *Educ Prim Care.* 2017;28(3):134–136.

19. Albert M, Hodges B, Regehr G. Research in medical education: balancing service and science. *Adv Health Sci Educ.* 2007;12(1):103–115.

20. Ringsted C, Hodges B, Scherpbier A. 'The research compass': an introduction to research in medical education: AMEE Guide no. 56. *Med Teach.* 2011;33(9):695–709.

21. van Enk A, Regehr G. HPE as a field: implications for the production of compelling knowledge. *Teach Learn Med.* 2018;30(3):337–344.

22. Whitehead B. A history of nurse education and the clinical nurse educator. In Dyson S, McAllister M, eds. *Routledge International Handbook of Nurse Education.* London and New York: Routledge; 2020: 3–20.

23. Institute of Medicine. *Dental Education at the Crossroads: Challenges and Change.* Washington, DC: National Academies Press; 1995.

24. Stewart D, Letendre DE. Chapter 2 – The pharmacy education: a historical perspective. In Fathelrahman AI, Mohamed Ibrahim MI, Alrasheedy AA, et al., eds. *Pharmacy Education in the Twenty First Century and Beyond.* London: Academic Press; 2018: 11–20.

25. Baernstein A, Liss HK, Carney PA, et al. Trends in study methods used in undergraduate medical education research, 1969–2007. *JAMA.* 2007;298(9):1038–1045.

26. Eva KW. Broadening the debate about quality in medical education research. *Med Educ.* 2009;43(4):294–296.

27. Kuper A, Albert M, Hodges BD. The origins of the field of medical education research. *Acad Med.* 2010;85(8):1347–1353.

28. Lee K, Whelan JS, Tannery NH, et al. 50 years of publication in the field of medical education. *Med Teach.* 2013;35(7):591–598.

29. Monrouxe LV, Liu GR-J, Yau S-Y, et al. A scoping review examining funding trends in health care professions education research from Taiwan (2006–2017). *Nurs Outlook.* 2020;68(4):417–429.

30. Palmquist E, Ricard C, Chen L. Review of surgical education research trends in North America. *J Surg Educ.* 2019;76(6):1476–1483.

31. Rotgans JI. The themes, institutions, and people of medical education research 1988–2010: content analysis of abstracts from six journals. *Adv Health Sci Educ.* 2012;17(4):515–527.

32. Ackel-Eisnach K, Raes P, Hönikl L, et al. Is German medical education research on the rise? An analysis of publications from the years 2004 to 2013. *GMS Z Med Ausbild.* 2015;32(3):Doc30.

33. Azer SA. The top-cited articles in medical education: a bibliometric analysis. *Acad Med.* 2015;90(8):1147–1161.

34. Engel JD, Filling CM. Research approaches in health professions education: problems and prospects. *Eval Health Prof.* 1981;4(1):13–20.

35. Graham AC, McAleer S. An overview of realist evaluation for simulation-based education. *Adv Simul (Lond).* 2018;3:13.

36. Jenkins TM, Underman K, Vinson AH, et al. The resurgence of medical education in sociology: a return to our roots and an agenda for the future. *J Health Soc Behav.* 2021;62(3):255–270.

37. Kaae S, Traulsen JM. Qualitative methods in pharmacy practice research. In Babar Z-U-D, ed. *Pharmacy Practice Research Methods.* Cham: Springer International Publishing; 2015: 49–68.

38. Lee CH, Chen PJ, Lai HY, et al. A scoping review of medical education research for residents in radiation oncology. *BMC Med Educ.* 2020;20(1):13.

39. Maggio LA, Costello JA, Norton C, et al. Knowledge syntheses in medical education: a bibliometric analysis. *Perspect Med Educ.* 2021;10(2):79–87.

40. Maggio LA, Ninkov A, Costello JA, et al. Knowledge syntheses in medical education: meta-research examining author gender, geographic location, and institutional affiliation. *PLoS One.* 2021;16(10):e0258925.

41. Nabeiei P, Amini M, Ghanavati S, et al. Research priorities in medical education at Shiraz University of Medical Sciences: categories and subcategories in the Iranian context. *J Adv Med Educ Prof.* 2016;4(1):26–32.

42. Rangel JC, Cartmill C, Kuper A, et al. Setting the standard: Medical Education's first 50 years. *Med Educ.* 2016;50(1):24–35.

43. Rosenthal M. Qualitative research methods: why, when, and how to conduct interviews and focus groups in pharmacy research. *Curr Pharm Teach Learn.* 2016;8(4):509–516.

44. Webster F, Krueger P, MacDonald H, et al. A scoping review of medical education research in family medicine. *BMC Med Educ.* 2015;15(1):79.

45. Eva KW. The more things stay the same, the more they change. *Med Educ.* 2016;50(1):1–2.

46. Cook DA, Bordage G, Schmidt HG. Description, justification and clarification: a framework for classifying the purposes of research in medical education. *Med Educ.* 2008;42(2):128–133.

47. Boet S, Sharma S, Goldman J, et al. Medical education research: an overview of methods. *Can J Anaesth.* 2012;59(2):159–170.

48. Ji YA, Nam SJ, Kim HG, et al. Research topics and trends in medical education by social network analysis. *BMC Med Educ.* 2018;18(1):222.

49. Schuwirth LW, Durning SJ. Educational research: current trends, evidence base and unanswered questions. *Med J Aust.* 2018;208(4):161–163.

50. Kelly AE, Lesh RA. Trends and shifts in research methods. In Kelly AE, Lesh RA, eds. *Handbook of Research Design in Mathematics and Science Education.* New York and London: Routledge; 2000: 35–44.

51. Norman G, Sherbino J, Varpio L. The scope of health professions education requires complementary and diverse approaches to knowledge synthesis. *Perspect Med Educ.* 2022;11(3):139–143.

52. Maggio LA, Ninkov A, Frank JR, et al. Delineating the field of medical education: bibliometric research approach(es). *Med Educ.* 2022;56(4):387–394.

53. Martimianakis M, Mylopoulos M, Woods N. Developing experts in health professions education research: knowledge politics and adaptive expertise. *Adv Health Sci Educ.* 2020;25(5):1127–1138.

The tree stands firm. Its roots deep and intertwined with the ground, as it reaches up to the sky. Just like the foundational principles of our research, although often hidden, the roots are central to the tree: nourishing, giving strength and protection

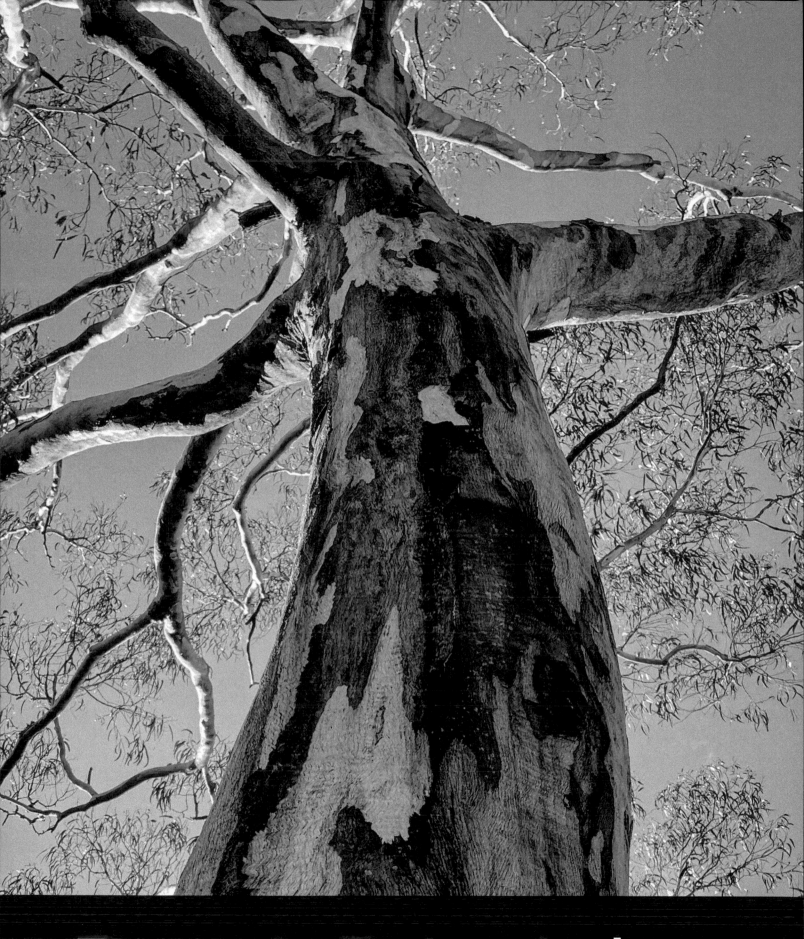

Part I: Principles

Theory in Health Professions Education Research

Charlotte E. Rees[1,2], Lulu Alwazzan[3], and Lisi J. Gordon[4]

[1] The University of Newcastle Callaghan, New South Wales, Australia
[2] Monash University, Clayton, Victoria, Australia
[3] Imam Mohammad Ibn Saud Islamic University, Riyadh, Saudi Arabia
[4] University of Dundee, Dundee, Scotland, UK

Box 2.1   Chapter 2 learning objectives: After reading this chapter you should be able to ...

- Explain what theory is in health professions education research (HPER)
- Outline the different purposes of theory in HPER
- Critique the challenges in applying theory to HPER
- Appraise how theory can be employed to improve HPER
- Reflect critically on theories relevant to your own HPER

2.1   INTRODUCING CHAPTER 2

> ... theory permeates almost every aspect of the study—even if the author does not recognize this influence [1 p. 1]

The term theory has different meanings in different contexts; in this chapter, we describe it as: 'an organized, coherent, and systematic articulation of a set of statements related to significant questions ... communicated in a meaningful whole' [2 p. 37]. Like Sutton and Staw, we see theory as different to: 'references, data, variables, diagrams, and hypotheses' [3 p. 371]. Whether you love or loathe theory, it matters. It is intrinsically intertwined with educational research data and practice [4–7]. While employing theory is not without its challenges, you can apply it variously to improve the integrity and rigour of your research. This chapter serves to help you better understand theory and plan for its optimal use within

---

Foundations of Health Professions Education Research: Principles, Perspectives and Practices, First Edition. Edited by Charlotte E. Rees, Lynn V. Monrouxe, Bridget C. O'Brien, Lisi J. Gordon, and Claire Palermo.
© 2023 John Wiley & Sons Ltd. Published 2023 by John Wiley & Sons Ltd.

your studies (see Box 2.1). In section 2.2, we unpack diverse understandings of theory in educational research, and in section 2.3, we consider its multiple purposes in HPER. We consider the challenges of employing theory in section 2.4, and in section 2.5, we outline the various approaches to its application. We bring these issues to life throughout this chapter by discussing four case studies. These include studies exploring postgraduate nursing objective structured clinical examinations (OSCEs) [8], medical students' intimate examination dilemmas [9], senior medical trainees' transitions [10, 11], and women in academic medicine [12]. See Box 2.2 for a brief overview of these cases. Sometimes, early career researchers and those new to theory express challenges employing theory, as well as difficulties with theory-related terminology [13]. Consequently, this chapter may take you longer to digest but we encourage you to persevere. We hope this chapter helps you: develop your understanding, think about theory critically, and plan for theory in your HPER.

Box 2.2   Case studies: An overview

Postgraduate nursing OSCEs [8]: We conducted 15 focus groups with Australian postgraduate nursing OSCE candidates (n=42), examiners (n=20), and simulated patients (n=17) to better understand the importance of OSCE materials (e.g., objects, technologies, spaces) for candidate performance. Candidate unfamiliarity with materials and missing/malfunctioning materials were thought to negatively impact their performance during OSCEs. Participants reported making micro-adjustments to materials during the OSCE to make the OSCE work as a high-stakes performance assessment.

Intimate examination dilemmas [9]: We conducted 54 group or individual interviews with 200 medical students from three schools (UK, Australia) to better understand their professionalism dilemmas. In 71/833 narratives collected, students narrated being instructed to observe/perform intimate exams without valid patient consent. In 58 narratives, students reported complying with instructions (employing 349 compliance explanations) and in 13 narratives, they reported refusing instructions (using 84 refusal explanations). Compliance explanations (e.g., 'had to') significantly downplayed student intentionality, whereas refusal explanations emphasised intentionality.

Transitions to trained doctors [10, 11]: We undertook a longitudinal diary study (including entrance and exit interviews and repeated diaries over 7–10 months) with 18 Scottish doctors to understand their trainee-trained (specialty) doctor transitions. Doctors experienced multiple transitions in various contexts (role, work, home, education), affecting them and their significant others in multiple domains (psychological, physical, social, cultural) [10]. Additionally, trainees reported feeling 'betwixt and between' different identities [11].

Women in academic medicine [12]: We interviewed 25 female clinical academics in five Saudi Arabian medical schools. Through interviews, we explored females' career progression and leadership including the influence of context, intersecting identities, and language use. Women's career progression and leadership seemed influenced by intersecting identities (e.g., gender and motherhood), varying according to career progression, organisational cultures, and specialties.

2.2   DIFFERENT WAYS OF UNDERSTANDING THEORY

There are diverse ways of understanding theory with little consensus [3, 14]. This is unsurprising when you consider the range of implicitness/explicitness with which theory is employed and the multiple ways it is classified [15]. Some use unique metaphors to describe theory in educational research and its purposes, for example, as a tool-shed: 'a repository, a way of tidying the various bodies of knowledge and analytical instruments that might be used' [14 p. 78], or a narrative protagonist: a 'character with a role within a research story' [16 p. 447]. However, most literature classifies theory depending on its size/scope, philosophical foundations, disciplinary underpinnings, belongingness to theoretical clusters, types, and where it sits on a continuum [1, 14, 17–20]. While these classifications imply that theories can be neatly packaged, they do not always fit easily; with fuzzy boundaries between categories. Please see our book glossary for definitions of theory-related terms used throughout this chapter.

2.2.1   Theory by Size/Scope

Theory can vary from grand to macro and micro [1, 15, 16, 18, 21]. Grand theories are relatively abstract general approaches (e.g., constructionism), which provide scaffolding, typically theorising all aspects of something such as being (ontology), knowing (epistemology), and learning at a societal level, and are applicable to many different situations [14, 18, 19, 22]. Conversely, macro and micro theories can be applied to specific circumstances and/or components of a learning environment, with macro theories focusing on local systems including cultural/contextual aspects, and micro theories focusing on individual level action or interaction in context [18, 21, 22]. For example, Samuel et al. [22] explored context-specificity in clinical reasoning in the simulated environment through a series of experiments, drawing on situated cognition theory (constructed as macro theory), as well as cognitive load theory and self-regulated learning theory (constructed as micro theories). Furthermore, Rees et al. [23] explored power in family medicine bedside teaching encounters through video observation, drawing on social constructionism (constructed as grand theory) and symbolic interactionism, Foucault's capillary power, and Goffman's dramaturgy theory (constructed as micro theories). A quick search of HPER journals (*Academic Medicine*, *Advances in Health Sciences Education*, *Medical Education*, *Medical Teacher*) for papers including the terms theory/theories/theoretical illustrates considerable heterogeneity over the last decade, with about forty different theories identified in around two hundred papers. The most identified theory at a macro level is cultural–historical activity theory (CHAT: from a sociomaterial cluster) [24], and at a micro level is generalisability theory (from a measurement theory cluster) [25], and self-determination theory (from a motivation theory cluster) [26]. Box 2.3 provides brief outlines of these commonplace theories.

Box 2.3   Brief description of three common theories in HPER in the last decade

Cultural–historical activity theory (CHAT) [24]: A sociomaterial theory at the macro level, CHAT provides a conceptual/methodological framework to consider practice-based social learning mediated through non-human materials [27]. With the activity system or interacting activity systems (including the activity's object,

(continued)

(continued)

subject, tools, rules, communities, and divisions of labour) as the basic analytic unit [27, 28], CHAT sensitises researchers to different aspects of sociomaterial learning, privileging cultural features and the historicity of the activity system [29]. It also highlights contradictions within and between activity systems (e.g., student learning versus patient care), with a view to resolving such tensions through new ways of (expansive) learning [27, 28].

Generalisability theory (GT) [25]: A measurement theory at the micro level, GT provides a conceptual/analytical framework for test reliability [30]. An extension of classical test theory (CTT), it examines the relative contribution of a measurement's object (e.g., student performance in an OSCE), so-called person variance, compared with multiple sources of error variance (so-called facets of generalisation) simultaneously (e.g., rater, station, circuit, occasion) [30, 31]. A generalisability study unpacks the observed score variance into different parts attributable to different sources of score variability (variance components related to facets). Furthermore, those variance component estimates can be used in a decision study, where variance components and measurement reliability can be estimated for different assessment designs (e.g., estimating how many stations are required for a reliable OSCE).

Self-determination theory (SDT) [26]: A motivation theory at the micro level, SDT theorises individuals as growth-orientated with three inborn needs (autonomy, competence, and relatedness) determining growth [32]. The theory posits that motivation can range from none (amotivation) to external motivation (driven by external rewards and punishment) to intrinsic motivation (driven by self through interest and satisfaction), with a process of internalisation occurring whereby external motivation shifts to intrinsic through satisfying autonomy, competence, and relatedness needs [32]. High intrinsic motivation is thought to lead to better learning through autonomous self-regulation [32]. Such autonomous self-regulation however can be found in two examples of extrinsic motivation—identified regulation (where learners understand the significance of others' rules) and integrated regulation (where learners connect others' rules to their own norms and values) [32].

2.2.2   Theory by Philosophical Foundations

Often seen as grand theories (non-specific and abstract), all HPER is underpinned by theories or views about the nature of reality (ontology), knowing (epistemology), how to access/construct knowledge (methodology), and what is most valued in terms of reality, knowledge, and coming to know (axiology) [33, 34]. Ontology refers to the assumptions that we make about what is real, with different grand theories (e.g., scientific, realist, interpretivist, critical, or pragmatic approaches) ascribing to different conceptualisations of reality; for example, is there a single reality that exists independent of human interaction (as in scientific realism), or are there multiple versions of reality (as in relativism) (see Table 2.1) [35]? Aligned with ontology, these grand theories will have a particular epistemology, which relates to our assumptions about what we can know about reality and what knowledge is; for example, is reality viewed as objective (as in the scientific approach) or is it subjective (as in the interpretivist approach) [35]? Furthermore, ontological and epistemological assumptions will be aligned to understandings about the ways in which we can access or create knowledge, known as methodology (e.g., experimental designs, ethnography, or a raft of other methodologies).

Research approaches covered in the book					
Grand theories (research approaches)	Scientific (Chapter 5)	Realist (Chapter 6)	Interpretivist (Chapter 7)	Critical (Chapter 8)	Pragmatic (Chapter 9)
Purpose	To explain/predict patterns	To understand how/when complex things work	To understand	To emancipate	To improve/change
Ontology	Scientific realism	Scientific or critical realism	Relativism or critical realism	Historical realism	Pluralism
Epistemology	Objectivity	Objectivity or subjectivity	Subjectivity	Collectivity	Intersubjectivity
Methodology	Experimental/survey research, empirical observation, hypothetico-deductive model, quantitative methods, research conducted from outside (e.g., dualism)	Whatever quantitative, qualitative, or mixed methods that suit developing/refining programme theory (e.g., realist synthesis, realist evaluation), research conducted from outside or inside	Qualitative research (e.g., ethnography, phenomenology, narrative enquiry), research conducted from inside (e.g., co-construction)	Participatory qualitative research conducted alongside partici-pants (e.g., co-design, decolonising)	Any quantitative, qualitative or mixed methods that align with research goals (e.g., action research)
Axiology	Empiricism, quantifiable data, facts, objectivity, dualism, validity, reliability, generalisability	Stratified reality, emergence, complexity, generative mechanisms, context, theory, trust-worthiness, coherence, configurational analysis	Language, social interaction, context, depend-ability, credibility, confirmability, transferability, reflexivity	Democracy, egalitarianism, emancipation, change, depend-ability, credibility, confirmability, transferability, reflexivity	Action, application, improving human experience
Theoretical perspectives	Positivist, post-positivist	Programme theory, middle-range theory	Interpretivist	Critical enquiry, feminism, postcolonialism	Pragmatist

TABLE 2.1   Summary of grand theories underpinning HPER approaches. Adapted from [34].

Finally, all realities (ontologies) and ways of knowing (epistemologies) are under-pinned by sets of values (axiology) which guide and shape all aspects of our research [33, 34]. We present a summary of the grand theories underpinning the five HPER approaches covered in Part II of this book in Table 2.1. Read the philosophical stand-point sections of Chapters 5-9 for more details.

2.2.3   Theory by Disciplinary Underpinnings

HPER is underpinned by eclectic foundational disciplines such as psychology, soci-ology, education, biomedical sciences, mathematics, economics, and management [7]. Theories can and do arise from these different discipline-specific domains but can also be interdisciplinary in nature [1, 18, 36]. For example, CHAT is interdisci-plinary, whereas generalisability theory is founded within mathematics and self-deter-mination theory within psychology. Furthermore, these disciplinary foundations influence educational practices; with three common disciplinary lenses identified in the HPER literature. Two of these are psychological in orientation – cognitive-behavioural, focusing on thinking and action, and humanistic, focusing on individu-als meeting their potential. The third is sociological in orientation – sociocultural, focusing on the social and cultural contexts of learning [16, 37].

2.2.4   Theory by Clusters

Specific macro or micro theories typically belong to higher-order theory clusters, such as behavioural, social, or practice theories [20]. These theory clusters outlined in the literature are often the starting point for selecting specific theories. For example, you would first identify a relevant theory cluster (based on your ontological and epistemological positioning), and then make sense of different theories within that cluster to select optimal theory/theories for your study [38]. For example, if you contemplate behavioural theories relating to assessment at the micro level, you might first think of measurement theory, before focusing on specific theories such as classical test theory, generalisability theory, or item-response theory [31, 39]. Alternatively, if you consider social theories relating to gender at the macro level, you might first think about feminism broadly, before focusing on specific theories like liberal, postcolonial, or intersectional feminism [40]. Finally, if you think about practice theories foregrounding human–material relationships at the macro level, you might initially ponder sociomateriality before narrowing to specific theories such as actor–network theory (ANT), complexity theory, or CHAT [41].

2.2.5   Theory by Types

Theories can be described as scientific or lay, with scientific theories also described as substantive and formal, and lay theories described as folk, common sense, or even conspiracy theories [1, 36, 42, 43]. Essentially, scientific theories can be differentiated from lay theories in their ability to be supported, refuted, or modified through rigorous research [42]. From a scientific research approach (see Chapter 5), theory is described as: 'an interrelated set of constructs (or variables) formed into propositions, or hypotheses, that specify the relationship among variables (typically in terms of magnitude or direction)' [15 p. 51]. Theory in quantitative studies is typically expressed as a series of hypotheses, or if-then logic statements expressing why independent (predictor) variables might cause dependent (outcome) variables, or visual models demonstrating causal pathways among variables [1, 15, 44]. Alternatively, theory in qualitative studies can be employed to shape the whole research process, helping to interpret data, or theory can be built, grounded in qualitative data [45].

2.2.6   Theory by Continua

Theory in education can be related to two intersecting continua: (1) theory versus practice, and (2) plural versus singular [14]. At the theory end of the theory–practice continuum, theory can be described as: 'an elegant description of knowledge' [14 p. 82], with theory being formally expressed as a series of statements, rather like the scientific theories mentioned in section 2.2.5 (e.g., self-determination theory). Moving to the mid-point of this theory–practice continuum, theory can be seen as hypotheses or hunches based on practical experience – something that can be tested in the loosest sense based on observation, as in initial programme theories within realist evaluation (see Chapter 6). Finally, the practice end of this continuum includes personal theory/craft knowledge (like lay theories mentioned in section 2.2.5). Regarding the plural–singular continuum, at the plural end, theory in education can be seen as: 'broadening bodies of knowledge or collations of cognate knowledge' [14 p. 83] (e.g., theory clusters like feminist theory), whereas at the singular end, theory can be viewed as: 'single formally stated ideas or loosely stated hypotheses' [14 p. 83] (e.g., a specific theory within the feminist cluster, like intersectionality). When unpacking theory by continua, you should consider theory in relation to both continua. For example, SDT as both scientific theory and singular, or sociomateriality theory as scientific theory and plural. Now read through the chapter cases to better understand theories at different levels in action (see Box 2.4), and pause and reflect on possible theories for your own HPER (see Box 2.5).

Box 2.4   Case studies: Theory use

Postgraduate nursing OSCEs [8]: We employed sociomateriality as a grand theory to explore OSCE stakeholders' perceptions of human–material interactions impacting on candidate performance. We drew on the basic ontological principles of sociomateriality: that materials and humans matter (symmetry); that materials shape human activity (agency); and that things emerge from sociomaterial assemblages. We did not employ a specific macro sociomaterial theory like CHAT (theory as plural). We did not ask participants interview questions about materials, but they volunteered data relevant to sociomateriality. So, we used sociomateriality at the data analysis stage, with it shaping all steps of our team-based qualitative analysis. We sensitised ourselves to human–material interactions and explored patterns between data regarding human–material interactions and candidate performance to answer our research question (theory at the mid-point of the theory–practice continuum).

Intimate examination dilemmas [9]: We employed Bertram Malle's folk conceptual theory of behavioural explanation as a micro and singular theory [46], and his associated coding scheme [47]. This theory helped us explore factors cited by students when narrating their compliance/refusal behaviours, and how they explained those behaviours to legitimise them. This micro theory therefore shaped our research questions and our expected findings (which could be considered hypotheses or predictions, although we did not term them as such in our paper) [9 p. 263]. We employed Malle's validated coding scheme to code students' explanations [47], and analysed these employing basic and descriptive statistics (at the theory end of the theory–practice continuum). Our findings supported Malle's theory [46], but only loosely guided our educational recommendations.

Transitions to trained doctors [10, 11]: We selected social constructionism as a grand theory to explore doctors' transitions. We employed Multiple and Multidimensional Transitions (MMT) theory as our macro theory to conceptualise transitions as ongoing, non-linear processes of adaptation (psychological, social, and educational) triggered by changing contexts, relationships, and identities [48]. Moreover, we employed identity work theory and conceptions of liminality [49, 50] as micro theories to explore participants' betwixt and between (liminality) experiences. Our findings made conceptual contributions to the interdisciplinary liminality literature, arguing against linear transitions (the theory end of the theory–practice continuum). Further, we introduced the notion of occupying liminality whereby participants rejected others' grants of their new trained doctor status [11].

Women in academic medicine [12]: Drawing on social constructionism as a grand theory [51], and intersectionality as a micro and singular feminist theory [52], we explored female clinical academics' views/experiences of career progression/leadership. This intersectionality micro theory helped shape our research questions

(continued)

> *(continued)*
>
> and methods. We were particularly interested in how participants talked about their career progression/leadership. During data analysis we looked beyond what participants said, to how they spoke including how they constructed their different personal (e.g., mother) and professional (e.g., physician) identities and how these multiple identities intersected. Using this intersectional lens, we interrogated content- (e.g., leadership) and process-related themes (e.g., metaphoric talk), thereby sitting at the mid-point of the theory–practice continuum.

Box 2.5 Pause and reflect: Think about possible theories for your research

Think about an HPER project you are currently conducting or planning to conduct.

- What grand theories might influence your approach to this project? What are your views about reality (ontology), how this reality can be known (epistemology), ways of accessing or constructing knowledge (methodology), and what is most valued (axiology)?
- What are the key concepts related to your project? What macro and/or micro theory clusters or specific theories might relate to these key concepts? (Identify these by exploring what theories others use in your area, or by searching the literature using search terms related to your concept(s) AND theor*).
- What might be the repercussions of selecting between different types of relevant theories? Or not explicitly articulating or developing theories for your research?
- Revisit this pause and reflect box once you have read other sections in Chapter 2 and further developed your ideas for theory in your own research.

2.3 DIFFERENT PURPOSES OF USING THEORY IN HPER

Through theory we can better understand and explain complex issues, such as how things work, social interactions, and different phenomena [1, 7, 22, 45, 53–56]. Some [19, 57] argue that the more complex the phenomenon, the more theory is required. When considering the multiple purposes of theory, it is helpful to tease out the key drivers for theory at the different levels such as grand versus macro/micro. For example, at the grand theory level, the purpose depends on the research approach [45, 54]. From scientific and realist approaches, theory primarily serves to facilitate causal explanation (albeit causality is viewed differently between the two approaches: see Chapters 5 and 6). From an interpretivist approach, theory typically serves to strengthen understanding (see Chapter 7). From a critical approach, it largely serves to challenge the status quo and facilitate emancipation (see Chapter 8). Finally, from a pragmatic approach, it primarily serves to guide action and further enquiry (see Chapter 9). Aligned with these different purposes, theory (especially grand theory) serves to shape the education research process in an internally coherent fashion [5, 15, 21, 22, 52], with underpinning philosophies (e.g., epistemology of objectivism) influencing the theoretical perspective chosen (e.g., positivism), the methodology (e.g., experiment) and the methods (e.g., quantitative scales) [51].

However, at the macro/micro levels, theory can have additional purposes. Brown et al. [16] identified six purposes in 23 general practice education papers published during 2013–2017. The papers employed various macro/micro theories to: (1) align with a position (to give credibility to the author's perspective or to sensitise the reader to the author's stance); (2) to identify a research problem; (3) to drive forward an idea; (4) to provide a methodological tool (e.g., data collection/analysis tool); (5) to interpret findings (especially helping to understand why); and (6) to represent an object of examination (in order to explore the utility of a theory, test theory, or build an extended theory). Brown et al. [16] also suggested that theory could have central or peripheral roles within papers. Central roles included providing methodological tools or serving as objects for examination, whereas peripheral roles included enabling credibility or driving forward ideas [16, 36]. Others have suggested that macro/ micro theory enables educational research projects to build on one another [7, 21, 53], thereby enhancing conceptual generalisability [18, 58]. Plus, given the theoretical eclecticism of HPER with diverse theories to address the same or different phenomena like learning [16, 19, 45], macro/micro theory can help foster innovations in interdisciplinary collaboration; arguably crucial in an education field with many diverse foundational disciplines [7]. In sections 2.3.1 to 2.3.3, we talk more about three central purposes of theory: shaping the research process; theory testing; and theory building. But before reading these sections, read Box 2.6.

Box 2.6   Case studies: An overview of the purposes of theory

Postgraduate nursing OSCEs [8]: We saw sociomaterial entanglements within OSCEs as complex phenomena, so employed general sociomateriality principles. Given the recent blossoming of HPER papers advocating sociomaterial approaches [59–62], we partly employed sociomateriality to give credibility to our approach. Our understanding of this grand theory (and previous work using specific macro sociomaterial theories like complexity theory [63] and CHAT [64, 65]) partly sensitised us to the problem of OSCE materials in our data post hoc and drove our idea that OSCE materials were central to candidate performance and thus examination fairness. We therefore analysed talk about materials and sociomaterial entanglements within our performance theme, drawing on sociomaterial concepts like tinkering/rupturing [59, 60]. Finally, our sociomaterial lens served to build on emerging conceptual literature on sociomateriality (specifically ANT) and OSCEs [66], thereby striving for conceptual generalisability.

Intimate examination dilemmas [9]: We saw students' compliance with or refusal of instructions to act unprofessionally as complex, so employed Malle's folk theory of behavioural explanation post hoc to better explain such behaviours [46]. At the grand theory level, our scientific purpose was to explain the factors cited in students' compliance/refusal explanations, and how they cited those factors. Malle's [46] theory partly sensitised us to the problem of intimate exam dilemmas in our data, as we had worked with this theory previously [67, 68]. It also drove our idea about why such long-standing behaviours in medical education continued to endure. Most importantly, the theory provided the methodological tools for the study (Malle's [47] validated framework) to develop our research questions/predictions and analyse our data. The theory also provided us with an object of examination that we could essentially test, with us finding evidence supporting Malle's theory [46].

(continued)

(continued)

Transitions to trained doctors [10, 11]: Our grand theory (social constructionism) and macro MMT theory were established at the study outset *(a priori)*, thereby shaping our research design, data collection, and analysis. Furthermore, we started thinking about doctors reporting being betwixt and between trainee-trained doctor identities while analysing our data, so our post hoc micro theories relating to identity work (and liminality) helped us further interpret our complex longitudinal data [49, 50]. These theories were also objects of examination, enabling us to extend existing theory [11].

Women in academic medicine [12]: For a deeper and more credible understanding of women's views/experiences of career progression/leadership, we used an *a priori* intersectional lens [52]. Through this intersectional lens we were sensitised to identities as multiple and dynamic, as well as constructed through participants' narratives; where no one identity (e.g., gender) was assumed more important than another (e.g., culture, parenthood). The theory shaped our study and our narrative data interpretation, thereby enhancing our understanding of often taken-for-granted cultural complexities.

2.3.1   Theory to Shape the Research Process

Grand theories (e.g., ontology/epistemology) inevitably shape the research process including: (1) helping to clarify epistemological dispositions; (2) selecting topics and developing research questions; and (3) shaping methodological/method choices [1, 13]. Such theoretical perspectives (e.g., positivism, constructionism) influence methodological choices respectively (e.g., experimental method, phenomenology). Furthermore, *a priori* macro/micro theories can also shape all stages of the research process influencing research questions, sampling strategies, and data collection/analysis. Various scholars [19] liken macro/micro theories to lenses allowing us to look at phenomena in certain ways, and suggesting different educational practice solutions [20]. Furthermore, *a posteriori* (or post hoc) macro/micro theories can be employed at the data analysis stage, especially for qualitative research, to make sense of data.

2.3.2   Research to Test Theory

The foundations of science include the processes: 'of theorizing, collecting evidence, testing theory, revising theory, and then working through the cycle again' [69 p. 1]. Researchers socialised into the scientific (and realist) approaches are typically accustomed to theory being something to be tested (see Chapters 5 and 6) [56]; theory informs experimentation, which subsequently informs the support, refutation, and/or modification of theory [56]. For example, theory developing/guiding a research programme, defining/prescribing how variables are measured, testing middle-range or substantive scientific theories, and providing rationales for relationships among variables [17]. Multiple benefits exist of theory-driven analysis in quantitative research, including: (1) it encourages researchers to make explicit their assumptions; (2) it holds them accountable to data, thus preventing poor statistical practices such as manipulation to find statistical significance (see Chapter 3); and (3) it helps develop knowledge cumulatively through identifying where a theory works or not, bridging between ours and others' studies in conceptual replication/generalisability [69]. Some talk about theory-informed quantitative data analysis as the translation of relationships between measured constructs into statistical models such as structural equation modelling [69]. While a statistical model is not a theory per se, it can be seen as representing theory [17]. For example, Piggott explains that: 'it takes complex thinking to examine a theory, break it down into testable parts, translate it into a testable statistical model, and then compare the results to what is predicted from the theory' [69 p. 13]. Although we typically associate deductive theory use with scientific approaches, which primarily aim to test hypotheses/theory, qualitative studies from other approaches such as interpretivism (see Chapter 7) can also deductively interrogate data from a theoretical perspective [15, 45, 54], as illustrated in Box 2.6. Although such qualitative research rarely labels the purpose as theory-testing, qualitative data analysis often supports, refines, or modifies *a priori* macro/micro theories.

2.3.3   Research to Build Theory

Theory can be the end point of inductive research, as in grounded theory [43], or the building of initial programme theories, as in realist approaches [70]. In the quick literature search of explicit theory use in papers from HPER journals in the last decade, grounded theory is relatively popular. Unlike other common theories mentioned in Section 2.2.1 (CHAT, generalisability theory, and SDT), grounded theory is better described as a methodology, serving to build theory from qualitative data [45]. Whether grounded theory is situated within a positivist-orientated approach pioneered by Glaser and Strauss [71], or the pragmatic and constructivist approach of Charmaz [72], the methodological fundamentals of this exploratory research include: (1) iterative cycles of sampling, data collection, and analysis with early analytical and conceptual insights shaping subsequent sampling (as in theoretical sampling) and data collection; (2) coding of data organised around key concepts or actions with an evolution of the coding framework as data collection continues, progressing to the development of broader categories including conceptual relationships (shifting from codes to categories to concepts); and (3) an analytical process of constant comparison – with important data (e.g., quotations) compared with other data to explore similarities and differences (see Chapter 9) [43]. While grounded theory is unlikely to generate new theory with explanatory or predictive power, it can provide: 'imaginative understanding' [72 p. 126] and generate hypotheses that can be tested with other methods [43]. Finally, initial programme theory (i.e., theories about why and how programmes work) common to realist approaches can be built through abstract theory [70], qualitative research with key stakeholders (e.g., interviews), and/or qualitative analysis of programme documentation (see Chapter 6). Before moving on to section 2.4, reflect critically on the different purposes of published research relevant to your chosen topic of enquiry (see Box 2.7).

Box 2.7   Stop and do: Identify different purposes of theory in published research

- Thinking about the same HPER project as Box 2.5, find up to four published studies relevant to your project. Identify: (1) a relevant quantitative study that serves to test/verify theory; (2) a relevant qualitative study that aims to build theory (e.g., grounded theory); (3) a relevant qualitative study that employs theory to shape the research process (e.g., influencing research

(continued)

(continued)

> questions, data collection/analysis); and (4) a relevant study you could describe as atheoretical (i.e., no explicit references to theory).
>
> - How would you describe these papers on Bradbury-Jones and colleagues' typology of levels of theory visibility: seemingly absent (level 1), implied (level 2), partially applied (level 3), retrospectively applied (level 4), or consistently applied (level 5) [36].
> - How is theory presented across the papers (e.g., as hypotheses, if-then logic statements, visual models, or something else)? Where is theory discussed (one or multiple sections or throughout the entire paper)? Is theory used explicitly enough and why? Is theory sufficiently defensible and why? Is theory aligned with the philosophical standpoint of the study?

2.4   THE CHALLENGES OF USING THEORY IN HPER

Employing theory in educational research is not without its challenges. While HPER has largely been criticised over recent decades for being insufficiently theoretical, some have stridently warned against overreliance on theory, and others still contend that when theory is employed in educational research it can be suboptimal (e.g., uncritical, underdeveloped, or shallow) [1, 3, 4, 16, 21, 73–75]. We consider these challenges next, but first read Box 2.8.

Box 2.8   Case studies: Challenges of using theory

Postgraduate nursing OSCEs [8]: Working with sociomateriality was time-consuming including reading books [76], and journal articles [61, 62], and making sense of the theory cluster (sociomateriality) in relation to specific macro theories. Regarding too little theory, we purposely did not employ any specific macro theories (e.g. CHAT, ANT, complexity theory), so we needed to justify our approach to employing grand sociomateriality theory in our paper. At this level, sociomateriality could be critiqued as too abstract and/or lacking in utility in terms of testability or prediction, although that was never our study aim. Sociomateriality might have blinded us to other findings relevant to OSCE candidate performance in our data (e.g., human–human interactions), plus we found what we were looking for in terms of theory (so could be critiqued for confirmation bias from a scientific standpoint).

Intimate examination dilemmas [9]: Regarding insufficient theory, we employed a post-positivist grand theoretical perspective but failed to make this explicit in our paper [34]. It was also extremely time-consuming to get to grips with Malle's theory – we needed to read and make sense of his book and validated coding framework [46, 47]. Concerning theoretical overreliance, we found what we were looking for in terms of the theory (so could be critiqued for confirmation bias), plus our use of this specific theory could have blinded us to alternative data interpretations. Our paper could also be criticised for lacking practical applications. Finally, in terms of suboptimal use of theory, probably the biggest criticism of Malle's [46] theory is that it lacks parsimony (it is complex and therefore challenging to describe and apply). We did not critique the theory in our published paper, largely because we focused on describing the theory and its relevance to our study.

Transitions to trained doctors [10, 11]: While our grand and macro theories were relatively easy to articulate and aligned comfortably with our research design and data collection/analysis, our fine-grained data analysis with our chosen micro theory required considerable time, discussion, and reading, as well as further data analysis (as evidenced by the three-year duration between our two papers). Further, our micro theory did not quite fit with our data, which left some questions unanswered and opened up an opportunity to extend theory [11]. Finally, our paper could be criticised for lacking practical application.

Women in academic medicine [12]: First, as the study was about multiple identities and identity construction, we needed a broader understanding of gender and identity theories, which the first author lacked at the time of her Masters study but developed through reading and discussions with her supervisor (second author). Second, although an intersectional lens [52] gave us a better understanding of women's views and experiences of career progression/leadership and ideas for more research, our findings did not easily lend themselves to specific practical applications. As a result, it was challenging to discuss the educational implications of our findings based on our data and theory.

2.4.1   Too Little Theory

Many scholars argue that atheoretical research does not exist because all research is imbued with grand theory (theories about reality and knowledge), even if this is not made explicit [19, 21]. However, HPER does not always draw on macro/micro theories and given the purposes of theory outlined in section 2.3, this can be problematic. Ignoring theory can be seen as overlooking the origins of problems that research seeks to address, can lead to findings that are difficult to transfer to other settings, can risk pursuing educational innovations that are ineffective, and ultimately, can prevent topics of enquiry or research fields from progressing [1, 4, 7, 22]. Some attribute the dearth of theory to lack of theoretical knowledge and/or motivation among some HPE researchers, with Ellaway going so far as calling this theoriaphobia: 'a fear, rejection or disengagement with theory' [77 p. 1]. James describes theoriaphobia in his remarks on an experienced teacher who complained that educational research was 'too theoretical' and lacked relevance to practice: 'For her [Margaret], most educational problems could be solved by the application of common sense coupled with a greater trust in professional teachers, so did not need "theory"' [6 p. 243]. Other scholars have provided alternative rationales behind the lack of theory in HPER, at both the individual (e.g., theories can be time-consuming to engage with, and challenging to apply) [7, 21], and discipline levels (e.g., publishing theoretically-rich accounts of research in applied HPER journals with tight word counts is challenging) [3, 7, 21].

2.4.2   Too Much Theory

Ellaway also introduced the term theoriaphilia within HPER, defined as the: 'tendency to overemphasize or overfocus on theoretical matters to the detriment of other parts of a study' [77 p. 2]. Such overreliance on theory can be thought to jeopardise, for example, the more practical aspects of studies like educational implications [22]. Furthermore, some criticise theory use in educational research, either because of its fragility [22], or because of its longevity and creed-like status despite insufficient evidence [14]. Thomas, perhaps the biggest faultfinder of theory in educational research, critiques theoretical hegemony as reinforcing educational methods and practices, that are: 'a means of controlling what is permitted to count as knowledge' [14 p. 86], which serves to discourage diversity of thought and inhibits creativity [14]. Furthermore, with an overreliance on specific macro/micro theories, researchers can run the risk of: (1) blindness (i.e., to findings inconsistent with the chosen theory), (2) confirmation bias (i.e., findings consistent with what they were looking for), and (3) straitjacketing (i.e., twisting their data to fit the chosen theory) [1, 14]. Various researchers have called for increased openness, a more ad hoc approach, thought experiments, and diversity in order to identify disruptive breakthroughs and enable revision of theory based on data and application to HPE settings [22, 69].

2.4.3   Not-Quite-Right Theory

Theory has been criticised for its peripheral/minimal use for suboptimal purposes (e.g., academic credibility) [14]. Such minimal use can include theory dropping (i.e., theory mentioned in the literature review but omitted from the rest of the paper) or theory positioning (i.e., theory being introduced within a paper but without citation) [78], leading to a lack of transparency [21]. However, the most pervasive and important criticism centres on uncritical use, including theory diversification (i.e., introducing multiple theories without making their relevance clear) [78]. While some have criticised grand theory for being too abstract and thus lacking utility in terms of testability and prediction (explaining everything and nothing) [17, 22], others have criticised specific macro/micro theories (e.g., cognitive load theory) for having central tenets impossible to falsify [79].

Some argue that theories are neither exclusively nor intrinsically right or wrong for any specific phenomenon [19, 56]. For example, Grant and Osanloo commented that for research students: 'No one perfect or right theory [exists] for a dissertation, but certain theories are popular within each discipline.' [13 p. 14] However, numerous scholars [22] have argued that macro/micro theories are not created equal, and consequently, there are numerous ways in which we can judge the quality of specific theories and their application from different research approaches. For example, thinking about a scientific approach (see Chapter 5), scientific theories can be evaluated based on various criteria: (1) their explanatory power (how well does theory explain data?), (2) predictive power (how well does theory predict data?), (3) scope (how well does theory generalise to other contexts?), (4) testability (how well can theory propositions be measured?), (5) falsifiability (how specific is theory to enable falsification?), (6) parsimony (how simple and clearly described is theory?), (7) pragmatic adequacy (is the utility of theory made clear?), (8) operational adequacy (how clear is the link between theory propositions and research methods?), (9) empirical adequacy (how congruent are collected data with theory?), and (10) cumulative nature (how many studies have contributed to theory development and refinement?) [3, 14, 17, 45, 69, 80, 81]. From a realist approach (see Chapter 6), the quality of programme theory has been judged according to four criteria: (1) the extent to which the programme theory explains phenomena at grand, macro, and micro levels (is it at an appropriate level of abstraction?), (2) its potential fit with the research topic and explanatory power, (3) its simplicity and ability to inspire further programme theory development, and (4) its compatibility with realist principles of generative causation [70]. Finally, from a grounded theory approach (see Chapter 9), theory should be: (1) understandable, (2) original, (3) fit data on which it is grounded (credibility), (4) fit research participants' and users' realities (resonance), (5) be reasonably general to be applied to various contexts (usefulness), and (6) provide the theory-user with sufficient control to bring about change [43].

Finally, and irrespective of research approach, internal coherence is a key criterion for judging the quality of theoretical application within any given study (see

Chapter 4 for more details) [34]. Ultimately, you should try to avoid theoretical mismatches within your study as these can jeopardise its integrity. Such mismatches can occur if you: (1) fail to focus on the real research problem or fail to understand the intricacies of theory or its key relevant aspects [17]; (2) misalign your study's underlying ontological and epistemological foundations with the ways in which you conduct your research [21]; (3) misalign theory with the problem, purpose, questions, and significance of your research [13]; and (4) employ multiple but misaligned theories from different domains or with different philosophical or theoretical standpoints, so they sit together awkwardly in your study [22]. Before you move on to the next section, stop and critically appraise theory use in a selected paper (see Box 2.9).

Box 2.9   Stop and do: Critically appraise the use of theory in an example paper

- Read the following open-access paper: Hindi AMK et al. Using communities of practice as a lens for exploring experiential pharmacy learning in general practice: are communities of practice the way forward in changing the training culture in pharmacy? *BMC Med Educ.* 2022;22:12 https://bmcmededuc. biomedcentral.com/articles/10.1186/s12909-021-03079-8 [82].

- Critically appraise the use of theory in this paper.

- Make a note of the following: (1) what explicit/implicit theories are used and for what purposes?; (2) is there too much, too little, and/or inappropriate use of theory? (if so, list all the ways); (3) what would you say is the biggest problem with the theory and/or its application in this paper and why?

- Click on the 'peer review reports' for this *BMC Medical Education* paper to see what the reviewers say about theory use in this paper. How do these compare with your notes?

- What have you learnt from critically appraising the theory in this HPER paper that you could apply to your own research?

2.5   APPLYING THEORY TO IMPROVE HPER

Skilled application of theory within HPER can be described as theoretical connoisseurship [83], that is, recognising: 'which theory might serve the research purpose in a given context and how that theory might be used for that purpose' [16 p. 445]. As an HPE researcher, you can develop your theoretical connoisseurship in general ways and in ways specific to projects. We provide you with advice based on the literature and our own experiences.

2.5.1   Developing General Theoretical Connoisseurship

Numerous scholars talk about the importance of HPE researchers developing their theoretical understandings and capabilities through self-directed learning (e.g., reading theory-orientated books and journals), participating in theory-orientated continuing professional development (e.g., courses, workshops, conferences), as well as conducting collaborative theory-orientated research [4, 21, 58, 75]. Inspired by Russell's [84] ten tips for developing wine connoisseurship, Box 2.10 provides tips for becoming a theory connoisseur.

Box 2.10   Ten tips for developing theoretical connoisseurship. Adapted from [84]

Ten tips for developing theoretical connoisseurship. Adapted from [84]

1. Improve your theoretical understanding with short bursts of focused learning, but remember that building theoretical expertise takes time and dedication.
2. Become a theory expert by working with different theories with various sizes/scopes and from diverse philosophical/disciplinary foundations (e.g., see how Varpio and colleagues [57] discuss four agency-related theories and their applications to interprofessional learning to tackle wicked problems).
3. Compare theories, teasing out their similarities and differences to make sense of them.
4. Fully engage your senses (seeing and hearing) to appreciate the different features of theory, drawing on feedback wherever possible.
5. Enhance your theoretical understanding by thinking about your embodied and sensory experiences of theory.
6. Theory connoisseurs are not just good at using theory, but have extensive knowledge about theory, understanding when a particular theory was developed and by whom, its foundations, and subsequent evolutions.
7. Develop your theoretical vocabulary, learning many terms describing theory and having theoretical conversations with academics/practitioners.
8. As a novice you may lack the theoretical processing abilities of experts, so it may take you longer to get to grips with a new theory, exploring how to apply it, but you can become theoretically skilled with practice.
9. Develop your connoisseurship through learning about high-quality theories and better understanding their foundational philosophies and disciplinary domains.
10. Even experts make mistakes about theory (e.g., misunderstanding or misapplying theory), so persevere and learn from mistakes.

2.5.2   Developing Theoretical Connoisseurship Specific to Projects

A powerful way of developing theoretical connoisseurship is through participation – conducting theoretically-orientated collaborative research [21, 75]. Attune to theory from the outset of your project, with some scholars [13] providing guidelines to dissertation students for selecting theoretical frameworks (see Box 2.11). The most common theory questions research students ask us pertain to what we call theoretical topping and tailing: at the top, how should I find theory?; at the tail, how should I disseminate theory? Given the diversity of HPE and its foundational domains, there can seem limitless possibilities for the use of macro/micro theories. As illustrated in Box 2.11, at a relatively early point in a specific project, you will need to identify macro/micro theories that are internally coherent with your philosophical standpoint and key concepts, alongside your developing ideas for research questions and methodologies/methods. You and your collaborators may have a relevant theory in mind based on previous research. If that is the case, we encourage you to remain open to identifying alternative theories. Through this, you might find an alternative theory more appropriate to your current study.

> **Box 2.11   Guidelines for selecting theory for dissertation research***
>
> 1. Identify your ontological and epistemological underpinnings (i.e., grand theories about being and knowing).
> 2. Identify macro/micro theories consistent with these philosophical underpinnings and expand your thinking to the key concepts of your study. What are the disciplinary roots of potential theories (e.g., psychology, sociology, education, economics, or something else)?
> 3. Develop your knowledge of relevant theories and reflect critically on why each theory is important. How well-developed are these theories?
> 4. Review the literature to gauge support for these theories. What are their benefits?
> 5. Review how others have applied the theories in HPER.
> 6. Critically appraise the theories. What are their weaknesses?
> 7. Think about how the theories connect with your study problem, purpose, significance, and design. Are the theories internally coherent with your methodological plan?
> 8. Select your theoretical framework to provide a blueprint for your study design. To what extent might your theories be employed *a priori* (from the start) or *a posteriori* (after collecting your data)?

*Adapted from Grant and Osanloo [13 p. 19].

2.5.2.1   Theory from the Top

We recommend searching for theory using a combination of Internet (in the early, rudimentary stages) and database searches (e.g., Medline, PubMed, CINAHL, PsycInfo, ERIC), as your ideas shape up. Booth and Carroll [85] developed the BeHEMoTh (Behaviour, Health, Exclusions, and Models or Theories) framework for specifying and identifying models and theories for systematic reviews, which we think could be applied in HPER. Although meant for systematic reviews involving behaviour change interventions, the BeHEMoTh procedures can help to identify relevant theory [85]. So, let's see how this framework could guide a literature search for HPER theory using an example question from the literature: "How is power constructed within family medicine bedside teaching?" [23 p. 157] For this research question, the behaviour (or concept) of interest is 'power' (and its synonyms), the health (or educational) context is 'bedside teaching' and/or 'family medicine' (and their synonyms), the exclusions might include 'statistical models', and the models or theories should include candidate terms like concept(s)/conceptual, framework(s), model(s), and theory/theories/theoretical (for more details about BeHEMoTh search processes see Booth and Carroll [85 p. 227–228]). Finally, alongside these electronic searches, we also suggest strategic hand-searching in theory-orientated textbooks [86], and theory-orientated journals, including *Medical Education's* cross-cutting edge papers, *Medical Teacher's* theory guides and theory special issues (e.g., CHAT special issue: 43(1), pp. 1–120), plus *Advances in Health Sciences Education's* theory column [19].

2.5.2.2   Theory at the Tail

In terms of disseminating theory-orientated research, Brown et al. [16] suggest that the role of theory should be clearly articulated in papers through early introduction and presentation throughout, including discussion sections. They liken theory to a character in a story that requires an entrance, development, and exit, with peripheral (so-called cameo appearances) risking being meaningless, confusing, or distracting [16]. Therefore, we encourage you to constantly attune yourself to theory in papers and conference presentations. Ask yourself the question: how do authors/presenters attend to theory in their outputs? And what does good dissemination of theory look like? Identify examples of well-articulated theory in papers from different journals/ dissertations and use these ideas to help guide your own theoretical dissemination. See how we applied theory in our case studies in Box 2.12. Next, try an example search of theory related to your own HPER (see Box 2.13).

Box 2.12   Case studies: How we applied theory

Postgraduate nursing OSCEs [8]: Although we had reasonable understandings of soci- omateriality based on prior research [64, 65] and extensive previous reading [59, 60, 76], we searched for more recent references using scientific databases [61, 62]. We also solicited feedback from sociomaterial scholars after data collection to solicit advice on sociomateriality's applicability to our OSCE data. These scholars provided further rec- ommended reading, which we incorporated into our write-up. Drawing on Brown et al. [16], we ensured that sociomateriality was a central character across our research paper (i.e., abstract, introduction, methods, results, and discussion). However, this was not the case in our original manuscript submission. One peer reviewer suggested that we needed to make stronger links between our study findings and sociomaterial- ity in our results section and we enacted this feedback in our revised manuscript.

Intimate examination dilemmas [9]: As alluded to earlier, we had worked with Malle's theory and coding framework [46, 47] for two previous studies [67, 68] and had reasonable understandings of the theory and its application. We had done extensive reading of the theory [46, 47], including getting advice directly from Malle on the application of his coding framework for naturalistic qualitative data for our earlier study [67]. Consistent with Brown et al. [16], Malle's [46] theory was central within our paper. While it was discussed in all sections of the manu- script, it was dominant in the introduction, methods, and results sections, but rather peripheral in our discussion. On reflection, its exit could have been improved.

Transitions to trained doctors [10, 11]: At the outset, we planned to draw on MMT theory [48] and we were fortunate to have the theory's originator (Jindal-Snape) as a team member. In our first paper [10], we talked about MMT theory in all sections of our paper, thereby giving the theory a central and consistent role across the paper. For the micro theories used in our second paper [11] (theories related to identity work and liminality [49, 50]), we went beyond the educational literature and into the social sciences literature, doing extensive reading and discussion to identify theories most relevant to our data [49, 50]. Again, these micro theories played prominent roles across all aspects of our paper, but especially in our discus- sion section as we were able to extend theory [11].

Women in academic medicine [12]: This was my earliest experience (as first author) conducting HPER drawing on gender-related theory for my Masters dissertation. However, my supervisor (second author) had experience working with intersec- tionality theory [87] and was simultaneously supervising other research students employing intersectionality theory [88, 89]. We engaged in considerable reading and discussion about intersectionality theory and its applicability. I also talked to other students using intersectionality theory to make sense of its benefits, challenges, and applications. Although the theory was present across the paper (mostly abstract, introduction, methods, and discussion), in some ways, it took a peripheral role in the paper given its relevance to only one-third of the research questions.

Box 2.13   Stop and do: Searching for theory relevant to your HPER. Adapted from [85]

- Thinking about the same HPER project as Box 2.5, develop a preliminary research question.
- Using the BeHEMoTh (Behaviour, Health, Exclusions, Models, Theories) framework [85], identify terms for your Behaviour/Concept(s) of interest, your Health/Educational context(s), your Exclusions (e.g., statistical models, models of care, disease models), and your Models and/or Theories.
- Using a relevant database, run a rudimentary search to see what theories you can identify. Are there any promising ones that you should explore further?
- Read Booth and Carroll's BeHEMoTh multistage search processes if you would like to conduct a more systematic search for theory [85].

2.6   CHAPTER SUMMARY

In this chapter, we have discussed different ways of understanding theory – by size/scope, philosophical foundations, disciplinary underpinnings, clusters, types, and continua. We provided an overview of multiple purposes of grand theory dependent on research approach – to explain/predict (scientific/realist), to understand (interpretivist), to emancipate (critical), and to improve (pragmatic), as well as unpacking different roles of macro/micro theory in shaping the research process and testing or building theory. We illustrated the challenges of working with theory, outlining three key common criticisms of HPER theory – that research has too little theory, too much theory, or employs theory suboptimally. We also highlighted common criteria for appraising the quality of theory and its application in HPER. Finally, we discussed general and specific ways of developing theoretical connoisseurship in HPER, with a smorgasbord of tips that all emphasise the importance of time, dedication, and collaboration. We hope this chapter has clearly outlined the foundations of theory in HPER and will help you reflect critically on your application of theory in HPER. We invite you to extend your learning about HPER theory by reading the suggested references in Box 2.14.

Box 2.14   Recommended reading for HPER theory

Brown J, Bearman M, Kirby C, et al. Theory, a lost character? As presented in general practice education research papers. *Med Educ*. 2019;53(5):443–457 [16].

Hean S, Anderson L, Green C, et al. Reviews of theoretical frameworks: challenges and judging the quality of theory application. *Med Teach*. 2016;38(6):613–620[81].

(continued)

(continued)

Rees CE, Monrouxe LV. Theory in medical education research: how do we get there? *Med Educ.* 2010;44(4):334–339 [21].

Samuel A, Konopasky A, Schuwirth LWT, et al. Five principles for using educational theory: strategies for advancing health professions education research. *Acad Med.* 2020;95(4):518–522 [22].

Varpio L, Paradis E, Uijtdehaage S, et al. The distinctions between theory, theoretical framework, and conceptual framework. *Acad Med.* 2020;95(7):989–994 [45].

REFERENCES

1. Collins CS, Stockton CM. The central role of theory in qualitative research. *Int J Qual Methods.* 2018;17(1):1–10.

2. Meleis AI. *Theoretical Nursing: Development and Progress*, 4th ed. Philadelphia: Lippincott Williams & Wilkins; 2007.

3. Sutton RI, Staw BM. What theory is not. *Adm Sci Q.* 1995;40(3):371–384.

4. Brosnan C. How and why social science theory can contribute to medical education research. *Med Educ.* 2013;47(1):5–7.

5. Burke CT. The biographical illumination: a Bourdieusian analysis of the role of theory in educational research. *Sociol Res Online.* 2011;16(2):1–9.

6. James D. Theory and educational research: toward critical social explanation. *Br J Sociol Educ.* 2010;31(2):243–248.

7. Gibbs T, Durning S, Van Der Vleuten C. Theories in medical education: towards creating a union between educational practice and research traditions. *Med Teach.* 2011;33(3):183–187.

8. Rees CE, Ottrey E, Barton P, et al. Materials matter: understanding the importance of sociomaterial assemblages for OSCE candidate performance. *Med Educ.* 2021;55(8):961–971.

9. Rees CE, Monrouxe LV. Medical students learning intimate examinations without valid consent: a multicentre study. *Med Educ.* 2011;45(3):261–272.

10. Gordon L, Jindal-Snape D, Morrison J, et al. Multiple and multidimensional transitions from trainee to trained doctor: a qualitative longitudinal study in the UK. *BMJ Open.* 2017;7(11):e018583.

11. Gordon L, Rees CE, Jindal-Snape D. Doctors' identity transitions: choosing to occupy a state of 'betwixt and between'. *Med Educ.* 2020;54(11):1006–1018.

12. Alwazzan L, Rees CE. Women in medical education: views and experiences from the Kingdom of Saudi Arabia. *Med Educ.* 2016;50(8):852–865.

13. Grant C, Osanloo A. Understanding, selecting and integrating a theoretical framework in dissertation research: creating the blueprint for your "house." *Adm Issues J.* 2014;4(2):12–26.

14. Thomas G. What's the use of theory? *Harv Educ Rev.* 1997;67(1):75–104.

15. Creswell JW. *Research Design: Qualitative, Quantitative, and Mixed Methods Approaches*, 3rd ed. Los Angeles: SAGE; 2009.

16. Brown J, Bearman M, Kirby C, et al. Theory, a lost character? As presented in general practice education research papers. *Med Educ.* 2019;53(5):443–457.

17. Kitchel T, Ball AL. Quantitative theoretical and conceptual framework use in agricultural education research. *J Agric Educ.* 2014;55(1):186–199.

18. Reeves S, Albert M, Kuper A, et al. Why use theories in qualitative research? *BMJ.* 2008;337(7670):a949.

19. Varpio L, Ellaway RH. Shaping our worldviews: a conversation about and of theory. *Adv Health Sci Educ.* 2021;26(1):339–345.

20. Kilminster S. Off the peg or made to measure: how does this theory fit? *Med Educ.* 2017;51(4):342–343.

21. Rees CE, Monrouxe LV. Theory in medical education research: how do we get there? *Med Educ.* 2010;44(4):334–339.

22. Samuel A, Konopasky A, Schuwirth LWT, et al. Five principles for using educational theory: strategies for advancing health professions education research. *Acad Med.* 2020;95(4):518–522.

23. Rees CE, Ajjawi R, Monrouxe LV. The construction of power in family medicine bedside teaching: a video observation study. *Med Educ.* 2013;47(2):154–165.

24. Engestrom Y. *Learning by Expanding: An Activity-Theoretical Approach to Developmental Research.* Cambridge: Cambridge University Press; 1987.

25. Cronbach LJ, Gleser GC, Nanda H, et al. *The Dependability of Behavioral Measurements: Theory of Generalizability for Scores and Profiles.* New York: Wiley; 1972.

26. Ryan RM, Deci EL. Self-determination theory and the facilitations of intrinsic motivation, social development and well-being. *Am Psychol.* 2000;55(1):68–78.

27. Qureshi SP. Cultural historical activity theory for studying practice-based learning and change in medical education. *Adv Med Educ Pract.* 2021;12:923–935.

28. Larsen DP, Nimmon L, Varpio L. Cultural historical activity theory: the role of tools and tensions in medical education. *Acad Med.* 2019;94(8):1255.

29. Frambach JM, Driessen EW, van der Vleuten CPM. Using activity theory to study cultural complexity in medical education. *Perspect Med Educ.* 2014;3(3):190–203.

30. Sawaki Y. Generalizability theory. In Salkind NJ, ed. *Encyclopedia of Research Design.* Thousand Oaks, California: SAGE; 2010: 533–537.

31. Bloch R, Norman G. Generalizability theory for the perplexed: a practical introduction and guide: AMEE Guide no 68. *Med Teach* 2012;34(11):960–992.

32. ten Cate O, Kusurkar RA, Williams GC. How self-determination theory can assist our understanding of the teaching and learning processes in medical education. AMEE Guide no. 59. *Med Teach.* 2011;33(12):961–973.

33. Varpio L, MacLeod A. Harnessing the multidisciplinary edge effect by exploring paradigms, ontologies, epistemologies, axiologies, and methodologies. *Acad Med.* 2020;95(5):686–689.

34. Palermo C, Reidlinger DP, Rees CE. Internal coherence matters: lessons for nutrition and dietetics research. *Nutr Diet.* 2021;78(3):252–267.

35. Al-Saadi H. *Demystifying Ontology and Epistemology in Research Methods.* Sheffield, UK: University of Sheffield; 2014. https://www.academia.edu/26531411/Demystifying_Ontology_and_Epistemology_in_research_methods (accessed 26 Oct 2022).

36. Bradbury-Jones C, Taylor J, Herber O. How theory is used and articulated in qualitative research: development of a new typology. *Soc Sci Med.* 2014;120:135–141.

37. Bleakley A, Bligh J, Browne J. *Medical Education for the Future: Identity, Power and Location.* London: Springer Science & Business Media; 2011.

38. Crawford LM. Conceptual and theoretical frameworks in research. In Burkholder GJ, Cox KA, Crawford LM, et al., eds. *Research Design and Methods: An Applied Guide for the Scholar-Practitioner.* Los Angeles: SAGE; 2020: 35–48.

39. De Champlain AF. A primer on classical test theory and item response theory for assessments in medical education. *Med Educ.* 2010;44(1):109–117.

40. Sharma M. Applying feminist theory to medical education. *Lancet.* 2019;393(10171):570–578.

41. Fenwick T, Nimmo GR. Making visible what matters: sociomaterial approaches for research and practice in healthcare education. In Cleland JC, Durning SJ, eds. *Researching Medical Education.* Chichester: Wiley Blackwell; 2015: 67–79.

42. Norman G. From the editors: research, theory and science in medical education. *Adv Health Sci Educ.* 1997;1(3):175–177.

43. Watling CJ, Lingard L. Grounded theory in medical education research: AMEE Guide no 70. *Med Teach*. 2012;34(10):850–861.

44. Saldana J, Omasta M. *Qualitative Research: Analyzing Life*. Thousand Oaks, Calif.: SAGE; 2017.

45. Varpio L, Paradis E, Uijtdehaage S, et al. The distinctions between theory, theoretical framework, and conceptual framework. *Acad Med*. 2020;95(7):989–994.

46. Malle BF. *How the Mind Explains Behavior: Folk Explanations, Meaning, and Social Interaction*. Cambridge, Mass.: MIT Press; 2004.

47. Malle BF, *F.Ex: A Coding Scheme for Folk Explanations of Behavior, Version 4.4*. Eugene: University of Oregon; 2007.

48. Jindal-Snape D. *A-Z of Transitions*. Basingstoke: Palgrave MacMillan; 2016.

49. Beech N. On the nature of dialogic identity work. *Organ Stud*. 2008;15(1):51–74.

50. Ybema S, Beech N, Ellis N. Transitional and perpetual liminality: an identity practice perspective. *Anthropol South Afr*. 2011;34(1–2):21–29.

51. Crotty M. *The Foundations of Social Research: Meaning and Perspective in the Research Process*. London: SAGE; 2003.

52. Crenshaw KW. Demarginalizing the intersection of race and sex: a black feminist critique of antidiscrimination doctrine, feminist theory and antiracist politics. *Univ Chic Leg Forum*. 1989;140(1):139–167.

53. Egbert J, Sanden S. *Foundations of Education Research: Understanding Theoretical Components*, 2nd ed. New York: Routledge; 2019.

54. Lingard B. Thinking about theory in educational research: fieldwork in philosophy. *Educ Phil Theory*. 2015;47(2):173–191.

55. Laksov KB, Dornan T, Teunissen PW. Making theory explicit – an analysis of how medical education research(ers) describe how they connect to theory. *BMC Med Educ*. 2017;17(1):18.

56. Norman G. Editorial – theory testing research versus theory-based research. *Adv Health Sci Educ*. 2004;9(3):175–178.

57. Varpio L, Aschenbrener C, Bates J. Tackling wicked problems: how theories of agency can provide new insights. *Med Educ*. 2017;51(4):353–365.

58. Willis K, Daly J, Kealy M, et al. The essential role of social theory in qualitative public health research. *Aust N Z J Public Health*. 2007;31(5):438–443.

59. Fenwick T. Sociomateriality in medical practice and learning: attuning to what matters. *Med Educ*. 2014;48(1):44–52.

60. Fenwick T, Dahlgen MA. Towards socio-material approaches in simulation-based education: lessons from complexity theory. *Med Educ*. 2015;49(4):359–367.

61. MacLeod A, Cameron P, Ajjawi R, et al. Actor-network theory and ethnography: sociomaterial approaches to researching medical education. *Perspect Med Educ*. 2019;8(3):177–186.

62. MacLeod A, Ajjawi R. Thinking sociomaterially: why matter matters in medical education. *Acad Med*. 2020;95(6):851–855.

63. Gordon L, Rees C, Ker J, et al. Using video-reflexive ethnography to capture the complexity of leadership enactment in the healthcare workplace. *Adv Health Sci Educ*. 2017;22(5):1101–1121.

64. Ajjawi R, Monrouxe LV, Rees CE. Learning clinical skills during bedside teaching encounters in general practice: a video-observational study with insights from activity theory. *J Workplace Learn*. 2015;27(4):298–314.

65. Kajamaa A, Mattick K, Parker H, et al. Trainee doctors' experiences of common problems in the antibiotic prescribing process: an activity theory analysis of narrative data from UK hospitals. *BMJ Open*. 2019;9(6):e028733.

66. Bearman M, Ajjawi R. Actor-network theory and the OSCE: formulating a new research agenda for a post-psychometric era. *Adv Health Sci Educ*. 2018;23(5):1037–1049.

67. Knight LV, Rees CE. "Enough is enough, I don't want any audience": exploring medical students' explanations of consent-related behaviours. *Adv Health Sci Educ*. 2008;13(4):407–426.

68. Monrouxe LV, Rees CE, Lewis NJ, et al. Medical educators' social acts of explaining passing underperformance in students: a qualitative study. *Adv Health Sci Educ.* 2011;16(2):239–252.

69. Pigott TD. The role of theory in quantitative data analysis. In Wyse D, Selwyn N, Smith E, et al., eds. *The BERA/SAGE Handbook of Educational Research: 2 Volume Set.* London: SAGE; 2017: 699–710.

70. Shearn K, Allmark P, Piercy H, et al. Building realist program theory for large complex and messy interventions. *Int J Qual Methods.* 2017;16(1):1–11.

71. Glaser BG, Strauss AL. *The Discovery of Grounded Theory: Strategies for Qualitative Research.* Chicago: Aldine; 1967.

72. Charmaz K. *Constructing Grounded Theory: A Practical Guide Through Qualitative Analysis.* London: SAGE; 2006.

73. Heng TT. Examining the role of theory in qualitative research: a literature review of studies on Chinese international students in higher education. *J Int Students.* 2020;10(4):798–816.

74. Tight M. Research into higher education: an atheoretical community of practice? *High Educ Res Dev.* 2004;23(4):395–411.

75. Teunissen PW. On the transfer of theory to the practice of research and education. *Med Educ.* 2010;44(6):534–535.

76. Fenwick F, Edwards R, Sawchuk P. *Emerging Approaches to Educational Research: Tracing the Sociomaterial.* London: Routledge; 2011.

77. Ellaway RH. Theoriaphobia, theoriaphilia, theoriamania. *Adv Health Sci Educ.* 2021;26(1):1–3.

78. Kumasi KD, Charbonneau DH, Walster D. Theory talk in the library science scholarly literature: an exploratory analysis. *Libr Inf Sci Res.* 2013;35(3):175–180.

79. Verkoeijen PPJL, Tabbers HK. Good research requires productive theories and guidelines. *Med Educ.* 2013;47(9):863–865.

80. Shoemaker PJ, Tankards Jr JW, Lasorsa DL. *How to Build Social Sciences Theories.* Thousand Oaks, Calif.: SAGE; 2004.

81. Hean S, Anderson L, Green C, et al. Reviews of theoretical frameworks: challenges and judging the quality of theory application. *Med Teach.* 2016;38(6):613–620.

82. Hindi AMK, Willis SC, Schafheutle EI. Using communities of practice as a lens for exploring experiential pharmacy learning in general practice: are communities of practice the way forward in changing the training culture in pharmacy? *BMC Med Educ.* 2022;22:12.

83. Biesta G, Allan J, Edwards R. The theory question in research capacity building in education: towards an agenda for research and practice. *Br J Educ Stud.* 2011; 59(3):225–239.

84. Russell A. Ten tips to become a wine expert. The University of Sydney; 2017. https://www.sydney.edu.au/news-opinion/news/2017/07/13/ten-tips-to-become-a-wine-expert.html (accessed 5 October 2022).

85. Booth A, Carroll C. Systematic searching for theory to inform systematic reviews: is it feasible? Is it desirable? *Health Info Libr J.* 2015;32(3):220–235.

86. Cleland JC, Durning SJ, (eds.) *Researching Medical Education.* Chichester: Wiley Blackwell; 2015.

87. Tsouroufli M, Rees CE, Monrouxe LV, et al. Gender, identities and intersectionality in medical education research. *Med Educ.* 2011;45(3):213–216.

88. Verma A. Intersecting identities in healthcare education: exploring the influence of gendered environments on healthcare students' workplace learning, retention and success. UK: University of Dundee; Unpublished PhD thesis; 2018.

89. Offiah G. Women in surgery: exploring stakeholders' lived experiences in the Irish and Scottish healthcare system. UK: University of Dundee; Unpublished PhD thesis; 2021.

Ethics in Health Professions Education Research

Lynn V. Monrouxe[1], Ghufran Jassim[2], and Bridget C. O'Brien[3]

[1] The University of Sydney, Camperdown, New South Wales, Australia
[2] Royal College of Surgeons in Ireland–Medical University of Bahrain, Bahrain
[3] University of California San Francisco, San Francisco, California, USA

Box 3.1   Chapter 3 learning objectives: After reading this chapter you should be able to ...

- Describe the key theoretical perspectives involved in ethical decision-making in health professions education research (HPER)
- Explain the scope and role of Institutional Review Boards and Human Research Ethics Committees
- Outline the key ethical considerations in human research
- Discuss issues of research integrity and how to maintain this in your own work
- Evaluate the range of ethical issues when publishing your research

---

3.1   INTRODUCING CHAPTER 3

> Multitasking, multidisciplinary work and multi-authored works ... [are] expected in order to ... move up the scientific ranks ... Complex relationships are accompanied with tough decisions regarding authorship, dicing the funding pie, and how to treat privileged data ... the temptation to cheat, cut corners, and misbehave seems to be at its zenith ... the best (or highly rewarded) science is compromised with seemingly endless ethical issues. [1 p. 2]

Ethics in research is the 'framework for creating a fabric of integrity' [1 p. 9]. Ethical considerations occur across all stages of research including design, applying for funding, data collection and analysis, dissemination, quality appraisals, and peer review [1–4]. But research ethics are far from simple. They focus on interrelationships

---

Foundations of Health Professions Education Research: Principles, Perspectives and Practices,
First Edition. Edited by Charlotte E. Rees, Lynn V. Monrouxe, Bridget C. O'Brien, Lisi J. Gordon, and Claire Palermo.

between context and the people involved: researchers, supervisors, participants, practitioners, patients, funders, and research users. These interrelationships can lead to variations in knowledge construction, with research ethics and your own decision-making playing key roles in your research integrity [5]. Challenging decisions and conflicting priorities can compromise research integrity, especially in our publish or perish academic climate [3, 6–8]. Thus, from a deficit perspective [9–11], scientific misconduct has been the subject of much writing. This highlights wide-ranging unethical researcher behaviours across six misconduct categories (data, methods, policy, outside influence, credit, and cutting corners) which we use to structure part of our chapter [10, 11].

In this chapter, we aim to help you consider the ethical issues you might encounter within HPER (see Box 3.1), supporting you as you face the hurdles along your research journey. See the book glossary for all ethics-related terms employed in this chapter. We begin by outlining key theoretical perspectives involved in ethical decision-making in section 3.2. In section 3.3, we turn to practical processes of doing ethics via Institutional Review Boards (IRBs) and Human Research Ethics Committees (HRECs). We consider six categories of misconduct in section 3.4, then summarise our chapter in section 3.5. As we highlight these interrelated ethical issues, we bring them to life through discussions of our own ethical conundrums (mostly de-identified) across multiple 'pause and reflect' boxes and a case study. By engaging in this chapter, we expect you to be better able to evaluate ethical issues as you undertake your HPER and prepare for decisions that lay ahead.

3.2 ETHICAL DECISION-MAKING: THEORETICAL CONSIDERATIONS

... ethics is a systematic approach to understanding, analyzing, and distinguishing matters of right and wrong ... [12 p. 23]

Ethics are not a static set of rules/procedures guiding behaviour; active participation in ethical action is required based on codes of conduct providing sound rationales for action. Ethical practice is underpinned by concerns around freedom of personal choice and obligations to others. As such, ethics have strong relational components: our ethical choices affect others. However, ethics are not black and white. Some actions considered ethical from one perspective might be thought unethical from another. A distinction has been made in the literature between procedural ethics and ethics in practice [13]. In this section, we begin by providing an overview of various ethical perspectives that inform research decision-making processes.

While numerous ethical standpoints exist [5], two key perspectives have been identified: Indigenous and Euro-Western [14]. Regarding Indigenous perspectives, ethical practices have their roots in the interrelational values of respect, connectivity, and reciprocity. While international differences in Indigenous perspectives exist, we focus on commonalities. Typically, ethics within an Indigenous framework recognises the importance of the intimate interconnections between Indigenous Peoples and their lands [14]. Core international principles include: relational accountability (to all, including colleagues, participants, ancestors, the land, and for some cultures, dreams), communality of knowledge (everyone contributes, knowledge is interrelational), reciprocity (taking just what you need and giving back), and benefit-sharing [14, 15]. Further, there is recognition that: 'within a relationship of unequal power, ethical safety is more likely to be achieved by developing interdependence and trust' [14 p. 27]. Euro-Western practices, on the other hand, are typically rooted in the philosophical traditions of deontology, utilitarianism, and virtue ethics. While deontology and utilitarianism drive decision-making processes around which action you should take, virtue ethics focus on the kind of person you should be.

Regarding deontology, Beauchamp and Childress [16] outline one perspective grounded in Euro-Western individualism and philosophy asserting that our actions are inherently right or wrong and ends cannot justify the means. In other words, this ethical stance asserts an individual action can be morally correct (or not), irrespective of any consequences and contexts. This perspective comprises the following four key obligatory universal principles (rules) to guide ethical decision-making (henceforth known as principlism): respect for autonomy (and decision-making capacities), non-maleficence (avoid causing harm), beneficence (providing benefit), and justice (fairness of benefit/risk distribution).

Utilitarianism instead draws on the principle of benefit-maximisation (and harm-minimisation). A cost–benefit analysis is considered around potential positive and negative impacts of research on all stakeholders before actions are decided [17]. This entails a majority rules approach where individuals are only a means to an end rather than the end itself. When considering research from a utilitarianism perspective, concepts such as informed consent and participant deception are key points: what if your research uncovers valuable insights into the ways in which we act in the world, but only if participants are deceived? [18]

Finally, virtue ethics are context dependent, open to interpretation [19], and can be influenced by religious teachings. For example, Islamic ethics (based on the Qur'ān) emphasise accountability to God, God's unity, and the notion of *maslahah* (public benefits) at its foundation. Here, ethical concepts are defined as: (1) positive, *sālihāt*, good behaviour (e.g., goodness, honesty, justice), and (2) negative, *sayyiāt*, bad behaviour (e.g., subjugation, dishonesty, misconduct) [20]. Others advocate different virtues, such as Confucianism with the interdependent virtues of *rén* (humanism) and *yì* (justice) that comprise the ethical system supported by *li* (respect for social etiquette), *shu* (empathy), and *zhì* (wisdom, knowing what is right) [21]. Work through Box 3.2 to explore these different ethics approaches to the well-known trolley problem.

Box 3.2 Pause and reflect: The trolley problem and three Euro-Western ethics approaches*

The trolley (train) problem can help us think through why we might take an action (or not) and whether all actions with the same consequences are equal. It is an important thought-dilemma, giving rise to issues around the differences between doing and allowing harm, and might provide insights into your own ethical stance.

Consider the following: You are standing by a lever near a rail track and along comes a trolley. On the track there are five workers (unbeknown to the trolley driver). You can divert the trolley to another line using the lever. However, there is someone working on that line too. If you pull the lever, one person will die. If you do not pull it, five people will die. What do you do? This video explains the situation and options: https://youtu.be/bOpf6KcWYyw.

Deontological: The most appropriate action is the moral (right/wrong) action. Is it right to kill someone even if the action results in saving five lives?

Utilitarian: The most appropriate action will achieve the greatest good. Would saving five lives be considered achieving the greatest good?

Virtue ethics: In some cultures, the most appropriate action is to pull the lever because saving more lives is what a virtuous person would do. However, in some cultures, a virtuous person might act differently. For example, in Daoism the concept of *Wu wei* (無為: inaction) gives priority to the natural way of the world. We cannot truly anticipate the consequences of our actions (the one person killed might later have gone on to save others' lives), so how can we intervene?

Reflect:

- What would you do and why?
- Think of a situation in your own HPER where the trolley problem might be relevant.

We omit Indigenous approaches here due to their wide-ranging perspectives and the lack of research from which we might draw.

Now that you have reviewed several ethical perspectives, take a moment to consider how these relate to your own ethical perspectives (see Box 3.3).

Box 3.3   Pause and reflect: Reflect on your sociocultural and ethical upbringing

- Which ethical perspective(s) resonates with you and why?
- Where do your ethical principles come from, and how strongly do you believe in them?
- What does this mean for you as a researcher?
- How will you maintain your ethical stance when working with others with different stances?

3.3   DOING ETHICS: PRACTICAL CONSIDERATIONS

Appreciating ethical perspectives is key to *doing* ethical research. But who oversees the ethical conception and progression of research? In this section, we consider the practical issues around developing and monitoring research guidelines.

3.3.1   Institutional Review Boards (IRBs) and Human Research Ethics Committees (HRECs)

If you have not already encountered institutional review boards (IRBs) or human research ethics committees (HRECs), you will soon (henceforth collectively called IRBs). In most countries, researchers undertaking work with humans are usually required to submit their research protocol to an IRB prior to data collection (so-called procedural ethics) [22]. While procedures are relatively well-established and similar across contexts, IRB procedures and criteria are newer to some world regions. For example, research examining Middle Eastern countries' ethics guidelines suggest that some do not yet have national guidelines (e.g., Syria, Iraq), some are silent on the issue (e.g., Oman, Palestine, Yemen), and some have up to three guidelines (e.g., Saudi Arabia) [23]. Furthermore, not all guidelines mention IRBs and the requirement for research to be passed by ethics committees. For simplicity, we therefore focus on processes of IRBs and codes of conduct within Euro-Western countries where things are relatively standardised. However, see Box 3.4 for an example of a region with newly established ethics guidelines.

IRBs typically comprise small committees with at least five people from mixed backgrounds (academic/lay) providing opinions regarding proposals' ethical status. Drawing primarily on deontological principles, the key concern of IRBs is to provide ethics review judging whether participant risks are offset by expected benefits. Furthermore, they ensure that consent, autonomy, relative confidentiality, and privacy in data management are ensured, alongside methodological robustness. IRBs' work is partly informed through international ethical obligations embodied in codes of conduct, national laws, and organisational constraints [24].

IRBs have a duty to provide systems ensuring that you stand by your ethical obligations set out in your approved protocol. That is, that you obtain informed consent, you notify the IRB of any protocol problems and significant changes, and so on. Within HPER, unlike clinical research, risks for participants are often relatively low [25]. Nonetheless, you must still consider all possible risks (e.g., coercion, psychological risks) and include ways to mitigate them.

> ## Box 3.4 Pause and reflect: IRBs and codes of conduct in Middle Eastern countries
>
> IRBs and codes of conduct are newly and slowly progressing processes in the Middle East. Although the number of Middle Eastern countries with ethics committees is gradually developing, ethical review of clinical trial proposals is still underdeveloped, with inconsistencies and omissions [23, 26]. As is often the case for non-Western countries, guidelines are initially based on Euro-Western ethical codes (e.g., Declaration of Helsinki, Nuremberg Code) without considering cultural/religious contexts. For example, there is an absence of discussion of the impact of Fatwa (decree from an Islamic religious leader) on the application of ethical principles. Furthermore, given that ethics reflect a mixture of cultural values, adherence to ethical frameworks is not straightforward. For example, established guidelines for informed participant consent are set by IRBs, yet research in the context of Lebanon and Qatar suggests the actual practice of obtaining consent is influenced by researchers' own ideas around what participants need: often providing information informally and waiving the requirement for signatures [27]. And while IRBs are making great progress in reviewing and maintaining minimal standards for ethical obligations such as consent, confidentiality, and robustness of methodology, extensive work is still needed in monitoring committees, and obtaining research status reports during and after completion, alongside processes around data credibility and scientific validity of research activities.
>
> Reflect:
>
> - Consider the status of IRBs in your region. Are they well established? Do they reflect your cultural values and norms?
> - Does the status of IRBs affect your intentions (or ability) to work internationally?
> - What steps would you take to ensure your international research is ethically monitored?

3.3.2 Codes of Conduct

Codes of conduct comprise institutional guidelines developed to ensure that researchers have clarity in how they should conduct their research, both in terms of virtues and actions [28]. Thus, codes of conduct are morally binding standards that guide, control, and sometimes regulate behaviours. Having said this, many codes are based around the ethics of principlism, which structures the review process to improve researcher accountability towards high-quality research, with participants' rights central [29].

There is no single overarching code of conduct for you as a researcher. Rather, it is your responsibility to find out which codes are relevant for your institutional context, professional body, collaborators, participants, and any international codes of practice. Thus, if you are researching with Indigenous colleagues and participants, you should seek out the relevant codes of conduct for doing so. For example, Australia's National Health and Medical Research Council developed ethical guidelines governing research with Aboriginal or Torres Strait Islanders that highlights core values of: 'spirit and integrity, cultural continuity, equity, reciprocity, respect, and responsibility' [30 p. 3]. Furthermore, it is important for you to be aware that considerable variation exists across different codes, potentially causing confusion (see Chapter 13). First, different terms might be used to mean similar things, such as intellectual freedom and academic freedom (both address your rights to an unobstructed search for knowledge, but the former applies to all people, and the latter is reserved for academics). Second, the same terms can mean different things, such as different meanings of responsibility, respect, and justice. It is therefore important that you consider the different contexts in which codes are situated, paying close attention to any definitions offered. Take a moment to consider the codes of conduct relevant to your research (see Box 3.5).

Box 3.5 Stop and do: Which code(s) of conduct should you consider?

Consider the different codes of ethical conduct that might apply to you and think about your organisation, professional body, research partners, and so on.

- What are the main commonalities across the documents?
- What (if any) differences exist between the codes?
- Are there omissions in the codes? If so, what are they?
- How do the codes fit with your own personal ethical codes?

If you are not sure which codes apply to your context, consider these general codes:

- British Educational Research Association [BERA] (2018) *Ethical Guidelines for Educational Research*, fourth edition, London. https://www.bera.ac.uk/researchers-resources/publications/ethical-guidelines-for-educational-research-2018 [accessed 17 September 2022].
- The PRO-RES Framework for Ethical Evidence (2019) https://prores-project.eu/ [accessed 17 September 2022].
- The American Educational Research Association (AERA) Code of Ethics (2011) https://www.aera.net/About-AERA/AERA-Rules-Policies/Professional-Ethics [accessed 17 September 2022].

(continued)

(continued)

- The Singapore Statement on Research Integrity (2010) https://wcrif.org/guidance/singapore-statement [accessed 17 September 2022].
- The Australian Code for the Responsible Conduct of Research (2018) https://www.nhmrc.gov.au/about-us/publications/australian-code-responsible-conduct-research-2018 [accessed 17 September 2022].

3.4   RESEARCH INTEGRITY

Despite well-articulated codes, ethical/integrity breaches are relatively common. In this section, we consider breaches in six domains: data, methods, policy, outside influence, credit, and cutting corners [10].

3.4.1   Data Breaches

Here we cover academic dishonesty that involves data manipulation. Data falsification occurs when researchers manipulate (or omit) data to achieve desired results (e.g., support preferred claims or favoured hypotheses). Falsification also includes image manipulation or presentation such as presenting graphical data using a distorted scale to exaggerate small differences, or visually distorting data through inappropriate use of colour gradients [31]. Other data manipulation practices include: omitting data from analyses (sometimes because they look wrong), overlooking flawed data or methods in others' research, fabricating data, and ignoring data that contradict previous research findings [10, 31, 32]. While these may seem like obvious practices to avoid, there are situations where ethical conduct is ambiguous. For example, consider survey results with missing data. You might choose to impute a mean for missing data to preserve sample size. Or, if you have a subgroup within a survey with a low response rate, you might consider excluding this group from your analysis. Pause and reflect on a data manipulation dilemma in Box 3.6.

Data manipulation applies to qualitative data as well as quantitative. For example, data manipulation can include intentional misrepresentation of research participants' talk or written data [33], or engaging in misrepresentation in neglectful (rather than purposeful) ways. Indeed, consider participants from marginalised or minority populations. How might you conduct your research ethically, given that your interpretation of participants' talk might not necessarily reflect participants' experiences and meaning? Your interpretation could misrepresent (albeit unintentionally) the phenomenon at hand, but might also serve to: 'significantly impact individuals that already experience discrimination and undue social stress' [34 p. 277]. There are ways in which you might mitigate these harms (see Chapters 7 and 8), so it is important that you are aware of such issues [35]. Furthermore, for Indigenous Peoples, the very word research can be offensive, and all research conducted on, rather than with, participants is considered unethical: leading to missed representations [36]. However, there are different viewpoints on data representation, some dependent upon research approaches taken (see Part II of this book). Recognising your duty to accurately represent your data throughout your research journey will help diminish any potential harms.

> **Box 3.6 Pause and reflect: Data manipulation dilemma**
>
> <u>Scenario 1</u>: You are working as a PhD student on a research project for which your supervisor won a grant. The research uses an experimental design to test an *a priori* null hypothesis (see Chapter 5). At the end of your pre-planned data collection cycle, you examine the descriptive results, then perform statistical tests. Your results are somewhat aligned with your desired outcome (i.e., almost reaching statistical significance to support your supervisors' developing theory), but there is another trend in the data that would contest this theory. Your supervisor tells you to continue your data collection until you reach the desired statistical significance, then stop (thereby avoiding a significant outcome for the unwanted trend).
> Reflect:
>
> - Is what the supervisor suggests ethical? What is your reasoning around your response?
> - How would you respond to your supervisor? Why?

3.4.2 Methods Breaches

Methods misconduct includes inadequate or inappropriate research design, substandard record/data management, and the non-reporting of key methodology features in protocols, grants, or articles [10]. Thus, within this section we ask the following questions [37]: Who does what, to whom, and why? What comprises data and what happens to it? How transparent are researchers when reporting their work?

In terms of who and why, we begin with participant–researcher power disparities. Some argue that ethical research entails matched researcher–participant groups (e.g., Indigenous researchers for Indigenous research questions, disability researchers for disability research questions) to ensure that people with lived experiences are adequately represented [38]. Regardless of whether this approach is optimal (or even feasible) for your research, it is important to attend to issues of power symmetries, decolonisation, inclusivity, and equality when designing and conducting your research (see Chapter 8).

Regarding what comprises data and how it is handled, whatever philosophical position you work within, and whether you decide to conduct an experiment (see Chapter 5) or interview (see Chapter 6–9), what is important is that: (1) it is suitable to the research question(s); and (2) it is managed appropriately. These aspects will be described in your research protocol and submitted to the appropriate IRB alongside your data management plan. Indeed, when undertaken correctly, your data management plan is the: 'ultimate data quality assessment tool' [39 p. 314], describing the expected data, how it fits with your research questions and approach, and how it will be managed (including storage, analysis, and disposal).

Transparency in methods and research reporting is also key: insufficient reporting of the methodological processes involved in your study makes critical appraisal processes impossible [40]. By using reporting guidelines, you can improve the value of your work and minimise omissions, ensuring your research is understood and/or can be replicated (see Chapter 4 for more on reporting guidelines, and Chapters 5–9 for approach-specific guidelines).

3.4.3 Policy Breaches

Policy misconduct includes bypassing or omitting aspects of human research requirements (e.g., informed consent, confidentiality, transparency, protecting vulnerable participants). We mainly associate this area of academic integrity with IRB processes. You are probably aware that you should monitor participant risks and burdens, minimising them to ensure benefits outweigh harms. Clear statements around these aspects are required when submitting your research to IRBs, so that committees can make their assessments. However, as with all human research, the risk–benefit analysis is dynamic and clear articulation of monitoring processes is necessary. When developing your plan, you need to consider the following: what are the risks? (risk identification), what is the probability that risks will occur? (risk estimation), and, should they occur, how much harm they will pose? (risk evaluation). All elements of the study should be evaluated for risk, alongside comments on any study benefits.

Many of our ethical considerations around human research are interrelated, which creates dilemmas for researchers. For example, informed consent, anonymity, and confidentiality can be problematic when undertaking research (especially qualitative participant-led) in small communities [41]. Furthermore, it is important to acknowledge the dynamic nature of these constructs during the conduct of your research. Consider the continuous nature of informed consent throughout the recruitment, data collection, and even dissemination phases of your research. These include knowledge sharing, power imbalances, communication of risks and benefits, and how consent is ascertained and recorded across each phase (e.g., written, orally, implied).

The act of gaining consent necessarily includes aspects around disclosure and comprehension of information, consent being voluntary (not coerced), and participants having the capacity to understand what they are consenting to [42]. You therefore need to disclose information to participants around what the research is about, why they have been invited to participate, what will happen to them and their data, and their right to withdraw at any time (and without having to explain why). These issues of disclosure and comprehension are often dealt with via participant information sheets and consent forms. However, disclosure of information does not mean that it has been adequately communicated. For example, research suggests that even if participants have signed consent forms, they rarely read sections on benefits, anonymity, and confidentiality [43]. Being present when information sheets and consent forms are read and signed can increase engagement [43], providing an opportunity for conversations about your study.

Viewing informed consent as a process, rather than a one-off (tick-box) occurrence, is especially important when you use qualitative methods. In qualitative research, the trajectory of the topic under investigation can rapidly change: in observational research, unexpected events might occur, and during interviews, the subject matter might drift or a participant might become distressed when discussing specific events. Thus, participants may need a break from the data collection process (e.g., turning off the recording device until they compose themselves), or even withdrawing from the study entirely. Approaching consent as an ongoing process facilitates negotiation and revision, providing participants with a more collaborative and autonomous decision-making role [44].

Other key human research ethical issues are the related constructs of participant confidentiality, anonymity, and de-identification. Confidentiality is your promise to neither ask participants for personal data without good reason, nor disclose identifying information about them: respecting their privacy, dignity, and autonomy [45]. Anonymisation is an essential aspect of your data collection, management, and (where appropriate) safe, responsible data-sharing [46, 47]. Although anonymisation and de-identification are often considered synonymous, their meaning varies internationally and legally. Thus, de-identification occurs when personal (formal) identifiers (e.g., name, gender, age, ethnicity, religiosity, professional group) are removed and sometimes replaced when reporting data. This is undertaken to ensure that participants cannot be directly identified from reading your article. Anonymisation, however, is associated with data protection legal frameworks that stipulate a person must not be identified directly or indirectly from information you disclose [46]. While the removal of direct identifiers is the first step, you might also need to take other steps to modify identifiers (e.g., the context in which your data were collected). For quantitative research, where your data are numerical, anonymisation is straightforward. However, if your research is qualitative, things become more complex. Deductive disclosure, or what Tolich [48] calls internal confidentiality, considers whether others from the same group, organisation, or research context can deduce your participants' identities. This issue is especially problematic where participants' interconnected relationships can be made visible through their talk (particularly narratives) and may require modification or omission of direct quotes to preserve anonymity.

Finally, confidentiality has its limits. For example, information might be disclosed during your data collection that legally or ethically needs to be communicated, thus revealing your participants' identities. Indeed, Bos [45] classifies confidentiality breaches according to four types: culpable, justifiable, and enforced breaches, and waivers. Culpable breaches comprise situations in which you fail to sufficiently consider all deductive disclosure aspects prior to publishing, leaving participants open to identification. Justifiable breaches are where you might be extremely concerned for others' welfare if you fail to act on information, despite this breaching participant confidentiality. Enforced breaches occur when, by law, you are asked to reveal the identity of your research participant(s). Such enforced breaches are rare, and this is highly unlikely in HPER. Finally, participants might waive their right to confidentiality, the most common type of breach. It can apply to research in which participants are also collaborators (e.g., co-participatory research designs: see Chapters 8 and 9) and research into sensitive areas where the limits of confidentiality are discussed upfront (see Box 3.7).

Box 3.7   Pause and reflect: Case study illustrating the limits of confidentiality

Scenario 2: Our research programme examining healthcare students' professionalism dilemmas included numerous narrative interview studies [49]. During these interviews, participants narrated hundreds of events occurring in clinical and university settings. Although we anticipated some types of events due to our knowledge of the literature and cultures in which students were learning, some events comprised shocking, pervasive, and harmful practices. We thought that if we intervened, we could potentially stop them, prevent future lapses, and even in some cases save lives. While we needed to make hard decisions about breaking participants' confidentiality, we informed participants upfront (verbally and through the studies' information sheets) around the limits of confidentiality. If

(continued)

(continued)

they told us something we believed was illegal or harmful and we thought we could do something to prevent it happening again, then we would talk with them about the appropriate course of action, possibly breaking confidentiality.

Three situations arose across our research programme where we decided to act. These involved allegedly illegal/unprofessional behaviours by a university-based lecturer (case 1), a student (case 2), and multiple practicing clinicians in a particular speciality (case 3). In all cases, we discussed our concerns with the relevant participant(s), explaining that we needed to act. Our key concern was that, despite them not revealing the perpetrator(s) name, it was possible for us to deductively discover who was being discussed. We explained that it was possible that action could directly prevent future harms to various people including students (case 1); peers, patients, and the university (case 2); and patients (case 3). In all situations we ascertained participants' agreement to raise concerns with key people/institutions, how we would share those concerns (and to whom), and whether they wanted involvement in the raising concerns processes. Once we acted, we gave them feedback on outcomes.

Regarding participant confidentiality breaches, in the first two cases participants voluntarily waived their right to confidentiality. But in the third case, confidentiality was partially breached (revealing participants' location and year of study, but not names), comprising a justifiable breach.

Reflect:

- What (if any) situations could occur in your own HPER that may require you to breach participant confidentiality?
- How might you plan for these situations as part of IRB processes?
- If breaches are necessary, what steps should you take to breach confidentiality in the most ethical manner?

3.4.4   Breaches Involving Outside Influences

Outside influence misconduct includes non-disclosure of conflicts of interest and the manipulation of study results due to funder or employer pressures. A conflict of interest (also called competing interest) happens when you take advantage of your position for personal benefit. This is not confined to financial interests, and can be: 'anything that interferes with, or could reasonably be perceived as interfering with, the full and objective presentation, peer review, editorial decision-making, or publication of research or non-research articles submitted to a journal' [50 p. 1]. The conflict itself is not misconduct; rather it becomes misconduct when you prioritise your own interests. Furthermore, the very act of non-disclosure is also considered misconduct. However, it has been argued that our decision-making capacities are ethically bounded, in that we consider ourselves to be good citizens, severely constraining our ability to recognise our own conflicts of interest (especially invisible conflicts including loyalty for our national/ethnic group) [51]. As Chugh et al. so eloquently put it: 'Ethical decisions are biased by a stubborn view of oneself as moral, competent, and deserving, and thus, not susceptible to conflicts of interest.' [51 p. 80] To overcome these issues, it might be useful to have competing interests conversations with your research team and/or supervisors in which you explore together potential conflicts and resolutions (see Box 3.8).

> **Box 3.8 Pause and reflect: Case scenario on possible conflicts of interest**
>
> <u>Scenario 3</u>: A technology company develops a new gaming software that can be used for educational purposes. The software seems promising and user friendly. The company approaches you as a researcher, offering a generous honorarium to study the utility of this software in education. They pay for your travel and accommodation to go to their headquarters to meet senior management. As part of a confidentiality agreement, the company instructs that any payment must not be disclosed. At the time, you were excited at the prospect of doing the work and did not give it much thought. After two years, the study is complete. You decide to publish in a peer-reviewed journal. The journal requests that you disclose any conflicts of interest.
>   Reflect:
>
> - What (if any) conflicts of interest exist in this scenario? If there are conflicts of interest, how would you manage these?
> - Discuss your thinking with your peers and/or supervisors.

3.4.5 Credit Breaches

Here we consider wide-ranging issues comprising credit misconduct to help you navigate potential pitfalls and facilitate your decision-making towards publishing ethically [10]. Generally, it has been identified that credit misconduct arises from the pressure to publish that all academics continually experience [52, 53]. This publish or perish phenomenon is where the number of outputs published is privileged, rather than the quality of those outputs. Such quantity metrics can be favoured as part of hiring decisions, promotion, tenure, grants, and even cash bonuses for researchers contingent on their publication records [8]. Indeed, it is these grey areas of publishing, rather than severe cases (e.g., data/results falsification, unscrupulous interpretation of statistics, fake peer review), where you may inadvertently slip up, and which comprise the most common ethical breaches in publishing [2, 10].

3.4.5.1 Plagiarism, Self-plagiarism, Duplication, and Recycling

Acts of plagiarism and self-plagiarism are not clear-cut. Furthermore, these constructs are contested across different countries and cultures (see Box 3.9) [54–56]. With so much subjectivity in this area, we emphasise that what we present here is not necessarily a how-to guide. Even if something is deemed technically adequate, such as recycling your words in a grant application, your work might be evaluated poorly if you go beyond acceptable practices in your field (due to the limited number of people in HPER).

There are multiple ways you might commit plagiarism, including passing off others' ideas as your own or copying and pasting others' sentences and even their phrases without adequate referencing. Indeed, it has been said that: 'to me, plagiarism is the most boring of ethical offences; largely borne of both academic laziness and ignorance' [1 p. 21]. Typically, any kind of plagiarism is an intentional act, albeit through laziness. However, at times it is unintentional. For example, cryptomnesia in research contexts is the phenomena where someone thinks they have created an idea or proposition, but they have previously encountered it, forgotten it, and now it is recalled as if it is their own work. Plagiarism via cryptomnesiatic writing is therefore unintended [57]. Further, plagiarism via ignorance is also unintentional, but not excusable.

Self-plagiarism comprises the copying of chunks of your own previously published writing into another document for publication or distribution. Although some might think that self-plagiarism is a strange concept, essentially stealing from yourself, in the context of copyright ownership, the notion of theft becomes more straightforward [58]. Thus, it is important to understand whether the publisher (more common) or the author holds the copyright. When the publisher holds the copyright, an author must request permission to cite large chunks of text or to reproduce figures or tables, even if they are the original author. Furthermore, when the copying of words, tables, and figures renders the second publication redundant, it can comprise a serious ethical breach [59, 60], running the risk of creating a duplicate publication (e.g., presenting the same or similar dataset and conclusions).

Is it ever acceptable for you to copy and paste your previously written works? For the method section of a publication, especially for longitudinal research with multiple publications, an almost verbatim description can sometimes be acceptable, as even journal editors find self-plagiarism slippery [61]. However, this strategy is risky. Likewise, reporting the same theoretical position across related articles can result in acceptable degrees of repetition [61]. It is also argued that recycling your conference material is generally allowable [1], because conference work tends to be where the inception of ideas is disseminated and presented to peers for feedback (see Chapter 11). Such work comprises the foundations of your peer-reviewed publication, rather than completed, published works. Some conferences also allow you to submit abstracts of work that has already been published, so long as the work has not previously been presented at the conference. The rationale is that conferences offer a different form of dissemination and can increase the visibility of published work. Other places in which your work might be recycled are book chapters and grant applications. Once again, care needs to be taken when working up your peer-reviewed publications as book chapters (e.g., re-writing prose, obtaining copyright permission to reproduce figures and tables). However, grant applications are different. Given that you are not disseminating original works; rather, you are making a case for new research, copying chunks of text (e.g., methods sections) is not considered self-plagiarism. However, plagiarising others in this context is unethical. Whether plagiarism, self-plagiarism, or recycling, the issue of duplication is complex. One argument for duplication is to make research available in other languages, although research suggests that this only comprises around one-fifth of cases [62].

Box 3.9   Pause and reflect: Perspectives on Confucian plagiarism

To understand the intent and meaning behind any act, you need to understand the actor and their culture. For example, Confucian-influenced societies (e.g., China, Japan, Korea, Taiwan, Vietnam) generally have a number of features attributed to their philosophy. Above all is the construct of *filial piety* (respect for parents, elders, and ancestors). This respect often includes using their words, because authors and texts are revered: 'to fulfill the ethical obligations of their cultural heritage' [54 p. 96]. This practice leads to copying rather than adopting a critical stance; maintaining a sense of harmony. Thus, (over)respect for seniority may sometimes mean there is a reluctance to critique seniors' points of view, or to challenge potential misconduct by senior researchers within unbalanced power relationships.

Reflect:

- If you were working as part of an international group, how could you better understand different perspectives on plagiarism and mitigate any risks?

3.4.5.2   Salami Slicing and Meat Extenders

Closely linked with self-plagiarism is the construct of salami slicing or data portioning: otherwise known as the 'least publishable unit' [63]. Salami slicing entails publishing multiple articles unnecessarily (i.e., when a more comprehensive paper could otherwise be published) [64]. Meat extenders comprise publications that take previously published data, add to them and create another publication. As a practice this might mean that key elements of the report (e.g., methods, theory, aims, rationale) are at risk of being self-plagiarised. However, there are legitimate reasons why multiple papers from the same dataset might be reported separately, including: stringent journal word limits, spreading knowledge across journals with different readership or language, presenting data through a different analytical lens, presenting different data from the same study to answer different research questions, ability to present more detailed information regarding the study, and the rapid dissemination of findings [64–66].

3.4.5.3   Authorship

> Used appropriately, authorship establishes accountability, responsibility, and credit for scientific information. [67 p. 222]

Responsible authorship is key within publication ethics [68]. It carries substantial privileges and is important for your career development, but there are also responsibilities and legal implications. Appropriate acknowledgement of contributors to manuscripts is not always straightforward [69, 70]. Misappropriation of authorship, however, undermines the trust we have in our publishing system and researchers' integrity. As you begin your own journey through the world of academic publishing (see Chapter 11), it is important that you are aware of the pitfalls around authorship processes. The practices and rationales you observe when deciding who to list as authors might not concord with international recommendations. This discord occurs because HPER is a rich multidisciplinary space, with each discipline bringing with it: 'the customs and traditions of their respective fields' [69 p.1171]. Thus, it is important for you to know that whether as a gift, or through perceived (or actual) coercion, adding authors to research publications, grant applications, and conference publications who have not contributed sufficiently to the research effort is unethical.

So, who is an author? Although there is no universally agreed definition of authorship, the International Committee of Medical Journal Editors (ICMJE) provides four criteria for authorship, all of which should be present in a responsible authorship situation. These comprise (1) substantial contribution to at least one of the following: research conception, design, acquisition, analysis, data interpretation; (2) manuscript drafting or critical intellectual revision; (3) final approval of submitted manuscript; and (4) accepting accountability for all elements of the research process [71].

Gift (or honorary) authorship occurs when someone is named as an author but has not contributed sufficiently to the article. Matters contributing to gift authorship include power imbalance, being dependent on a person for resources, and institutional/discipline/national culture and gender [72]. For example, as an early career researcher (ECR), you might feel pressure or obligation to name a senior colleague on your work (e.g., your section or department head, a scholar who has great standing in your area, a supervisor who has only made minor comments), perhaps to add credibility and increase the chances of getting published. Gifting also occurs as a way of thanking someone for support or advice, as a means of increasing publication productivity (i.e., the gift is repaid with a reciprocal gift), and sometimes as a result of coercion (e.g., the person enters the process as a co-author, fails to deliver, but strongly asserts they have significantly contributed). Ghost authorship occurs when someone who has made substantial intellectual contributions to the work is not listed as an author. Ghosts are frequently at the lower end of the power hierarchy (e.g., contract researchers, undergraduate students, outsourced scientists). A recent study of 46 international HPER directors and journal editors found that over 60% had encountered both gifting and ghosting authorship practices, despite 75% of them believing these to be undesirable practices [69].

Finally, issues around authorship order (who goes first, who is corresponding author) can also ensue. While authorship order conventions differ by discipline, HPER suggests that a high proportion of authors experience unethical pressure around authorship order [69]. More broadly across the academic publishing world, things can also get frenzied around authorship order: with PhD students being advised to avoid irritating their supervisors and sometimes published articles being withdrawn due to heated disputes [73]. Another ethical dimension of authorship order is the common use of alphabetising authors as a way of resolving disputes. However, this can disadvantage authors with last names beginning with letters at the end of the alphabet [74].

Whether by gifting, ghosting, or bumping oneself up the authorship order, the practice only benefits researchers themselves, bringing no benefits (and sometimes harms) to the field's advancement. Conversations around allotting authorship can be difficult, particularly in the case of power imbalances or promised contributions failing to materialise. However, we suggest bringing up issues early with your research teams to set realistic expectations around who contributes what and how authorship should be determined, with flexibility to change authorship and order depending on actual rather than planned contributions [75]. The National Information Standards Organization developed the Contributor Roles Taxonomy (CRediT) [76], comprising descriptors of 14 high-level roles often undertaken by contributors to research outputs. CRediT can be used by research teams to develop authorship statements, making everyone's contribution transparent. Look at Box 3.10 to consider what you might do when placed in authorship dilemma situations. Finally, as ECRs, it has been recommended that you also join the Open Researcher and Contributor Identification Database (ORCID) [77] to enhance transparency of your researcher identity [78].

Box 3.10   Pause and reflect: Authorship dilemmas

Scenario 4: You are a co-author on a paper that has been rejected from two journals (one without review, another with harsh reviews). The first author is determined to get the paper published. Although you invested considerable time on the research, you now have your doubts and feel that a lot more work needs to be done before you associate yourself with the manuscript. You contact the first author to tell them you are uncomfortable with resubmission, and the team needs to reconvene to decide on next steps to tackle reviewers' comments. The first author informs you that they have already submitted it to another journal (in exactly the same form as the previous submission).

Scenario 5: You are part of a large interprofessional team studying interprofessional learning. You have a memorandum of understanding including the principle that all professions will have a research member included as an author, based on the value: nothing about us, without us. All professions have been involved in designing the research, securing ethics approval, and recruiting participants.

However, one team member from one of the professions fails to adequately contribute to data analysis and writing of the article, despite multiple promises to do so. You discuss the situation with them and agree on further contribution requirements for authorship: they plan to approve the data analysis and write the paper's introduction. Unfortunately, their work is substandard, so you fully rewrite their introduction. They argue that they have still made a substantial contribution warranting authorship, but cannot entertain further work on the paper.
Reflect:

- What are the authorship integrity issues involved in these two scenarios?
- How might you best manage these situations?
- Discuss these issues with your peers and/or supervisors.

3.4.6 Breaches Involving Cutting Corners

We now turn to consider the issue of cutting corners [10, 11], also known as sloppy science. As Lowe so eloquently put it: 'Science is done by humans, and it's always going to have a fair amount of slop in it.' [79 p. 1] Sloppy science has been defined as: 'carefree and negligent research practices that include both intended and unintended violations of scientific norms' [45 p. 118]. We have already covered some of these practices above but here we consider unintended violations including carelessness when undertaking research (including inadequate project/team management possibly due to work overload) and scant or careless review of manuscripts or proposals.

3.4.6.1 Research Carelessness

Carelessness in research entails various encroachments of methodological principles that compromise the trustworthiness of research. This sloppiness can be an unintended outcome of not fully engaging with the philosophical underpinnings of your chosen methodology. Indeed, it is a widespread phenomenon, and especially problematic in HPER: drawing on social science research methodologies, the wide range of interpretations of what comprises each research approach can be a minefield for those both outside and inside the field (see Chapter 2 and Part II of this book). Furthermore, this lack of philosophical engagement can, in turn, create a greater degree of muddiness around the issue of what good science comprises. When published, a study becomes a sanctioned part of the body of literature in our field and is afforded a certain status by virtue of publication. As such, this carelessness has negative consequences in the field impacting on truth (what comprises valid knowledge) and on trust between researchers [80].

Bouter et al [80] identified 60 key intentional and unintentional careless practices in which researchers across multiple disciplinary fields engage. The most frequent acts of carelessness include: citing other work that enhances your own findings/convictions or to please editors, reviewers, or colleagues; poorly supervising junior colleagues; and demanding/accepting authorship when not meeting criteria. Furthermore, most frequently cited behaviours impacting on truth (valid knowledge) and trust include: inadequate reporting of study flaws/limitations; poor note-keeping of research processes; failing to raise concerns around others' integrity breaches; failing to adhere to simple quality assurance principles; and using others' ideas and wording without appropriate citation. Note that all these practices are preventable.

3.4.6.2   Ethics of Peer-review

Peer review is a key mechanism for upholding quality by checking that research has been undertaken ethically and rigorously. As such, it should pick up some issues raised earlier in the research integrity section. Yet, the peer-review system also has vulnerabilities and can be a site for unethical practice [10, 81]. Ethical behaviour and having an awareness of the ethical pitfalls in peer review are key to publication integrity [82]. There are a variety of stakeholders in the peer-review process: reviewers, editors, and authors.

Peer reviewers make important contributions to research ethics by checking research positioning, relevance, rigour, and coherence. Peer reviewers identify gaps in cited literature, detect flaws in research that can help prevent the publication of substandard work and any associated harms, and call attention to philosophical and methodological inconsistencies (see Chapters 2 and 4). Peer review, therefore, needs to be fair, comprehensive, and transparent. The construct of fairness in peer-review processes means that manuscripts are assessed ethically, without bias, being judged purely on the quality of work according to research approaches (rather than reviewer, editor, or journal ideologies), the rigour in which they have been conducted according to the approaches used, and the relevance and significance of the contribution to the field [83]. The comprehensiveness of reviews is an equally important ethical dimension. Scant reviews failing to comment on important aspects of quality can be considered substandard and, therefore, failing to uphold ethical standards. Yet comprehensiveness does not mean reviewers should comment on areas beyond their expertise, at least without acknowledging such gaps.

For transparency, reviewers must reveal bias and competing interests. Unmasking reviewers and editorial decision-makers can aid towards upholding an ethical stance within research and publishing (e.g., reducing opportunities for intended and unintended unethical practices: see Box 3.11). For example, there are moves towards greater transparency in peer review where authors, reviewers, and editors are made aware of each other's identities, sometimes being named in their roles within the publication itself, to facilitate the democratisation process and enhance accountability [82]. However, some argue that masking enables more honest, constructive reviews because there is reduced concern about author retaliation, especially in small research communities [84].

Box 3.11   Pause and reflect: Peer-review dilemma

Scenario 6: You receive a manuscript for peer review and spend several hours providing constructive feedback to the authors. You recommend rejecting the manuscript for this journal, but indicate that with some significant revisions and reframing, it might merit publication in a different journal. The editor rejects the manuscript. A few weeks later you receive an invitation to review the same manuscript for a different journal. It is identical to the one you initially reviewed (the authors did not incorporate any of your feedback).
  Reflect:

- What do you do and why?
- If you undertake the review, how much content from the prior review would you recycle?
- If you decline, would you give your rationale?

3.5   CHAPTER SUMMARY

In this chapter, we have discussed key considerations for ethical decision-making when designing, conducting, and publishing your research. We contrasted Indigenous ethical practices based on interrelational values of respect, connectivity, and reciprocity with Euro-Western practices grounded in philosophical traditions of deontology, utilitarianism, and virtue ethics [14]. Next we discussed procedural aspects of doing ethical research, including how IRBs (and HRECs) evaluate research protocols and how these committees draw on institutional and professional codes of conduct, national laws, and organisational constraints in their evaluation of ethical appropriateness. We then contemplated research integrity, considering areas prone to ethical pitfalls, namely data, methods, policy compliance, outside influence, crediting contributions, and cutting corners [9–11]. Throughout the chapter, we have stressed the contextual and dynamic nature of research ethics. What is right for one person in one situation may not be right for everyone, everywhere. This can bring about confusion, conflict, and/or confrontation when working interprofessionally and internationally, due to professionally and culturally developed assumptions and practices. Thus, you might sometimes feel like you are wading through a muddy pool of deep and sometimes treacherous water. However, we urge you to use your knowledge from this chapter and your further reading (see Box 3.12), to reflect on certain norms around the rights and wrongs of research ethics, to understand the origins of everyday ethical reasoning for you and your colleagues, and to develop greater clarity around your research endeavours. Through this process, you can become a virtuous researcher as our final quotation suggests. This treacherous muddy pool may then begin to clear. After all, the 'ideals of science are noble ideals that simply need to be executed with an ethic of integrity. This ethic of integrity combined with noble ideals should result in best practices.' [1 p. 180]

Box 3.12   Recommended reading for HPER ethics

Brooks R, te Riele K, Maguire M. *Ethics and Education Research*. London: SAGE; 2014 [19].

Committee on Publication Ethics (COPE) Council. COPE discussion document: handling competing interests. 2016: https://publicationethics.org—this comprehensive website has a plethora of information around publishing ethics, with wide-ranging real-life scenarios for you to explore (accessed 29 August 2022) [50].

Frandsen TF, Eriksen MB, Hammer DMG, et al. Fragmented publishing: a large-scale study of health science. *Scientometrics*. 2019;119(3):1729–1743 [64].

Higgins M, Kim E-JA. De/colonizing methodologies in science education: rebraiding research theory–practice–ethics with Indigenous theories and theorists. *Cult Stud Sci Educ*. 2019;14(1):111–127 [36].

Roshid MM, Alam Siddique MN, Sarkar M, et al. Doing educational research in Bangladesh: challenges in applying Western research methodology. In Zhang H, Chan PWK, Kenway J, eds. *Asia as Method in Education Studies: A Defiant Research Imagination*. London: Routledge; 2015: 129–143 [85].

REFERENCES

1. Stewart CN Jr. Research Ethics: The Best Ethical Practices Produce the Best Science. In Stewart CN Jr, ed. *Research Ethics for Scientists: A Companion for Students.* Chichester: John Wiley & Sons Ltd; 2011: 1–9.

2. D'Souza DM, Sade RM, Moffatt-Bruce SD. The many facets of research integrity: what can we do to ensure it? *J Thorac Cardiovasc Surg.* 2020;160(3):730–733.

3. Stewart CN Jr. How Corrupt is Science? In Stewart CN Jr, ed. *Research Ethics for Scientists: A Companion for Students.* Chichester: John Wiley & Sons Ltd; 2011: 11–20.

4. Poff DC, Ginley DS. Publication ethics. In Iphofen R, ed. *Handbook of Research Ethics and Scientific Integrity.* Cham: Springer International Publishing; 2020: 107–126.

5. Dahal B. Research ethics: a perspective of South Asian context. *Edukacja.* 2020; 152(1):9–20.

6. Maggio L, Dong T, Driessen E, et al. Factors associated with scientific misconduct and questionable research practices in health professions education. *Perspect Med Educ.* 2019;8(2):74–82.

7. Grimes DR, Bauch CT, Ioannidis JPA. Modelling science trustworthiness under publish or perish pressure. *R Soc Open Sci.* 2018;5(1):171511.

8. van Dalen HP, Henkens K. Intended and unintended consequences of a publish-or-perish culture: a worldwide survey. *J Assoc Inf Sci Technol.* 2012;63(7):1282–1293.

9. D'Amico TA. Commentary: scientists still behaving badly. *J Thorac Cardiovasc Surg.* 2020;160(3):734.

10. Godecharle S, Fieuws S, Nemery B, et al. Scientists still behaving badly? A survey within industry and universities. *Sci Eng Ethics.* 2017;24(6):1697–1717.

11. Martinson BC, Anderson MS, de Vries R. Scientists behaving badly. *Nature.* 2005;435(7043):737–738.

12. Butts JB, Rich KL. *Nursing Ethics: Across the Curriculum and into Practice*, 5th ed. Burlington: Jones & Bartlett Learning; 2020.

13. Guillemin M, Gillam L. Ethics, reflexivity, and "ethically important moments" in research. *Qual Inq.* 2004;10(2):261–280.

14. Kara H. *Research Ethics in the Real World: Euro-Western and Indigenous Perspectives.* Bristol: Policy Press; 2018.

15. Chilisa B. *Indigenous Research Methodologies.* Los Angeles: SAGE; 2019.

16. Beauchamp TL, Childress JF. *Principles of Biomedical Ethics*, 5th ed. New York: Oxford University Press; 2001.

17. Freakley M, Burgh G. *Engaging with Ethics: Ethical Inquiry for Teachers.* Katoomba: Social Science Press; 2000.

18. Oates J. Ethical considerations in psychology research. In Iphofen R, ed. *Handbook of Research Ethics and Scientific Integrity.* Cham: Springer International Publishing; 2020: 783–801.

19. Brooks R, te Riele K, Maguire M. *Ethics and Education Research.* London: SAGE; 2014.

20. Mogra I. Strengthening ethics: a faith perspective on educational research. *J Acad Ethics.* 2017;15(4):365–376.

21. Monrouxe LV, Rees CE, Ho M-J, et al. Professionalism dilemmas across national cultures. In Monrouxe LV, Rees CE, eds. *Healthcare Professionalism: Improving Practice through Reflections on Workplace Dilemmas.* Chichester: John Wiley & Sons, Ltd; 2017: 187–206.

22. World Medical Association. World Medical Association Declaration of Helsinki: ethical principles for medical research involving human subjects. *JAMA.* 2013;310(20):2191–2194.

23. Alahmad G, Al-Jumah M, Dierickx K. Review of national research ethics regulations and guidelines in Middle Eastern Arab countries. *BMC Medic Ethics.* 2012;13(1):34.

24. Carpentier R, McGillivray B. Protecting participants in clinical trials through research ethics review. In Iphofen R, ed. *Handbook of Research Ethics and Scientific Integrity*. Cham: Springer International Publishing; 2020: 91–106.

25. World Medical Association. WMA Declaration of Helsinki – ethical principles for medical research involving human subjects https://www.wma.net/policies-post/wma-declaration-of-helsinki-ethical-principles-for-medical-research-involving-human-subjects (accessed 29 August 2022).

26. Silverman H, Sleem H, Moodley K, et al. Results of a self-assessment tool to assess the operational characteristics of research ethics committees in low- and middle-income countries. *J Medic Ethics*. 2015;41(4):332–337.

27. Nakkash R, Qutteina Y, Nasrallah C, et al. The practice of research ethics in Lebanon and Qatar: perspectives of researchers on informed consent. *J Empir Res Hum Res Ethics*. 2017;12(5):352–362.

28. Freckelton I. Research misconduct. In Iphofen R, ed. *Handbook of Research Ethics and Scientific Integrity*. Cham: Springer International Publishing; 2020: 159–180.

29. Hunter D. *The SAGE Handbook of Qualitative Research Ethics*. London: SAGE; 2018.

30. National Health and Medical Research Council. Ethical conduct in research with Aboriginal and Torres Strait Islander peoples and communities: guidelines for researchers and stakeholders. Commonwealth of Australia. Canberra: 2018. https://www.nhmrc.gov.au/about-us/resources/ethical-conduct-research-aboriginal-and-torres-strait-islander-peoples-and-communities (accessed 29 August 2022.)

31. Armond ACV, Gordijn B, Lewis J, et al. A scoping review of the literature featuring research ethics and research integrity cases. *BMC Medic Ethics*. 2021;22(1):50.

32. Crameri F, Shephard GE, Heron PJ. The misuse of colour in science communication. *Nat Commun*. 2020;11(1):5444.

33. Artino AR, Driessen EW, Maggio LA. Ethical shades of gray: international frequency of scientific misconduct and questionable research practices in health professions education. *Acad Med*. 2019;94(1):76–84.

34. Thorpe A. Queering fieldnote practice with queer, trans, and non-binary populations. In Burkholder C, Thompson JA, eds. *Fieldnotes in Qualitative Education and Social Science Research: Approaches, Practices and Ethical Considerations*, New York: Routledge; 2020: 277–278.

35. Varpio L, Ajjawi R, Monrouxe LV, et al. Shedding the cobra effect: problematising thematic emergence, triangulation, saturation and member checking. *Med Educ*. 2017;51(1):40–50.

36. Higgins M, Kim E-JA. De/colonizing methodologies in science education: rebraiding research theory–practice–ethics with Indigenous theories and theorists. *Cult Stud Sci Educ*. 2019;14(1):111–127.

37. Iphofen R, Ethical issues in research methods: introduction. In Iphofen R, (eds.) *Handbook of Research Ethics and Scientific Integrity*. Cham: Springer International Publishing; 2020: 371–379.

38. Ní Chianáin L, Fallis R, Johnston J, et al. Nothing about me without me: a scoping review of how illness experiences inform simulated participants' encounters in health profession education. *BMJ Simul Technol Enhanc Learn*. 2021;7(6):611–616.

39. Gans Combe C. Research ethics in data: new technologies, new challenges. In Iphofen R, ed. *Handbook of Research Ethics and Scientific Integrity*. Cham: Springer International Publishing; 2020: 305–321.

40. Simera I, Altman DG, Moher D, et al. Guidelines for reporting health research: the EQUATOR Network's survey of guideline authors. *PLoS Med*. 2008;5(6):e139.

41. Heslop C, Burns S, Lobo R. Managing qualitative research as insider-research in small rural communities. *Rural Remote Health*. 2018;18(3):4576.

42. Faden RR, Beauchamp TL, King NMP. *A History and Theory of Informed Consent*. New York: Oxford University Press; 1986.

43. Douglas BD, McGorray EL, Ewell PJ. Some researchers wear yellow pants, but even fewer participants read consent forms: exploring and improving consent form reading in human subjects research. *Psychol Methods.* 2021;26(1):61–68.

44. Houghton CE, Casey D, Shaw D, et al. Ethical challenges in qualitative research: examples from practice. *Nurse Res.* 2010;18(1):15–25.

45. Bos J. Introduction. In Bos J, ed. *Research Ethics for Students in the Social Sciences.* Cham: Springer International Publishing; 2020: 1–5.

46. Mackey E. A best practice approach to anonymization. In Iphofen R, ed. *Handbook of Research Ethics and Scientific Integrity.* Cham: Springer International Publishing; 2020: 323–343.

47. Mozersky J, McIntosh T, Walsh HA, et al. Barriers and facilitators to qualitative data sharing in the United States: a survey of qualitative researchers. *PLoS One.* 2021;16(12):e0261719.

48. Tolich M. Internal confidentiality: when confidentiality assurances fail relational informants. *Qual Sociol.* 2004;27(1):101–106.

49. Monrouxe LV, Rees CE. *Healthcare Professionalism: Improving Practice through Reflections on Workplace Dilemmas.* Chichester: John Wiley & Sons; 2017.

50. Committee on Publication Ethics (COPE) Council. COPE discussion document: handling competing interests. 2016:https://publicationethics.org—this comprehensive website has a plethora of information around publishing ethics, with wide-ranging real-life scenarios for you to explore (accessed 17 March 2023).

51. Chugh D, Bazerman MH, Banaji MR. Bounded ethicality as a psychological barrier to recognizing conflicts of interest. In Cain DM, Moore DA, Loewenstein G, et al., eds. *Conflicts of Interest: Challenges and Solutions in Business, Law, Medicine, and Public Policy.* Cambridge, UK: Cambridge University Press; 2005: 74–95.

52. Paruzel-Czachura M, Baran L, Spendel Z. Publish or be ethical? Publishing pressure and scientific misconduct in research. *Res Ethics.* 2021;17(3):375–397.

53. Desmond H. Professionalism in science: competence, autonomy, and service. *Sci Eng Ethics.* 2019;26(3):1287–1313.

54. Lund JR. Plagiarism. *J Relig Theol Inf.* 2004;6(3–4):93–101.

55. Chien S-C. Taiwanese college students' perceptions of plagiarism: cultural and educational considerations. *Ethics Behav.* 2017;27(2):118–139.

56. Haitch R. Stealing or sharing? Cross-cultural issues of plagiarism in an open-source era. *Teach Theol Relig.* 2016;19(3):264–275.

57. Marsh R, Landau J. Item availability in cryptomnesia: assessing its role in two paradigms of unconscious plagiarism. *J Exp Psychol Learn Mem Cogn.* 1995;21(6):1568–1582.

58. Eaton SE, Crossman K. Self-plagiarism research literature in the social sciences: a scoping review. *Interchange.* 2018;49(3):285–311.

59. Teixeira da Silva JA. Copy-paste: 2-click step to success and productivity that underlies self-plagiarism. *Sci Eng Ethics.* 2017;23(3):943–944.

60. Committee on Publication Ethics (COPE) Council. Redundant (duplicate) publication in a published article https://publicationethics.org/resources/flowcharts/redundant-duplicate-publication-published-article (accessed 29 August 2022).

61. Bruton SV, Rachal JR. Education journal editors' perspectives on self-plagiarism. *J Acad Ethics.* 2015;13(1):13–25.

62. Errami M, Garner H. A tale of two citations: are scientists publishing more duplicate papers? An automated search of seven million biomedical abstracts suggests that they are. *Nature.* 2008;451(7177):397–399.

63. Ding D, Nguyen B, Gebel K, et al. Duplicate and salami publication: a prevalence study of journal policies. *Int J Epidemiol.* 2020;49(1):281–288.

64. Frandsen TF, Eriksen MB, Hammer DMG, et al. Fragmented publishing: a large-scale study of health science. *Scientometrics.* 2019;119(3):1729–1743.

65. Hicks R, Berg JA. Multiple publications from a single study: ethical dilemmas. *J Am Assoc Nurse Pract.* 2014;26(5):233–235.

66. Refinetti R. In defense of the least publishable unit. *FASEB J.* 1990;4(1):128–129.

67. Flanagin A, Carey LA, Fontanarosa PB, et al. Prevalence of articles with honorary authors and ghost authors in peer-reviewed medical journals. *JAMA*. 1998;280(3):222–224.

68. Schroter S, Montagni I, Loder E, et al. Awareness, usage and perceptions of authorship guidelines: an international survey of biomedical authors. *BMJ Open*. 2020;10(9):e036899.

69. Uijtdehaage S, Mavis B, Durning SJ. Whose paper is it anyway? Authorship criteria according to established scholars in health professions education. *Acad Med*. 2018;93(8):1171–1175.

70. Konopasky A, O'Brien BC, Artino AR, et al. I, we and they: a linguistic and narrative exploration of the authorship process. *Med Educ*. 2021;56(4):456–464.

71. International Committee of Medical Journal Editors (ICMJE). Defining the role of authors and contributors. https://www.icmje.org/recommendations/browse/roles-and-responsibilities/defining-the-role-of-authors-and-contributors.html (accessed 29 August 2022).

72. Maggio LA, Artino Jr. AR, Watling CJ, et al. Exploring researchers' perspectives on authorship decision making. *Med Educ*. 2019;53(12):1253–1262.

73. Grove J. What can be done to resolve academic authorship disputes? *Times Higher Education*. 2020; https://www.timeshighereducation.com/features/what-can-be-done-resolve-academic-authorship-disputes (accessed 29 August 2022).

74. Edwards B. Race, ethnicity, and alphabetically ordered ballots. *Elect Law J*. 2014;13(3):394–404.

75. Regehr G. When names are on the line: negotiating authorship with your team. *Perspect Med Educ*. 2021;10(4):197–199.

76. National Information Standards Organization. Contributor roles taxonomy (CRediT). https://credit.niso.org (accessed 29 August 2022).

77. ORCID. ORCID: connecting research and researchers. https://orcid.org (accessed 29 August 2022).

78. ten Cate O. The ethics of health professions education research: protecting the integrity of science, research subjects, and authorship. *Acad Med*. 2022;97(1):13–17.

79. Lowe D. Sloppy science. *Science*. 2012; https://www.science.org/content/blog-post/sloppy-science (accessed 29 August 2022).

80. Bouter LM, Tijdink J, Axelsen N, et al. Ranking major and minor research misbehaviors: results from a survey among participants of four World Conferences on Research Integrity. *Res Integr Peer Rev*. 2016;1(17):17.

81. Committee on Publication Ethics (COPE) Council. Ethical guidelines for peer reviewers: english, version 2 https://publicationethics.org/resources/guidelines/cope-ethical-guidelines-peer-reviewers (accessed 29 August 2022).

82. Roberts J, Overstreet K, Hendrick R, et al. Peer review in scholarly journal publishing. In Iphofen R, ed. *Handbook of Research Ethics and Scientific Integrity*. Cham: Springer International Publishing; 2020: 127–158.

83. Button KS, Bal L, Clark A, et al. Preventing the ends from justifying the means: withholding results to address publication bias in peer-review. *BMC Psychol*. 2016;4(1):59.

84. Regehr G, Bordage G. To blind or not to blind? What authors and reviewers prefer. *Med Educ*. 2006;40(9):832–839.

85. Roshid MM, Alam Siddique NM, Sarkar M, et al. Doing educational research in Bangladesh: challenges in applying Western research methodology. In Zhang H, Chan PWK, Kenway J, eds. *Asia as Method in Education Studies: A Defiant Research Imagination*. London and New York: Routledge; 2015: 129–143.

Quality in Health Professions Education Research

Bridget C. O'Brien[1], Eliot L. Rees[2,3], and Claire Palermo[4]

[1] University of California San Francisco, San Francisco, California, USA
[2] Keele University, Staffordshire, UK
[3] University College London, London, UK
[4] Monash University, Clayton, Victoria, Australia

> **Box 4.1   Chapter 4 learning objectives: After reading this chapter you should be able to ...**
>
> - Discuss different ways of conceptualising quality in health professions education research (HPER)
> - Explain a framework for quality in HPER
> - Describe the difference between reporting guidelines and critical appraisal tools
> - Identify reporting guidelines and critical appraisal tools that align with the five research approaches discussed in this book
> - Discuss the strengths and weaknesses of different tools for reporting and critical appraisal
> - Appraise the quality of a research report using appropriate tools and provide feedback to report authors

4.1   INTRODUCING CHAPTER 4

> Criteria for evaluating research depend on who forms them and what purposes he or she invokes. [1 p. 337]

As researchers in health professions education (HPE) we all strive to produce high quality research. What does high quality actually mean? Some may base their judgement of quality on the rigour of the research methods (see Chapters 5–9), the ethical

Foundations of Health Professions Education Research: Principles, Perspectives and Practices,
First Edition. Edited by Charlotte E. Rees, Lynn V. Monrouxe, Bridget C. O'Brien, Lisi J. Gordon, and Claire Palermo.

conduct of the research (see Chapters 3 and 7), or the alignment between philosophy, methodology, and method (see Chapter 2) [2]. Others may evaluate quality according to the relevance and potential impact of the research (see Chapter 12), the novelty of the research, or the clarity and persuasiveness of the writing. Ideally, we may expect all these features to be present in high-quality research, though in reality we often prioritise some over others based on our roles, values, philosophical orientations, and available resources. In this chapter, we aim to help you navigate the complex world of quality in HPER so you can clarify your own standards of quality and become familiar with various tools available to guide you in critically appraising your own and others' research (see Box 4.1).

Discussions of quality often orient towards different roles in research. That is, quality considerations may be different for a researcher conducting research (e.g., AMEE Guides [3–5]), a peer reviewer of research (e.g., AAMC Review Criteria for Research Manuscripts [6]), or a consumer or reviewer of a body of evidence (e.g., Critical Appraisal Skills Programme: CASP) [7]. While there is much overlap in the guidance for people with these roles, the different purposes yield slightly different formats (e.g., general questions or specific scoring criteria) and scope (e.g., consideration of clarity of writing, logical argumentation versus focus on technical details and methodology). In this chapter, we focus our discussion primarily on your role as an author. This means that quality includes both how you conduct your research as well as how you write about and report on your research (see Chapter 11). Learning about quality from this perspective will also assist you in reviewing others' research for peer-review purposes and as a research consumer.

In this chapter, we begin with a general discussion of various ways of conceptualising quality in HPER (section 4.2). In section 4.3, we discuss eight dimensions of quality that we see as most relevant to HPER. The eight dimensions constitute a framework based on a synthesis of various resources and discussions regarding quality in HPE, general education, and social sciences research [2, 6, 8–20]. This framework extends beyond technical or methodological standards of quality because we endorse a more holistic view of quality. Some of the dimensions are inherently contextual and subjective, which means they are not amenable to standardised ratings or checklists. As you will read in greater depth in Part II of this book, each research approach sets different standards for quality and uses customised tools to guide reporting and appraise quality. In section 4.4, we share some of the most common reporting guidelines and critical appraisal tools for approaches covered in this book, and we discuss the strengths and limitations of these tools and guidelines in section 4.5. In section 4.6, we talk about peer review as a way to develop your own sense of quality across the eight dimensions, and to build and refine your critical appraisal skills. Finally, in section 4.7, we summarise the chapter. Before proceeding to the next section, we invite you to pause and reflect on Box 4.2.

Box 4.2   Pause and reflect: Identify your own quality criteria

Before moving on, reflect on some of the features you associate with quality research. Write these down now and have them ready to compare with the eight dimensions discussed later in this chapter.

4.2   IDENTIFYING QUALITY INDICATORS

Think about the last time you ate at a restaurant you consider to be high quality. If you wanted to convince a friend to try this restaurant, what indicators of quality would you use? Your ability to articulate these indicators is important to ensure a shared understanding of what quality means and to facilitate discussion about the importance and value of each indicator. For example, if you value the ethical sourcing of ingredients, the aesthetics of the presentation, and the unique flavour combinations, while your friend values the restaurant ambience, efficiency of service, and freshness of the food, you may have very different views on the quality of the same restaurant. If you did not know what indicators you each had in mind, you would be perplexed about your disagreement and decide not to trust one another's restaurant recommendations.

Much like restaurants, HPER serves many purposes and audiences (as discussed in Chapters 1 and 2). As an HPE researcher, you want your research to improve education and ultimately health and well-being. Your ability to achieve these goals hinges on how well you can meet the appropriate quality standards and effectively communicate how your work aligns with these standards for the type of research you conduct. Your success also depends on how others evaluate the quality of your work, which means they must know what quality indicators to use based on the type of approach and goals of your research. Knowing common indicators of quality in HPER is critical to your ability to secure funding for your research (see Chapter 10), disseminate your research (see Chapter 11), build networks and collaborations with other researchers, and use your work to advance knowledge and change practice (see Chapter 12). While we view the influence on practice, policy, and theory as important goals of research, we acknowledge that evidence of such influence is challenging to produce and not necessarily a reliable indicator of quality.

Several articles have helped to elucidate quality indicators in HPER by clarifying editors' expectations and suggestions [11, 12, 18–20], and sharing observations about shortcomings [21–25]. There are three areas flagged as most in need of attention in HPER:

- conceptualisation of the problem and description of the guiding conceptual framework [21, 25];
- positioning of the work relative to existing literature (e.g., building on what is already known, filling a gap) [22, 23, 26];
- and methodological rigour (e.g., design aligns with research question, sample size or sufficiency, robust tools or techniques used to collect and/or analyse data) [2, 27, 28].

Conducting quality research requires time, resources, and training – all of which have been identified as lacking due to insufficient funding for HPER [29, 30]. While concerns about funding persist, most HPE journals have seen significant increases in submissions in recent years and low acceptance rates (see Chapter 13) [18, 31, 32]. These low acceptance rates may reflect rising standards for quality and/or higher quality research. The number of programmes offering advanced degrees in HPER has also grown substantially [33–35], which also likely contributes to increasing numbers of submissions. Authors in HPER have advanced knowledge through high-quality research in key areas such as assessment, feedback, professionalism, professional identity, and continuing professional development (see Chapter 1). This knowledge has influenced educational practice as evident in curricular reforms, innovations, and shifts in our approaches to assessment [35]. The thirst for quality research is clear in the continued calls for evidence-informed approaches in HPE [36], and the exponential rise in knowledge syntheses in recent decades (see Chapter 1) [37]. Now more than ever, it is crucial to know how to produce high-quality research.

4.3   DIMENSIONS OF QUALITY

After several fierce debates about what constitutes quality in HPER [8–10, 12, 14, 16, 17], the field now generally values multiple research approaches and types of evidence. Hierarchies of evidence common in clinical research that place highest value on evidence produced through meta-analyses of randomised controlled trials are widely recognised as problematic standards of quality for HPER [14, 27, 28]. Our approach to quality in HPER must be sensitive to the purposes, contexts, and philosophical orientations of researchers and research approaches (see Chapters 5–9). Evaluators of study quality must first identify which dimension(s) of quality are most relevant to the situation at hand (e.g., whether you are appraising for peer review, systematic review/knowledge synthesis, application to practice, study design), and then select appropriate indicators and standards for the relevant dimensions. In this section, we describe eight dimensions and offer questions you can use to consider quality in each dimension. The questions are written for retrospective evaluation, though they can also be used prospectively to design for quality in your own research (see Chapter 10). Box 4.3 summarises the dimensions, and Boxes 4.4 and 4.5 provide examples of how three published studies meet these eight dimensions of quality. The dimensions are loosely organised by the order in which you might consider them when planning a study. They also align with many chapters in this book (i.e., Chapters 5–9), as noted. See our book glossary for definitions of quality-related terms.

> **Box 4.3   Summary of eight dimensions of quality relevant to HPER**
>
> 1. Framing: Establishes the conceptual framework, problem statement, and research question.
> 2. Positioning: Situates the research within the existing literature.
> 3. Relevance: Addresses the needs and problems that matter to the target audience and context.
> 4. Ethics: Demonstrates that research was conducted responsibly, with integrity, and in ways that honour the rights of human participants in research.
> 5. Internal coherence: Demonstrates alignment of ontology, epistemology, axiology, methodology, and methods.
> 6. Rigour: Aligns with established methodological practices and criteria for credibility.
> 7. Presentation: Reports all key elements of the research, conveys information in a clear, logical way (well written, appropriate visuals).
> 8. Impact: Discusses interpretations and implications in a way that has potential influence on education practice, policy, and theory.

4.3.1   Framing

High-quality studies typically begin by identifying the problem, concern, or observation that the study addresses and explaining the researcher's orientation to that problem. The orientation includes the conceptual framework [21, 38], relevant theories (see Chapter 2), level of focus [39], and philosophical underpinnings or approach. The conceptual framework tells the reader how the researcher views the problem or phenomenon under investigation and outlines existing evidence, gaps in this evidence, and the methodological underpinnings of the research [38]. This framework can draw from theories, principles, evidence, or models [21]. In framing research, we must clearly indicate the level of focus of the problem, for example, whether the research aims to work at the level of individuals, interpersonal interactions, cultures, systems, or environments. The philosophical approach to the study lays the foundation for the study design, methodology, methods, presentation, interpretation of data, and implications (see Chapter 2).

Questions to consider in framing include:

- What problem or phenomenon does the study address?
- How is the problem or phenomenon conceptualised? What is the conceptual framework?
- What is the level of focus (e.g., individual, interactional, cultural, systems, environmental)?
- What philosophical assumptions and approach guide the study?
- Do the study aims and/or research question(s) align with all of the above?

4.3.2   Positioning

A quality study rarely exists in isolation from the broader literature. Instead, it adds to a developing story by connecting with and building on prior studies, which may mean challenging prior assumptions, framing the problem in a new way, or taking a different approach to studying the problem or phenomenon. Positioning has been described as joining a scholarly conversation – that is, you need to know what others are talking about before you jump into the conversation, you need to offer a new insight or perspective to advance the conversation, and what you offer needs to matter so that people remain engaged [26]. You do not want to jump into the conversation uninformed about what others have already written about the topic. In positioning a study, it is important to avoid rehashing everything that is known. Instead, aim for a balance that both establishes your credibility as a scholar by demonstrating your knowledge of the topic and carefully curates the literature to present an argument that shows the need for your study [40]. Positioning is also important when interpreting the findings of a study and describing its implications. A quality study advances theory, knowledge, and/or practice (see Chapter 1). This may mean filling in a piece of the puzzle as anticipated at the outset of the study, or it may mean finding something surprising or unanticipated – new pieces or pieces that do not seem to fit. Any of these can occur in a quality study – the key is clearly mapping back to the literature and explaining where and how the findings do or do not fit.

Questions to consider for positioning include:

- What scholarly conversations does the study speak to?
- How does the study use the literature to build an argument for the study aims and/or research questions?

- How do the study findings connect to existing literature and practice? In what ways do they support, refute, advance, or suggest new possibilities for what we currently think, know, and do?

4.3.3   Relevance

Quality is not an inherent property of a study; it will always be judged in context. Relevance considers the relationship between a study's anticipated implications and important contextual factors such as audience, setting, current events, and priorities [18, 41, 42]. A study can be well designed and methodologically strong, yet fail to be considered a quality study if its relevance to the audience and field is unclear. Relevance considers the importance and value of the study's goals and gauges whether the study is likely to yield findings that address needs and problems that matter to the desired audience (e.g., educators, researchers, learners, patients, funders, journal editors). You cannot assume that others will automatically recognise the relevance of your study. You must actively persuade them, particularly if your study falls in an area that has already received considerable attention and may feel a little stale, overly familiar, or does not speak to the hot topics or trends in the field.

Questions to consider for relevance include:

- Who is the desired audience of the study?
- Why will this study matter to them?
- What might change as a result of this study and why are these changes important?
- How may context influence the study?

4.3.4   Ethics

As discussed in the previous chapter, a quality study must be conducted in an ethical way. This includes procedures to protect the rights of humans involved in research, which are typically reviewed by institutional review boards (IRBs) or human research ethics committees (HRECs), and practices more generally associated with research integrity and the responsible conduct of research [43–45]. Several recent studies have revealed ethical shades of grey, or ambiguities, in HPER – most commonly around authorship and citation practices [46–48]. In a survey of 590 HPE researchers, 90% reported engaging in at least one questionable research practice [46]. Concerns about upholding ethical principles also arise around informed consent, privacy/confidentiality, anonymity, conflicts of interest, and incentives, particularly when conducting multinational and/or multicultural research as ethical standards can vary across contexts. This ambiguity underscores the importance of familiarising yourself with policies and guidelines (e.g., International Committee of Medical Journal Editors (ICMJE) criteria for authorship [49], local/national codes of conduct for the protection of human research participants [50, 51]), as well as local standards and cultural norms around the responsible conduct of research. For more on ethics in HPER, see Chapter 3.

Questions to consider for ethics include:

- What procedures were used to recruit and obtain informed consent from participants, protect participants' privacy, and ensure confidentiality?

- What processes were used to demonstrate trustworthiness and maintain integrity throughout the research process?
- How are the contributions of authors represented and are these consistent with authorship criteria?

Before moving on to the remaining four criteria, read through Box 4.4 to consider the application of framing, positioning, relevance, and ethics in three case studies.

Box 4.4   Case studies: An overview of three case studies and how each addresses four dimensions of quality (framing, positioning, relevance, ethics)

Survey of HPE authors' journal choices [52]: It is important for clinical educators to conduct scholarly activity and to make their scholarship public (framing). Advice is often provided on how to choose which journal to submit one's work to, but this is not based on any empirical evidence (framing). Our initial literature review left us wondering if different priorities in journal choice are associated with greater success at acceptance (positioning). Previous qualitative work suggests that authors balance journal prestige against other factors such as intended audience and perceived quality of the work (positioning). Numerous opinion pieces and commentaries offer factors to consider when making journal choices (positioning). We adopted a scientific approach enabling us to recruit a large and diverse sample to quantify the importance of different journal factors and test for associations between these factors and publication success. Understanding how authors make choices regarding journal submissions and the consequences of these choices enabled us to offer evidence-based guidance to newer scholars (relevance). Our research proposal was approved by an HREC (ethics). Participants were identified from corresponding authors on published articles, allowing us to do direct recruitment. Participants completed an online consent form before the survey (ethics).

Qualitative study of how students offer value to organisations through work-integrated learning [53]: Placements are an essential part of preparing health professionals for practice, yet there are shortages of quality experiences (framing). Little is known about the benefits of placements to organisations, over and above the education of students (framing). Previous systematic reviews have shown that placements increased students' patient care activities, interactions with patients, and service time (positioning). Additionally, students on placement support health professionals' knowledge and skills, and encourage them to learn and reflect on their practice. This evidence is from students on placements in hospital settings – other settings have not been explored (positioning). Conceptualising placements as a social exchange with multiple benefits for multiple stakeholders may create new opportunities and increase placement capacity (relevance). We sought HREC approval for interviews and use of assessment artefacts (ethics). Our research team was made up of those with experience of placements in other settings, as well as qualitative research.

Instrumental case study of health system outcomes from medical students' improvement projects [54]: Many HPE programmes engage students in health systems improvement (HSI) efforts (framing). Evaluation of these programmes tends to focus on learning outcomes and achievement of specific project goals rather than on systems-level outcomes and impact (framing). Our study sought to identify and evaluate systems-level outcomes of medical students' involvement in HSI efforts. We anticipated that our findings could be used by HPE programmes to expand evaluation in ways that would provide more comprehensive evidence of impact than reported in most published evaluations of programmes (positioning). We selected a pragmatic approach given our commitment to addressing a problem (how to gather more actionable indicators of programme value and opportunities for improvement) and including stakeholders in the research process (relevance). Our research team included faculty who coached students in HSI, HSI curriculum leaders, and health system leaders. We obtained permission to conduct the study from our IRB and from medical school curriculum leaders who provided staff resources and access to data needed for this study (ethics).

4.3.5 Internal Coherence

Internal coherence is an important marker of quality as it 'makes clear the conventions of the research to support interpretations' [2 p. 253]. In a study with internal coherence, the philosophy, methodology, and methods of research align [2, 55], as do the theories employed within the research such as grand, macro or micro theories (see Chapter 2) [39, 56]. Misalignment in any of these aspects can result in the research aims not being fully realised or the findings and limitations being misinterpreted [2]. There may be times when a study appears to lack alignment, typically due to lack of reporting of philosophical underpinnings or details of methodology but is nonetheless a strong study. Some approaches, such as pragmatic approaches (see Chapter 9) place less emphasis on alignment given the focus on outcomes. Some types of problems or questions may benefit from thoughtful and intentional mixing of theories or approaches [57]. If this occurs, it is critical to explain why a lack of alignment exists and how this was accounted for.

Questions to consider for internal coherence include:

- What philosophical approach guides the study and do the methodology and methods align with this approach?
- What theories have been used and are they aligned with the philosophical approach?
- If there appears to be misalignment, does the study address this or provide a rationale?

4.3.6 Rigour

When people think of quality, rigour is often the first dimension that comes to mind. The prevalence of critical appraisal tools for most types of research designs and methodologies reflects the strong emphasis on methodological rigour as a quality standard. However, the criteria for rigour vary by approach and methodology, meaning the criteria used must align with the methodology. In a study examining the meaning of rigour, researchers analysed 62 social science articles with rigour in the title and found much variation in the meaning and application of the term [58]. They characterised rigour in two ways: (1) compliance-based, with emphasis on the selection of appropriate research methodology, adherence to methodological conventions or accepted practices in execution of the methodology, and complete reporting of the methodology; and (2) criterion-based, with emphasis on global attributes of the research that can be customised to suit particular research approaches and methodologies, with less concern for rigid adherence to prescribed methodological practices and more tolerance for deviations when justified [58]. In this chapter, we opt for a criterion-based approach to rigour that considers five general elements of rigour pertaining to the research approaches described in the book (see Chapters 5–9 for more detail).

The five elements are:

- **Assumptions**: The philosophical orientation of the study with respect to ontology (the nature of reality) and epistemology (ways of understanding this reality). Stating these is necessary to ensure these assumptions are consistent throughout the study and are not violated.
- **Researcher positioning:** The perspective the researcher brings to the study, their role in the study, and the nature of their interaction with the data is clear and consistent with the assumptions of the approach and methodology [59–62].
- **Credibility**: The study adheres to widely accepted practices for data collection and analysis for the stated approach, methodology, and conceptual framework or theory, and the researchers explain the choices made when designing and conducting the study [63].
- **Sampling and power**: The researchers' process and rationale for choosing who or what to include as data sources and how much data to collect meets the standards or principles for the selected approach and methodology.
- **Application/Applicability**: Appropriate use and interpretation of the study findings, particularly considering sensitivity to users and context.

For examples of how these elements play out in the different approaches, see Box 4.5 and Chapters 5–9 later.

Questions to consider for rigour include:

- What perspectives do researchers bring to the study and how are these taken into account?
- How does the study earn the reader's confidence in the findings? (i.e., credibility, sampling, and applicability)?
- Does the study discuss implications that are reasonable and not overstated given the assumptions and methodology?

4.3.7   Presentation

The presentation of the research and organisation of ideas sends readers a message about the quality of the research. A solid study with valuable insights will not fare well in peer review if ideas are not presented in a clear and compelling way, and if key elements of methodology and methods are not reported. Several excellent resources exist to assist you with writing [64, 65], graphics [66], and thorough and transparent reporting [67]. Finding colleagues who are willing to do a constructive peer review prior to submission helps you to identify confusing passages, leaps of logic, and missing methodological details that you might not have noticed.

Additionally, you must select journals and other forms of knowledge mobilisation (e.g., conference presentations, podcasts, social media campaigns, infographics) that are a good fit for your research [52, 68]. See Chapter 11 for more details.

Questions to consider for presentation include:

- Are ideas presented clearly, using language and visuals appropriate for the anticipated audience?
- Is the study presented in a way that aligns with author guidelines for the selected journal and with reporting guidelines that match the approach, methodology, or methods?

4.3.8   Impact

Impact describes the effect research can have on practice, policy, theory, and other research [69]. In this book, we describe research impact as, 'the good that researchers can do in the world' [70 p. 15], with particular focus on the positive effects research can have outside of academia. Most often, the impact of HPER pertains to practitioners and the delivery of professional services, and to health and well-being [71]. While you rarely know the full impacts of your research at the outset of a study, you must be able to offer some realistic possibilities and specific strategies to enhance impact. Such possibilities might include suggested improvements to pedagogical techniques in particular content areas, new approaches to assessment or standard-setting, or identifying gaps in curricula. Having plans at the outset helps make the case for the value of your research. When presenting and disseminating findings from research, audiences will be eager to hear how they can use the findings in their own educational practices or to advocate for organisational or systems-level changes. Research that fares well on all indicators of rigour but offers the audience little sense of the potential or actual impacts of the research will likely suffer in overall quality evaluations. See Chapter 12 for more information about research impact.

Questions to consider for impact:

- What type(s) of impact is/are anticipated from this research in the short and long term?
- Who or what will benefit from this research?
- What evidence can demonstrate impacts?

Before moving on to section 4.4, read through Box 4.5 to consider the application of internal coherence, rigour, presentation, and impact in the chapter case studies.

Box 4.5   Case studies: How the authors addressed four quality dimensions (internal coherence, rigour, presentation, impact)

Survey of HPE authors' journal choices [52]: In line with our post-positivist approach, we conducted a quantitative study using an electronic survey (internal coherence). We ensured rigour by using best-practice guidance in the design of our survey instrument [72] and inviting a large, international random sample of individuals who had published HPER in the preceding two years (rigour). In preparing our manuscript, we followed the journal's instructions for authors and endeavoured to construct a compelling problem/gap/hook to persuade readers of its

(continued)

(continued)

importance (presentation) [26]. We chose an open-access journal to ensure those without institutional subscriptions would be able to access the article. We submitted the manuscript to a special themed issue regarding meta-research in medical education, so that it would be read by those with an interest in the topic. The journal editor commissioned an invited commentary, further helping to draw attention to our article. We have used the findings of our study in workshops and individual discussions with new researchers, aiming to support others in achieving impact with their work (impact).

Qualitative study of how students offer value to organisations through work-integrated learning [53]: We stated our philosophical position in the manuscript as interpretivism and aligned our methods, interviews, and documentary analysis of assessment artefacts with this positioning (internal coherence). We enhanced rigour by obtaining a complete sample of all educators involved in the placement under investigation and described our method of content and thematic document analysis in depth (rigour). We followed journal instructions for authors and used the CASP checklist [7] to ensure relevant elements of quality were clearly stated in the manuscript (presentation). Trust between universities, organisations, and students was found to support mutual benefits for all parties in work-integrated learning, and therefore may be fundamental for advancement of work-integrated learning in HPE. The findings have impact given the limited literature in non-hospital placement settings and use of a new theory which supports the translation of these findings to other disciplines and settings. We also achieved impact through publishing in a high-quality HPE journal, as well as engaging social media to share key messages (impact).

Instrumental case study of health system outcomes from medical students' improvement projects [54]: Consistent with our pragmatic approach, we selected instrumental case study methodology and included several data sources giving us multiple perspectives and insights into systems-level outcomes and impacts of student engagement in HSI efforts. We used a combination of literature review, consultation with education and health system leaders, and expertise of our research team to guide study design – including our choice of evaluation framework, data sources (students' written descriptions of their projects, students' poster presentations, surveys of faculty and staff coaches and partners in students' projects), and development of data extraction forms and surveys (internal coherence). Some of the ways we attended to rigour included meeting regularly as a team to share information and perspectives that provided context for the study, and this helped to illuminate various assumptions to be questioned and helped us clarify the goals of the study. We also used recommended procedures for survey development [5], and chose parameters for our case study that balanced data sufficiency (to support identification of actionable and transferable indicators) with the need to choose an optimal time frame and to contextualise our findings. We acknowledged study limitations, noting the importance of implementing our proposed framework of systems-level outcomes and indicators in other programmes to evaluate the framework's transferability and workability (rigour). As we prepared our study for publication, we followed suggestions from papers on case study research [73–75], reviewed case studies published in HPER journals and followed the author guidelines for our target journal (presentation). We planned for impact by sharing our published manuscript on social media, sharing our findings with education leaders at our institution, working with our local curriculum evaluation team to include systems-level outcomes in routine evaluation of the programme, and contributing to subsequent studies inspired by ours (impact).

Before moving on to the next section, take a moment to pause and reflect on these eight dimensions of quality (see Box 4.6) and compare them to the list of quality considerations you generated at the beginning of the chapter (see Box 4.2).

Box 4.6 Pause and reflect: Which dimensions of quality do you tend to emphasise?

- Which of the eight dimensions of quality are most important to you in your own research?
- How do you demonstrate quality in these dimensions when writing up your work?
- What changes will you make to your authoring based on this chapter?
- Which of the eight dimensions of quality do you emphasise as a peer reviewer?
- How do you evaluate quality in these dimensions?
- What changes will you make to your peer-reviewing based on this chapter?

In the next section, we will discuss the translation of these dimensions into resources such as reporting guidelines and critical appraisal tools.

4.4 OVERVIEW OF RESOURCES: REPORTING GUIDELINES AND CRITICAL APPRAISAL TOOLS

Reporting guidelines and critical appraisal tools are commonly used by authors to assist with manuscript preparation and by peer reviewers and researchers conducting literature reviews to evaluate several quality dimensions already described. While the two go hand in hand, reporting guidelines and critical appraisal tools serve distinct purposes. Reporting guidelines are designed to ensure that essential information is included in a manuscript so that others can critically appraise the research and make informed choices about how to use the study's findings (e.g., the applicability or transferability of the findings and conclusions to their own context) [67]. Critical appraisal tools, on the other hand, generally include a list of questions or criteria to enable systematic examination and evaluation of the trustworthiness, value, and relevance of research in a particular context [76, 77]. Both reporting guidelines and critical appraisal tools tend to be tailored to specific approaches and methodologies.

Many of the tools created to assist with evaluating research quality originated in clinical research, to help practitioners evaluate evidence and decide to what extent it should inform their decisions. The rise of evidence-based practice and efforts to review and synthesise existing knowledge also emphasised the need for tools to assess the quality of evidence[78].

As scholars attempted to employ these tools, they realised many published research articles lacked essential and comparable information needed to evaluate study quality and compare findings across studies. This problem led to the development of reporting guidelines as necessary precursors to critical appraisal [78].

As you plan and conduct your research, we encourage you to identify reporting guidelines and critical appraisal tools that align with your research approach. Box 4.7 includes guidelines and tools commonly used in HPER, although these are not the only ones. You can find additional reporting guidelines on the EQUATOR Network

Box 4.7 Reporting guidelines and critical appraisal tools for each approach

Reporting guidelines	Critical appraisal tools

Scientific approaches (see Chapter 5)

For randomised controlled trials:

- CONsolidated Standards Of Reporting Trials (CONSORT) [81]

For observational studies:

- STrengthening the Reporting of OBservational studies in Epidemiology (STROBE) [82]

For systematic reviews and meta-analyses:

- Preferred Reporting Items for Systematic Reviews and Meta-Analyses (PRISMA) [83]
- STructured apprOach to the Reporting In healthcare education of Evidence Synthesis (STORIES) [84]

For economic evaluations:

- Consolidated Health Economic Evaluation Reporting Standards (CHEERS) [85]

For methodologies associated with scientific approaches:

- Medical Education Research Study Quality Instrument (MERSQI) [86]
- Quality assessment criteria for evaluating primary research papers from a variety of fields [87]
- Critical Appraisal Skills Programme (CASP) checklists – Randomised Controlled Trial, Systematic Review, Cohort Studies, Case Control Studies, Economic Evaluations [7]

Realist approaches (see Chapter 6)

For reviews:

- Realist And Meta-narrative Evidence Synthesis: Evolving Standards (RAMESES) [88]

For evaluations:

- RAMESES II [89]

None available but many researchers use reporting guidelines to facilitate critical appraisal.

Interpretivist approaches (see Chapter 7)

For general qualitative research:

- Standards for Reporting Qualitative Research (SRQR) [90]

For interviews and focus groups:

- COnsolidated criteria for REporting Qualitative research (COREQ) [91]

For systematic reviews of qualitative studies:

- ENhancing Transparency in REporting the synthesis of Qualitative research (ENTREQ) [92]

For methodologies associated with interpretivist approaches:

- Quality assessment criteria for evaluating primary research papers from a variety of fields [87]
- Critical Appraisal Skills Programme (CASP) checklists—Qualitative Studies [7]

Critical approaches (see Chapter 8)

Many studies using critical approaches use qualitative methodologies, so guidelines mentioned under interpretivist approaches may apply.

For quality improvement studies:

- Standards for QUality Improvement Reporting Excellence (SQUIRE) [93]
- Standards for QUality Improvement Reporting Excellence in Education (SQUIRE-EDU) [94]

Co-design and patient/public/community involvement in research is an important part of quality in critical research, so we offer tools to consider how and when patients/public/community members are engaged:

- Public and Patient Engagement Evaluation Tool [95]
- Guidance for Reporting Involvement of Patients and the Public (GRIPP2) [96]
- Statement on consumer and community health involvement in research [97]

Reporting guidelines	Critical appraisal tools
Pragmatic approaches (see Chapter 9)	
Many studies using pragmatic approaches use methodologies associated with other approaches. See above for additional guidelines that may apply.	Many studies using pragmatic approaches use methodologies associated with other approaches. See above for additional tools that may apply.
For mixed methods studies:	For mixed methods studies:
• Good Reporting of A Mixed Methods Study (GRAMMS) [98]	• Mixed Methods Appraisal Tool (MMAT) [99]
	For action research:
	• Quality Choice Points in Education Action Research [100 p. 26–27]
	For constructivist-grounded theory studies:
	• Criteria for Constructivist Grounded Theory Studies [1 p. 337–338]

website [67], and additional critical appraisal tools on various library websites such as this one from Duquesne University (see https://guides.library.duq.edu/critappraise) [79]. Few HPER journals require authors and reviewers to use these guidelines to evaluate quality and we do not recommend their use as a rigid checklist or scoring system [80]. Instead, we recommend them as a resource that can help you think through key aspects, many of which are associated with rigour. They can also assist you in documenting key information and decisions that will likely be important when writing up your research. Most important is making sure to select guidelines and tools that match your research approach – otherwise there is a risk of using criteria that will cause readers and reviewers to question the credibility of your research (e.g., reporting inter-rater reliability statistics when using an interpretivist approach; citing lack of a representative sample as a limitation of critical research). Reviewing the selected journal's guidelines for authors is also critical as the journal may have specific requirements for how to report findings and format the manuscript (see Chapter 11) [11].

4.5 STRENGTHS AND LIMITATIONS OF USING REPORTING GUIDELINES AND CRITICAL APPRAISAL TOOLS TO EVALUATE QUALITY

Use of reporting guidelines and critical appraisal tools is more controversial for some research approaches than others. In scientific approaches, there is widespread agreement that certain study designs, methodologies, and procedures are more robust than others and therefore likely to produce higher quality evidence (e.g., randomised controlled trials compared to cohort or case-control studies) [101–103]. Transparency is valued for the purposes of study replication and verification of findings. Correspondingly, reporting guidelines and critical appraisal tools are widely accepted and used in peer review and knowledge syntheses for clinical research. However, the value of reporting guidelines and critical appraisal tools faces more scepticism in interpretivist, critical, and pragmatic approaches, where the goal is rarely replication or evaluation of rigour, and more often nuanced understandings of contexts, processes, and researcher discernment [104, 105]. Some of the key concerns about use of reporting guidelines and critical appraisal tools in interpretivist approaches include the diversity of methodologies (each with different underpinning assumptions and techniques), the heavy reliance on researcher insight and judgment (often requiring flexibility rather than standardisation), and the risk of uncritical application of criteria without considering context and nuance (e.g., looking for key terms like 'member checking' or 'saturation' as evidence of trustworthiness rather than seeking to understand how these procedures actually occurred in the research: see Chapter 7 for further details) [13, 105–108].

There are a range of strengths and limitations to reporting guidelines and critical appraisal tools. The strengths are that these resources help authors know what reviewers, editors, and thesis examiners will likely expect to see in research. They can be used with discretion to decide how to address these expectations. For example, to report what is expected or explain that some expectations are not appropriate (e.g., stating a guiding theory and hypothesis is not appropriate for a grounded theory study; requiring authors to cite a lack of comparison group as a study limitation is inappropriate for many interpretivist and critical approaches; see Part II of this book for more examples) [108]. Ultimately, these resources can enhance transparency and clarity in the description of the research process and findings (see Chapter 11). Using these resources can also increase the likelihood that research will be included in reviews and knowledge syntheses, since the authors of such studies often use reporting guidelines and critical appraisal tools in their screening processes and inclusion/exclusion criteria [86, 109].

The limitations of reporting guidelines and critical appraisal tools largely relate to the risk of viewing them as rigid and prescriptive rather than as flexible and context-sensitive. While several of these resources state that they should not be used in such ways [90], a journal may ask authors and/or reviewers to submit a completed checklist based on reporting guidelines. In these cases, there is a risk that the omission of information could be misconstrued as a sign of poor-quality research rather than appreciated as a legitimate decision. If an item on a required checklist or a suggestion from a reviewer does not align with the philosophical orientation or methodology of your study, you do not need to make changes, but you do need to explain why you are not checking a box or making changes (see Chapter 11). An additional risk is that fear of rigid application of critical appraisal criteria may stymie creativity and innovation (see Chapter 13). Authors may fear that deviation from conventional procedures represented in critical appraisal tools may reduce their chances of publication. HPER journals are generally receptive to innovation and unconventional research processes, so long as the rationale, key decisions, and procedures are well described [57].

4.6   APPRAISING QUALITY VIA PEER REVIEW

An excellent way to calibrate your personal quality barometer is to contribute to the peer-review process [110]. You can do this by volunteering to review for HPER journals, conferences, and grants; attending education scholarship works-in-progress sessions available at many institutions; and offering to provide feedback on colleagues' work pre-submission. After completing a review for a journal, you typically receive an email with the editor's decision and all reviewer comments. You can compare these reviews to your own and use them as a source of feedback, noting which dimensions of quality each reviewer addressed, what critical and reinforcing feedback they provided, and what suggestions they offered. Additionally, you may find it helpful to perform a group peer review of an article [111, 112], or to complete a mentored review with an experienced colleague who can provide feedback on your review. You can use the activity in Box 4.8 to practise peer-reviewing a manuscript.

When you review a journal article, conference submission, or grant proposal your review serves two purposes. First, it critically appraises the article to help editors or selection committees decide how to proceed with the submission. If the submission moves forward, there are often items authors must fix or address to ensure the work meets quality standards. These items should be clearly stated so editors and authors know what to prioritise. Second, your review gives authors valuable feedback for improvement. If their submission is not accepted, they can use the feedback to revise their work before submitting elsewhere.

There are many excellent articles and resources that provide guidance to peer reviewers [6, 20, 113–116]. We encourage you to use these along with reviewer guidelines provided by the journal, conference, or grant agency, and appropriate reporting guidelines and critical appraisal tools mentioned in Box 4.7. For more on peer review, see Chapters 3 and 11.

Box 4.8   Stop and do: Critical appraisal of an article

Read the abstract of at least one of the following open-access HPER papers. Each paper aligns with one of the five approaches covered in this book.

Scientific approach: Buchanan H, et al. Measuring evidence-based practice knowledge and skills in occupational therapy—a brief instrument. *BMC Med Educ.* 2015;15:191. https://bmcmededuc.biomedcentral.com/articles/10.1186/s12909-015-0475-2

Realist approach: Crampton P, et al. Realist evaluation of UK medical education quality assurance. *BMJ Open.* 2019;9(12):e033614. https://bmjopen.bmj.com/content/9/12/e033614

Interpretivist approach: Hayashi M, et al. Ambivalent professional identity of early remedial medical students from Generation Z: a qualitative study. *BMC Med Educ.* 2022;22:501. https://bmcmededuc.biomedcentral.com/articles/10.1186/s12909-022-03583-5

Critical approach: Giuliani M, et al. A critical review of representation in the development of global oncology curricula and the influence of neocolonialism. *BMC Med Educ.* 2020;20:93. https://bmcmededuc.biomedcentral.com/articles/10.1186/s12909-020-1989-9

Pragmatic approach: Webb KL, et al. A mixed-methods evaluation of the Educational Supervision Agreement for Wales. *BMJ Open.* 2017;7(6):e015541. https://bmjopen.bmj.com/content/7/6/e015541

- Based on your reading of the abstracts, which reporting guidelines and critical appraisal tools best suit each paper? Why?
- Now use the selected reporting guideline and/or critical appraisal tool to review one of these papers in full. After you finish, compare your reviews to the published peer reviews. (For *BMJ Open*, click Publication History from the menu on the left and click the Review History link to view the reviews; for *BMC Medical Education*, the link for the peer-review reports appears after the abstract).

(continued)

(continued)

- How did your appraisals compare to those of the peer reviewers?
- What challenges did you encounter in using the guideline and tool you selected?
- Would another guideline or tool be more appropriate for this review?

You could also do this activity as a group peer review [111, 112], or ask a colleague or mentor to provide feedback on your review.

4.7   CHAPTER SUMMARY

[O]ur efforts to appraise the quality of education research tend to focus on technical aspects of research design ... Although the rigor of research design is critical for all types of education studies, it is insufficient for improving the quality of our education research. [15 p. viii]

In HPER, we strive to produce high-quality research that matters to learners, educators, and institutions. Yet what constitutes high-quality research varies by context, approach, and audience. In this chapter, we discussed quality as a multidimensional construct. As you plan, conduct, and write up your research, we encourage you to attend to eight dimensions of quality (framing, positioning, relevance, rigour, internal coherence, presentation, ethics, and impact) by challenging yourself to answer the questions posed for each dimension. You may also find it helpful to take the perspective of a peer reviewer or member of your intended audience as a way of critiquing your work. We presented reporting guidelines and critical appraisal tools commonly used in HPER as resources that can assist you in taking these perspectives. We highlighted the strengths and limitations of these guidelines and tools so you feel confident in deciding how they may be best used to guide and report your research, as well as how to use them when you serve as a peer reviewer of others' research. We hope this chapter, coupled with the chapters in Part II of this book, gives you a strong foundation to design your next research study. We also invite you to read the items listed in Box 4.9 to delve deeper into the concept of quality in HPER.

Box 4.9   Recommended reading for quality in HPER

Durning SJ, Carline JD. *Review Criteria for Research Manuscripts*, 2nd ed. Washington, DC: Association of American Medical Colleges; 2015 [6].

Majid U, Vanstone M. Appraising qualitative research for evidence syntheses: a compendium of quality appraisal tools. *Qual Health Res.* 2018;28(13):2115–2131 [13].

O'Brien BC, West CP, Coverdale JH, et al. On the use and value of reporting guidelines in health professions education research. *Acad Med.* 2020;95(11):1619–1622 [80].

Palermo C, Reidlinger DP, Rees CE. Internal coherence matters: lessons for nutrition and dietetics research. *Nutr Diet.* 2021;78(3):252–267 [2].

Varpio L, Driessen E, Maggio L, et al. Advice for authors from the editors of Perspectives on Medical Education: Getting your research published. *Perspect Med Educ.* 2018;7(6):343–347 [18].

REFERENCES

1. Charmaz K. *Constructing Grounded Theory*, 2nd ed. Thousand Oaks, Calif.: SAGE; 2014.
2. Palermo C, Reidlinger DP, Rees CE. Internal coherence matters: lessons for nutrition and dietetics research. *Nutr Diet.* 2021;78(3):252–267.
3. Ringsted C, Hodges B, Scherpbier A. 'The research compass': an introduction to research in medical education: AMEE Guide no. 56. *Med Teach.* 2011;33(9):695–709.
4. Watling CJ, Lingard L. Grounded theory in medical education research: AMEE Guide no 70. *Med Teach.* 2012;34(10):850–861.
5. Artino AR, La Rochelle JS, Dezee KJ, et al. Developing questionnaires for educational research: AMEE Guide no. 87. *Med Teach.* 2014;36(6):463–474.
6. Durning SJ, Carline JD. *Review Criteria for Research Manuscripts*, 2nd ed. Washington, DC: Association of American Medical Colleges; 2015.
7. Critical Appraisal Skills Programme. CASP Checklist. https://casp-uk.net/casp-tools-checklists (accessed 1 September 2022).
8. Bligh J, Brice J. What is the value of good medical education research? *Med Educ.* 2008;42(7):652–653.
9. Dornan T, Peile E, Spencer J. On 'evidence'. *Med Educ.* 2008;42(3):232–234.
10. Dornan T, Peile E, Spencer J. In defence of the existing strengths of medical education research. *Med Educ.* 2009;43(4):391.
11. Ellaway RH. Journal standards. *Adv Health Sci Educ.* 2022;27(1):1–5.
12. Eva KW. Broadening the debate about quality in medical education research. *Med Educ.* 2009;43(4):294–296.
13. Majid U, Vanstone M. Appraising qualitative research for evidence syntheses: a compendium of quality appraisal tools. *Qual Health Res.* 2018;28(13):2115–2131.
14. Monrouxe LV, Rees CE. Picking up the gauntlet: constructing medical education as a social science. *Med Educ.* 2009;43(3):196–198.
15. Pigott TD, Tocci C, Ryan AM, et al. Introduction – quality of research evidence in education: how do we know? *Rev Res Educ.* 2021;45(1):vii–xii.
16. Thistlethwaite J, Davies H, Dornan T, et al. What is evidence? Reflections on the AMEE symposium, Vienna, August 2011. *Med Teach.* 2012;34(6):454–457.
17. Todres M, Stephenson A, Jones R. Medical education research remains the poor relation. *BMJ.* 2007;335(7615):333–335.
18. Varpio L, Driessen E, Maggio L, et al. Advice for authors from the editors of Perspectives on Medical Education: getting your research published. *Perspect Med Educ.* 2018;7(6):343–347.
19. West DC, Miller KH, Artino AR. Foreword: characteristics of RIME papers that make the cut. *Acad Med.* 2016;91(11):Si–Siii.
20. [No authors listed]. Good advice from the deputy editors of Medical Education: the sequel. *Med Educ.* 2022;56(5):468–469.
21. Bordage G. Conceptual frameworks to illuminate and magnify. *Med Educ.* 2009;43(4):312–319.
22. Cook DA, Beckman TJ, Bordage G. Quality of reporting experimental studies in medical education: a systematic review. *Med Educ.* 2007;41(8):737–745.
23. Meyer HS, Durning SJ, Sklar DP, et al. Making the first cut: an analysis of academic medicine editors' reasons for not sending manuscripts out for external peer review. *Acad Med.* 2018;93(3):464–470.
24. Norman G. Data dredging, salami-slicing, and other successful strategies to ensure rejection: twelve tips on how to not get your paper published. *Adv Health Sci Educ.* 2014;19(1):1–5.
25. Regehr G. It's NOT rocket science: rethinking our metaphors for research in health professions education. *Med Educ.* 2010;44(1):31–39.

26. Lingard LA. Joining a conversation: problem/gap/hook heuristic. *Perspect Med Educ.* 2015;4(5):252–253.
27. Norman G. RCT = results confounded and trivial: the perils of grand educational experiments. *Med Educ.* 2003;37(7):582–584.
28. Norman G. Is experimental research passé. *Adv Health Sci Educ.* 2010;15(3):297–301.
29. Archer J, McManus C, Woolf K, et al. Without proper research funding, how can medical education be evidence based? *BMJ.* 2015;350:h3445.
30. Gruppen LD, Durning SJ. Needles and haystacks: finding funding for medical education research. *Acad Med.* 2016;91(4):480–484.
31. Eva KW. Publishing during COVID-19: lessons for health professions education research. *Med Educ.* 2021;55(3):278–280.
32. Roberts LW, Coverdale J. Editorial decision making for Academic Medicine, 2021. *Acad Med.* 2021;96(1):1–4.
33. Sethi A, Schofield S, McAleer S, et al. The influence of postgraduate qualifications on educational identity formation of healthcare professionals. *Adv Health Sci Educ.* 2018;23(3):567–585.
34. Tekian A. Doctoral programs in health professions education. *Med Teach.* 2014;36(1):73–81.
35. ten Cate O. Health professions education scholarship: the emergence, current status, and future of a discipline in its own right. *FASEB Bioadv.* 2021;3(7):510–522.
36. Thomas A, Bussières A. Leveraging knowledge translation and implementation science in the pursuit of evidence informed health professions education. *Adv Health Sci Educ.* 2021;26(3):1157–1171.
37. Maggio LA, Costello JA, Norton C, et al. Knowledge syntheses in medical education: a bibliometric analysis. *Perspect Med Educ.* 2021;10(2):79–87.
38. Varpio L, Paradis E, Uijtdehaage S, et al. The distinctions between theory, theoretical framework, and conceptual framework. *Acad Med.* 2020;95(7):989–994.
39. Young M, LaDonna K, Varpio L, et al. Focal length fluidity: research questions in medical education research and scholarship. *Acad Med.* 2019;94(11S):S1–S4.
40. Lingard LA. Writing an effective literature review. Part I: mapping the gap. *Perspect Med Educ.* 2018;7(1):47–49.
41. Miller KH, O'Brien B, Karani R. Foreword: the role of relevance in medical education research. *Acad Med.* 2018;93(11S):Si–Siii.
42. Pangaro L, McGaghie W. Chapter 8: Relevance. In Durning SJ, Carline JD, eds. *Review Criteria for Research Manuscripts*, 2nd ed. Washington, DC: Association of American Medical Colleges; 2015: 25–27.
43. The American Educational Research Association (AERA). Professional ethics. AERA; 2011. https://www.aera.net/About-AERA/AERA-Rules-Policies/Professional-Ethics(accessed 29 August 2022).
44. British Educational Research Association (BERA). *Ethical Guidelines for Educational Research*, 4th ed. London: BERA; 2018. https://www.bera.ac.uk/researchers-resources/publications/ethical-guidelines-for-educational-research-2018 (accessed 29 August 2022).
45. World Conference on Research Integrity. *Singapore Statement on Research Integrity.* Singapore: World Conference on Research Integrity; 2010. https://wcrif.org/guidance/singapore-statement (accessed 29 August 2022).
46. Artino AR, Driessen EW, Maggio LA. Ethical shades of gray: international frequency of scientific misconduct and questionable research practices in health professions education. *Acad Med.* 2019;94(1):76–84.
47. Maggio LA, Artino AR, Watling CJ, et al. Exploring researchers' perspectives on authorship decision making. *Med Educ.* 2019;53(12):1253–1262.
48. Uijtdehaage S, Mavis B, Durning SJ. Whose paper is it anyway? Authorship criteria according to established scholars in health professions education. *Acad Med.* 2018;93(8):1171–1175.

49. International Committee of Medical Journal Editors (ICMJE). Defining the role of authors and contributors. ICMJE; 2022. https://www.icmje.org/recommendations/browse/roles-and-responsibilities/defining-the-role-of-authors-and-contributors.html (accessed 29 August 2022).

50. National Health and Medical Research Council (NHMRC). Ethical conduct in research with Aboriginal and Torres Strait Islander peoples and communities: guidelines for researchers and stakeholders. Australian Government: Canberra; 2018. https://www.nhmrc.gov.au/about-us/resources/ethical-conduct-research-aboriginal-and-torres-strait-islander-peoples-and-communities (accessed 29 August 2022).

51. National Health and Medical Research Council (NHMRC). Australian Research Council (ARC), and Universities Australia. National Statement on Ethical Conduct in Human Research; Australia: NHMRC; 2018. https://www.nhmrc.gov.au/about-us/publications/national-statement-ethical-conduct-human-research-2007-updated-2018#block-views-block-file-attachments-content-block-1 (accessed 26 October 2022).

52. Rees EL, Burton O, Asif A, et al. A method for the madness: an international survey of health professions education authors' journal choice. *Perspect Med Educ.* 2022;11(3):165–172.

53. Kemp C, van Herwerden L, Molloy E, et al. How do students offer value to organisations through work integrated learning? A qualitative study using social exchange theory. *Adv Health Sci Educ.* 2021;26(3):1075–1093.

54. O'Brien BC, Zapata J, Chang A, et al. Bridging medical education goals and health system outcomes: an instrumental case study of pre-clerkship students' improvement projects. *Perspect Med Educ.* 2022;11(4):179–186.

55. Carter SM, Little M. Justifying knowledge, justifying method, taking action: epistemologies, methodologies, and methods in qualitative research. *Qual Health Res.* 2007;17(10):1316–1328.

56. Johnston J, Bennett D, Kajamaa A. How to... get started with theory in education. *Clin Teach.* 2018;15(4):294–297.

57. Varpio L, Martimianakis MA, Mylopoulos M. Qualitative research methodologies: embracing methodological borrowing, shifting and importing. In Cleland J, Durning S, eds. *Researching Medical Education.* Oxford: Wiley Blackwell; 2015: 245–256.

58. Gill TG, Gill TR. What is research rigor? Lessons for a transdiscipline. *Inf Sci: The Int J Emerg Transdiscipline.* 2020;23:47–76.

59. Buetow S, Zawaly K. Rethinking researcher bias in health research. *J Eval Clin Pract.* 2022;28(5):843–846.

60. Hopkins RM, Regehr G, Pratt DD. A framework for negotiating positionality in phenomenological research. *Med Teach.* 2017;39(1):20–25.

61. Olmos-Vega FM, Stalmeijer RE, Varpio L, et al. A practical guide to reflexivity in qualitative research: AMEE Guide no. 149. *Med Teach.* 2022;1–11. https://pubmed.ncbi.nlm.nih.gov/35389310. Epub ahead of print.

62. Varpio L, O'Brien B, Rees CE, et al. The applicability of generalisability and bias to health professions education's research. *Med Educ.* 2021;55(2):167–173.

63. Stenfors T, Kajamaa A, Bennett D. How to ... assess the quality of qualitative research. *Clin Teach.* 2020;17(6):596–599.

64. Lingard LA, Watling C. *Story, Not Study: 30 Brief Lessons to Inspire Health Researchers as Writers.* Cham: Springer; 2020.

65. Coverdale JH, Roberts LW, Balon R, et al. Writing for academia: getting your research into print: AMEE Guide no. 74. *Med Teach.* 2013;35(2):e926–934.

66. Asif A, Burton O. Comic Sans or common sense? Graphic design for clinical teachers. *Clin Teach.* 2021;18(6):583–589.

67. EQUATOR Network. Enhancing the QUAlity and Transparency Of health Research. Reporting Guidelines for Main Study Types; https://www.equator-network.org (accessed 29 August 2022).

68. Ginsburg S, Lynch M, Walsh CM. A fine balance: how authors strategize around journal submission. *Acad Med.* 2018;93(8):1176–1181.

69. Fleming JI, Wilson SE, Hart SA, et al. Open accessibility in education research: enhancing the credibility, equity, impact, and efficiency of research. *Educ Psychol.* 2021;56(2):110–121.

70. Reed MS. *The Research Impact Handbook*, 2nd ed. Aberdeenshire: Fast Track Impact; 2018.

71. Research Excellence Framework (REF). Guidance on submissions. Annex C. UK: REF; 2021. https://www.ref.ac.uk/media/1447/ref-2019_01-guidance-on-submissions.pdf (accessed 22 March 2023).

72. Dillman DA, Smyth JD, Christian LM. *Internet, Phone, Mail, and Mixed-Mode Surveys: The Tailored Design Method*, 4th ed. Hoboken: Wiley; 2014.

73. Bunton SA, Sandberg SF. Case study research in health professions education. *Acad Med.* 2016;91(12):e3.

74. Cleland J, MacLeod A, Ellaway RH. The curious case of case study research. *Med Educ.* 2021;55(10):1131–1141.

75. Yazan B. Three approaches to case study methods in education: Yin, Merriam, and Stake. *Qual Rep.* 2015;20(2):134–152.

76. Buccheri RK, Sharifi C. Critical appraisal tools and reporting guidelines for evidence-based practice. *Worldviews Evid Based Nurs.* 2017;14(6):463–472.

77. Critical Appraisal Skills Programme (CASP). Critical appraisal. https://casp-uk.net/glossary/critical-appraisal (accessed 1 September 2022).

78. Altman DG, Simera I. A history of the evolution of guidelines for reporting medical research: the long road to the EQUATOR Network. *J Roy Soc Med.* 2016;109(2):67–77.

79. Critical appraisal tools: introduction. Duquesne University; https://guides.library.duq.edu/critappraise (accessed 3 September 2022).

80. O'Brien BC, West CP, Coverdale JH, et al. On the use and value of reporting guidelines in health professions education research. *Acad Med.* 2020;95(11):1619–1622.

81. Altman DG, Schulz KF, Moher D, et al. The revised CONSORT statement for reporting randomized trials: explanation and elaboration. *Ann Intern Med.* 2001;134(8):663–694.

82. von Elm E, Altman DG, Egger M, et al. The strengthening the reporting of observational studies in epidemiology (STROBE) statement: guidelines for reporting observational studies. *PLoS Med.* 2007;4(10):e296.

83. Page MJ, McKenzie JE, Bossuyt PM, et al. Updating guidance for reporting systematic reviews: development of the PRISMA 2020 statement. *J Clin Epidemiol.* 2021;134:103–112.

84. Gordon M, Gibbs T. STORIES statement: publication standards for healthcare education evidence synthesis. *BMC Med.* 2014;12:143.

85. Husereau D, Drummond M, Petrou S, et al. CHEERS good reporting practices task force. consolidated health economic evaluation reporting standards (CHEERS)—explanation and elaboration: a report of the ISPOR health economic evaluation publication guidelines good reporting practices task force. *Value Health.* 2013;16(2):231–250.

86. Cook DA, Reed DA. Appraising the quality of medical education research methods: the Medical Education Research Study Quality Instrument and the Newcastle–Ottawa Scale-Education. *Acad Med.* 2015;90(8):1067–1076.

87. Kmet LM, Lee RC, Cook LS. HTA Initiative #13 Standard quality assessment criteria for evaluating primary research papers from a variety of fields. Alberta Heritage Foundation; 2004.

88. Wong G, Greenhalgh T, Westhorp G, et al. RAMESES publication standards: meta-narrative reviews. *BMC Med.* 2013;11:20.

89. Wong G, Westhorp G, Manzano A, et al. RAMESES II reporting standards for realist evaluations. *BMC Med.* 2016;14(1):96.

90. O'Brien BC, Harris IB, Beckman TJ, et al. Standards for reporting qualitative research: a synthesis of recommendations. *Acad Med.* 2014;89(9):1245–1251.

91. Tong A, Sainsbury P, Craig J. Consolidated criteria for reporting qualitative research (COREQ): a 32-item checklist for interviews and focus groups. *Int J Qual Health Care.* 2007;19(6):349–357.

92. Tong A, Flemming K, McInnes E, et al. Enhancing transparency in reporting the synthesis of qualitative research: ENTREQ. *BMC Med Res Methodol.* 2012;12:181.

93. Goodman D, Ogrinc G, Davies L, et al. Explanation and elaboration of the SQUIRE (Standards for Quality Improvement Reporting Excellence) guidelines V.2.0: examples of SQUIRE elements in the healthcare improvement literature. *BMJ Qual Safe.* 2016;25(12):e27.

94. Ogrinc G, Armstrong GE, Dolansky MA, et al. SQUIRE-EDU (Standards for Quality Improvement Reporting Excellence in Education): publication guidelines for educational improvement. *Acad Med.* 2019;94(10):1461–1470.

95. Abelson J, Li K, Wilson G, et al. Supporting quality public and patient engagement in health system organizations: development and usability testing of the Public and Patient Engagement Evaluation Tool. *Health Exp.* 2016;19(4):817–827.

96. Staniszewska S, Brett J, Simera I, et al. GRIPP2 reporting checklists: tools to improve reporting of patient and public involvement in research. *BMJ.* 2017;358:j3453.

97. National Health and Medical Research Council (NHMRC). Statement on consumer and community involvement in health and medical research. https://www.nhmrc.gov.au/about-us/publications/statement-consumer-and-community-involvement-health-and-medical-research (accessed 22 March 2023).

98. O'Cathain A, Murphy E, Nicholl J. The quality of mixed methods studies in health services research. *J Health Serv Res Policy.* 2008;13(2):92–98.

99. Hong QN, Pluye P, Fàbregues S, et al. Mixed Methods Appraisal Tool (MMAT), version 2018. Registration of Copyright (#1148552); Industry Canada: Canadian Intellectual Property Office; 2018.

100. Bradbury H, Lewis R, Embury DC. Education action research: with and for the next generation. In Mertler CA, ed. *The Wiley Handbook of Action Research in Education.* Hoboken: John Wiley & Sons, Inc.; 2019: 7–28.

101. Evans D. Hierarchy of evidence: a framework for ranking evidence evaluating healthcare interventions. *J Clin Nurs.* 2003;12(1):77–84.

102. Greenhalgh T. How to read a paper: getting your bearings (deciding what the paper is about). *BMJ.* 1997;315(7102):243–246.

103. Guyatt GH, Sackett DL, Sinclair JC, et al. Users' guides to the medical literature. IX. A method for grading health care recommendations. *JAMA.* 1995;274(22):1800–1804.

104. Barbour RS. Checklist for improving rigour in qualitative research: a case of the tail wagging the dog? *BMJ.* 2001;322(7294):1115–1117.

105. Morse J. Why the Qualitative Health Research (QHR) review process does not use checklists. *Qual Health Res.* 2021;31(5):819–821.

106. Wharton T. Rigor, transparency, and reporting social science research: why guidelines don't have to kill your story. *Res Soc Work Pract.* 2017;27(4):487–493.

107. Barbour RS, Barbour M. Evaluating and synthesizing qualitative research: the need to develop a distinctive approach. *J Eval Clin Pract.* 2003;9(2):179–186.

108. Varpio L, Ajjawi R, Monrouxe LV, et al. Shedding the cobra effect: problematising thematic emergence, triangulation, saturation and member checking. *Med Educ.* 2017;51(1):40–50.

109. Haile ZT. Critical appraisal tools and reporting guidelines. *J Hum Lact.* 2022;38(1):21–27.

110. Eva KW. Altruism as enlightened self-interest: how helping others through peer review helps you. *Med Educ.* 2021;55(8):880–882.

111. Dumenco L, Engle DL, Goodell K, et al. Expanding group peer review: a proposal for medical education scholarship. *Acad Med.* 2017;92(2):147–149.

112. Richards BF, Cardell EM, Chow CJ, et al. Discovering the benefits of group peer review of submitted manuscripts. *Teach Learn Med*. 2020;32(1):104–109.

113. Azer SA, Ramani S, Peterson R. Becoming a peer reviewer to medical education journals. *Med Teach*. 2012;34(9):698–704.

114. Durning SJ, Sklar DP, Driessen EW, et al. "This manuscript was a complete waste of time": reviewer etiquette matters. *Acad Med*. 2019;94(6):744–745.

115. Eva KW. The reviewer is always right: peer review of research in medical education. *Med Educ*. 2009;43(1):2–4.

116. Yarris LM, Gottlieb M, Scott K, et al. Academic Primer Series: key papers about peer review. *West J Emerg Med*. 2017;18(4):721–728.

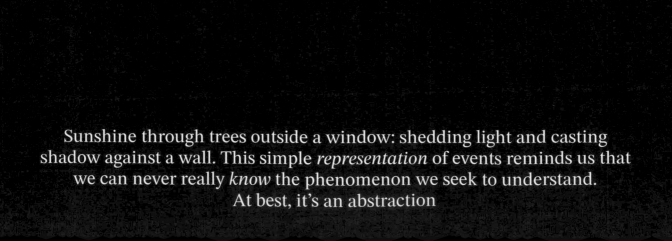

Sunshine through trees outside a window: shedding light and casting shadow against a wall. This simple *representation* of events reminds us that we can never really *know* the phenomenon we seek to understand. At best, it's an abstraction

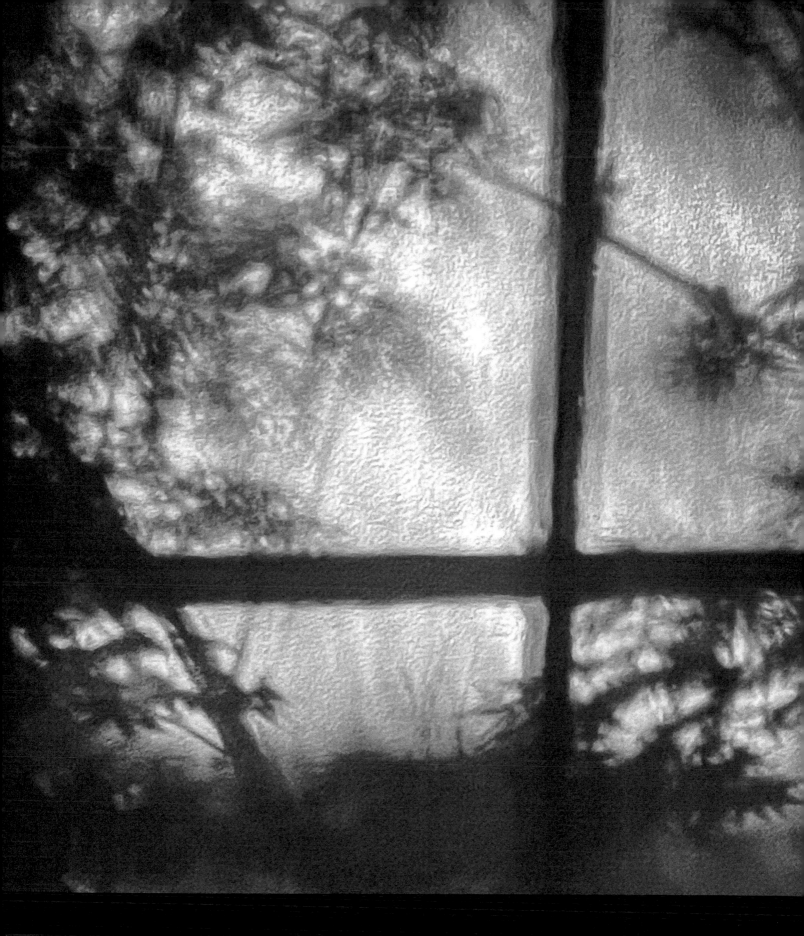

Part II: Perspectives

Introducing Scientific Approaches in Health Professions Education Research

Charlotte E. Rees[1,2], Jeffrey J.H. Cheung[3], Jonathan Foo[2], and Claire Palermo[2]

[1] The University of Newcastle, Callaghan, New South Wales, Australia
[2] Monash University, Clayton, Victoria, Australia
[3] University of Illinois at Chicago, Chicago, Illinois, USA

Box 5.1   Chapter 5 learning objectives: After reading this chapter you should be able to ...

- Describe the philosophical underpinnings (ontology, epistemology, and axiology) of scientific approaches
- Summarise common scientific methodologies in health professions education research (HPER)
- Identify key principles of scientific methods in HPER (sampling, data collection, and data analysis)
- Explain the main indicators of quality employed in scientific approaches
- Evaluate the strengths and challenges of scientific approaches for HPER
- Reflect on the applicability of scientific approaches to your own HPER

5.1   INTRODUCING CHAPTER 5

> the 'science' of medical education [has] the goal of demonstrating 'evidence' or proof for a set of simple, generalisable 'truths', which ultimately should be relevant to applied education practices. [1 p. 32]

Many people use the term scientific in health professions education research (HPER) as a synonym for rigorous, empirical, or systematic. In this chapter, however, we employ the term *scientific approaches* to reflect enquiry typically founded in the

---

Foundations of Health Professions Education Research: Principles, Perspectives and Practices,
First Edition. Edited by Charlotte E. Rees, Lynn V. Monrouxe, Bridget C. O'Brien, Lisi J. Gordon, and Claire Palermo.
© 2023 John Wiley & Sons Ltd. Published 2023 by John Wiley & Sons Ltd.

traditional sciences such as physics, biology, and chemistry, and then latterly the social sciences [2]. Scientific approaches aim to explain or predict regularities in the natural world based on relationships between variables and cause–effect inferences: hypothesis testing, randomisation, control, replicability, impartiality, predictive validity, and other features are therefore common in these approaches. This chapter will help you consider the applicability of scientific approaches to HPER. For example, are the methods used to conduct a randomised controlled trial (RCT) similarly appropriate to studies of educational interventions? In this chapter, we aim to help you think through the hows and whys of applying scientific approaches to HPER (see Box 5.1). What we present in this chapter reflects our reading of the scientific literature, as well as our own (and varied) experiences conducting and reviewing scientific approaches in HPER. In section 5.2, we describe the philosophical underpinnings of scientific approaches (crucial to improving the rigour of your research and for avoiding philosophical challenges), and in section 5.3, we summarise common scientific methodologies and methods used in HPER. We discuss the key markers of quality in scientific research in section 5.4, and in section 5.5, we evaluate the challenges and strengths of scientific approaches for HPER. We try to bring these issues to life throughout this chapter by illustrating details associated with four case studies based on our own research employing different scientific methodologies: a systematic review [3], an RCT [4], a non-experimental observational study [5],and a psychometrics study [6] (see Box 5.2 for a brief overview). We hope this chapter helps you decide if a scientific approach is appropriate for your research, plus prepares you for any challenges you may encounter along the way.

Box 5.2   Case studies: An overview

Systematic Review [3]: We conducted a systematic review involving comprehensively searching, reviewing, and appraising the literature on simulation in dietetics and how simulation was used to prepare dietetics students for practice.

Randomised Controlled Trial [4]: We explored the relationships between instructional design, medical trainees' conceptual knowledge, and their ability to demonstrate transfer of learning. Based on previous clinical reasoning research demonstrating the learning benefits of cognitive integration (where learners create conceptual connections between different types of knowledge) [7, 8], we answered the questions: (1) Does instruction designed to support cognitive integration improve trainees' learning and transfer for simulation-based procedural skills? (2) Is there a relationship between integrated instruction, conceptual knowledge, and procedural skills performance?.

Non-experimental Observation [5]: We examined the additional economic costs associated with physiotherapy student placement failure, and how these costs are distributed among stakeholders to inform the design of clinical education, remediation, and support structures.

Psychometrics [6]: We examined the reliability and cost of a newly designed Objective Structured Clinical Examination (OSCE) for postgraduate nurses to determine the optimal OSCE design (e.g., station number and duration) to cover the assessment blueprint.

5.2   PHILOSOPHICAL UNDERPINNINGS OF SCIENTIFIC APPROACHES

Understanding philosophies underpinning your chosen research approach is crucial if you are to understand its relevance, rigour, strengths, and limitations (see Chapter 2). You should also be mindful of your personal philosophies and how they intersect with your research approach, and how such personal philosophies might evolve over time and with different research projects: what do you think is the nature of reality? (ontology), what does knowledge and knowing mean to you? (epistemology), how do you think you can access this knowledge? (methodology), and, finally, what do you most value in terms of reality, knowledge, and coming to know? (axiology) [9, 10]. In our experience, many challenges in the research process – whether those reside within an individual researcher or within a research team (e.g., a research student and their supervisors) – can be traced back to philosophical misunderstandings (e.g., not being sure about the philosophies underpinning your chosen approach) or mismatches (either between researchers' different personal philosophies, or between personal philosophies and those underlying the research approach). Therefore, by understanding the philosophical foundations of a chosen research approach, both novice and experienced researchers alike can work to ensure: (a) rigour through the integrity and transparency of research philosophy [11], and through that internal coherence concept discussed in Chapters 2 and 4 [12, 13]; (b) understanding of the relevance of research within an interdisciplinary field approaching science in different ways; and (c) a smoother collaborative research journey (especially within interdisciplinary teams). Furthermore, Veen and Cianciolo remind us that: 'philosophy can be seen as the fundamental approach to pausing at times of complexity and uncertainty to ask basic questions about seemingly obvious practices so that we can see (and do) things in new ways'[14 p. 338]. See Box 5.3 for a summary of the case studies' philosophical underpinnings.

Box 5.3   Case studies: A summary of their philosophical underpinnings

Systematic Review [3]: We embraced a post-positivist theoretical perspective privileging realist ontology. We aimed to uncover facts about dietetics simulation practice, drawing on objectivist epistemology to generate knowledge independent from us, while acknowledging that what we uncovered was likely to be incomplete. In terms of axiology, we valued the inclusion of studies recognising the testability and quantification of the quality of simulation experiences.

Randomised Controlled Trial [4]: We adopted a realist ontology and objectivist epistemology, acknowledging the existence of cognitive phenomena (e.g., memory) external to ourselves. We thought that such phenomena could be inferred through experimental comparisons designed to control confounders (e.g., time on task). However, from a post-positivist standpoint, we recognised the challenges of accurately and reliably operationalising these phenomena through our interventions, study design, and assessment tools. Thus, we believed our findings could only approximate the truth.

Non-experimental Observation [5]: Although we did not give any explicit considerations to our philosophical underpinnings at the time of the study, we implicitly assumed that reality was singular, tangible, and measurable (realist

(continued)

(continued)

ontology), and that the nature of knowing was objective (objectivist epistemology). Aligned with post-positivism, we objectively quantified the cost of student failure, but in the belief that we could only arrive at an approximation of cost through careful empirical study. This study valued objectivity, quantifiable regularities, and reproducibility.

Psychometrics [6]: While our large interdisciplinary research team did not discuss research philosophies at the time, our quantitative evaluation served to triangulate reliability and cost; therefore, looking for one single point of convergence to determine the optimal number of OSCE stations. Underpinned by a realist ontology and objectivist epistemology, our study could be described as post-positivist as we recognised the fallibility of our methods, and the partiality of our findings. However, we still valued empiricism, facts, and objectivity.

5.2.1   Realist Ontology

As described in Chapter 2, ontology relates to the nature of reality. Realist ontology typically underpins scientific approaches [15], with both positivist and post-positivist theoretical perspectives suggesting that reality is: 'static and fixed ... [with the world being] ordered according to an overarching objective truth'[11 p. 361]. Positivism has, for example, been described as asserting: 'a single-objective, external, tangible, measurable reality'[16 p. 695]. See our book glossary for all key terms relating to scientific approaches in this chapter, including brief definitions of positivism and post-positivism. While positivism embraces the scientific method (discussed in section 5.2.3) as a way of knowing the world, post-positivists recognise that reality remains incomplete and probabilistic, and can only be inferred through observation [16, 17].

5.2.2   Objectivist Epistemology

Underpinning scientific approaches is objectivism that privileges facts (objective truth) rather than values, believing that objects exist independently of our consciousness of them [18]. While positivism suggests that there is an objective existence of reality [19], post-positivism postulates that there may be a truth that can be measured but such measurements will be imperfect [16]. With scientific approaches privileging objectivity, dualism is favoured [19]. Here, the scientific researcher strives to keep themselves separate from their research participants or objects of study in the belief that it will help maintain value-free, neutral, objectivity and thus minimise bias [19–22]. In this way, research can be described as conducted and reported 'from the outside'[21]. For example, scientific language employing the third person (e.g., 'The authors ...') downplays researcher involvement in studies and communicates dispassionate neutral observation [22, 23]. This is different to the use of first person singular 'I' or plural 'we', commonly preferred in other research approaches privileging subjectivity, for example interpretivism (see Chapter 7).

5.2.3   Scientific Methodology

Seeking to explain and predict universal features of humanhood, society, and the natural world, scientific approaches embrace empirical observation, privilege the hypothetico-deductive model, and value the measurement of variables to explain and predict patterns including causality [1, 11, 14, 19, 24, 25]. When we think about scientific approaches, we often first think of experimental research aligned with the hypothetico-deductive model [24]. This model has been described as a circular process starting with evidence-based theory to create testable hypotheses (often about causality such as X causes Y), then designing and conducting experiments manipulating independent variables to determine the effects on one (or more) dependent variable(s), while controlling for systematic errors through design features like randomisation and blinding, and thereby testing and developing theory [19, 26–28]. From a positivist perspective the aim is to verify theory, whereas post-positivism aims to refute theory (or accept or reject the null hypothesis) [16, 19]. Experiments can be described as explanatory, exploring whether interventions work in controlled, 'ideal' environments (often positivist), or pragmatic, exploring whether interventions work in real life and for whom (often post-positivist) [26, 28]. However, not all scientific HPER asks the question 'what works?' Therefore, non-experimental scientific approaches (often post-positivist) such as descriptive and observational questionnaire studies are common.

5.2.4 Scientific Axiology

Given that the purpose of scientific research is to explain or predict regularities and consistencies, it comes as no surprise that these approaches value empiricism – empirical observation, testability, and replication, as well as quantifiable data that can be reduced to quantifiable natural laws [2, 19, 22, 24, 29]. Scientific approaches also privilege facts (i.e., value-free neutrality), rather than values, beliefs, and subjectivities [2, 22, 30]. Linked with this, scientific approaches also value objectivity and dualism, as discussed in section 5.2.2 [19, 21]. Although this is the case with positivism and post-positivism alike, post-positivism typically acknowledges the impact of the researcher on the research process, recognising that bias is likely [16].

5.3 COMMON SCIENTIFIC METHODOLOGIES AND METHODS IN HPER

Scientific approaches underpinned by positivism and post-positivism are still considered dominant in HPER [1, 11, 21, 22, 25]. They are thought to dominate in two ways: (1) there is considerable research conducted through these approaches; and (2) other approaches to HPER, such as interpretivist approaches are often erroneously judged from a scientific standpoint [21, 22]. While considerable variety exists regarding the study designs employed within scientific approaches, as well as diversity in terms of how scholars categorise the different types of scientific approaches, in this chapter we focus on the most common scientific methodologies. We organise them in the following way: systematic reviews [15]; experimental studies [31, 32]; and non-experimental studies (see case studies) [3–6].

5.3.1 Systematic Reviews

Systematic reviews are literature reviews that: 'identify, select, appraise, extract and synthesise all high-quality research evidence relevant to a given question'[15 p. 747]. Privileging quantitative syntheses of results, they are traditionally underpinned by positivism [15]. While clinical medicine systematic reviews (e.g., Cochrane reviews) have focused questions and syntheses concentrating on justification/effectiveness, health education systematic reviews often have broader questions depending on context and syntheses focused on justification and descriptive clarification [33, 34]. Systematic reviews often use a question guided by the format of PICO (Participants, Interventions, Comparison, Outcomes) [35].A quick search of the HPER journals (*Academic Medicine, Advances in Health Sciences Education, Medical Education, Medical Teacher*) for the last decade (2011–2021) identified 200 papers with the word 'systematic review' in the title. These systematic reviews cover wide-ranging topics including learning (e.g., self-regulated learning), teaching (e.g., teaching empathy), assessment (e.g., open versus closed book), curriculum (e.g., Indigenous curriculum), faculty development, mentoring, and leadership. Although systematic reviews in HPER often include qualitative data and employ narrative (rather than quantitative) syntheses, they are still systematic in their approach to data searching and collation to adopt a reproducible, unbiased approach [36]. In terms of quantitative studies included in systematic reviews, sometimes meta-analyses are conducted as part of systematic reviews employing statistical methods to pool the quantitative results of included studies [37]. They determine the best estimate of effect across studies exploring similar questions, conceptual frameworks, interventions, measures, and outcomes [37]. They are however less frequent in HPER (46 were identified in the same search for the last decade), although their popularity seems to be growing recently.

5.3.2   Experimental Studies

Experimental approaches, like the RCT, serve to answer questions about what works for healthcare learning and assessment, and potentially why. They are relatively popular and enduring in HPER [37, 38]. For example, a quick search of the same four journals within the last decade identified 102 papers with the word 'trial' or 'experiment' in the title. Experimental studies aimed to compare formal education approaches (e.g., online learning, video-enhanced learning, simulation, games-based learning, case-based learning, seminars, adaptive learning) or informal interventions (e.g., mentoring, role-modelling, coaching, shadowing) on a multiplicity of outcomes for healthcare students or faculty (e.g., clinical reasoning, clinical skills, communication skills, cognitive skills including mindfulness, empathy, and reflection), while controlling for confounding variables.

5.3.3   Non-experimental Studies

Non-experimental scientific approaches in HPER are also widespread, and include observational investigations such as correlational questionnaire studies, and exploratory work including descriptive questionnaires and measurement psychometrics [39]. For example, the same four journals for the last decade revealed 483 papers with the word 'questionnaire' in the abstract, and 132 papers with the term 'psychometrics' in the abstract. Descriptive questionnaire studies typically outline learners' motivations about, perceptions of, or attitudes towards something educationally relevant (e.g., specialty choice, preparedness for practice, providing Indigenous healthcare). The observational studies typically explore correlations between multiple variables, sometimes making quasi-causal claims such as gender predicting burnout, personality type predicting specialty choice, or demographics predicting assessment performance. The psychometric studies, on the other hand, mostly focus on the reliability and validity of assessment approaches within health professions education including admissions tests (e.g., multiple mini-interview, situational judgement test), examinations of knowledge (e.g., multiple choice questions) or clinical competence (e.g., OSCE, long case), or workplace-based assessments (e.g., multisource feedback). Finally, the psychometrics studies also include the development and validation of scales to measure a wide range of concepts relating to learners/learning (e.g., tolerance of ambiguity, empathy, readiness for interprofessional learning, attitudes towards online learning) or teachers/teaching (e.g., readiness for curriculum change, teaching styles inventory). See Box 5.4 for a summary of the case studies' methodologies/methods.

Box 5.4   Case studies: A summary of their methodologies and methods

Systematic Review [3]: We used a reproducible search aligned with Cochrane guidelines for systematic reviews [33].We used scientific databases, as well as targeted searches of international dietetics journals and simulation industry organisations. Aligned with our scientific philosophies, our synthesis was guided by strict inclusion criteria focusing on simulation-based learning with simulated patients prior to dietetics students having any placement learning. The synthesis focused on measuring simulation-based learning outcomes and quality against simulation-based learning standards [40].

Randomised Controlled Trial [4]: We compared two instructional videos to teach lumbar puncture (LP) skills: (1) teaching the relevant procedural steps, and (2) teaching the same steps but including conceptual knowledge explaining why the steps were performed (e.g., anatomy). To minimise bias, we randomised participants into each group and controlled for confounders (e.g., time on task). After training, participants were tested on written knowledge tests and LP performance tests administered immediately after training, and one week later (retention and transfer tests). We used regression to test statistically significant relationships between three variables of interest: group (intervention vs control), conceptual knowledge test scores, and LP performance. Effectiveness of our instructional videos was inferred through group differences in participants' conceptual knowledge and LP performance tests.

Non-experimental Observation [5]: We modelled our design on 'burden of disease' studies common in clinical medicine. We utilised a non-experimental observational methodology with a cross-sectional design in which the dependent variable (cost) was measured at the same time as the independent variable (student performance). Privileging objectivity and reproducibility, we employed published values wherever possible, so they could be easily verified by others. Where published values did not exist, we conducted quantitative primary data collection and analysis using clearly defined statistical methods.

Psychometrics [6]: Our cross-sectional observational study involved collecting quantitative data pertaining to the reliability of the OSCE (i.e., all examiner marking sheets measuring OSCE candidate performance) and cost (i.e., measuring the volume of resource items identified for the OSCE and assigning monetary prices to the resource items). We conducted various univariate and multivariate statistics to establish the reliability of the OSCE, as well as estimate its reliability with different numbers of stations. We also calculated the total cost of the OSCE and the cost per candidate for 150 implementation alternatives varying, among other things, the number of OSCE stations. We triangulated the reliability and cost data to determine the optimal number of stations.

5.3.4   Scientific Sampling, Data Collection, and Analysis Methods

Given that scientific research aims to explain or predict regularities, consistencies, and laws, and that generalisability is a central value (more on that in section 5.4), random sampling is privileged to obtain study samples that are representative of broader populations [41]. Furthermore, in the case of experimental designs, random allocation is thought to be the most appropriate way to enhance the probability that any differences between experimental and control groups are due to interventions rather than other characteristics like learner demographics [27]. Data collection methods within experimental and non-experimental scientific HPER typically involve quantitative measures such as student performance data (e.g., OSCE results), validated scales (e.g., attitude scales), or questionnaire surveys [10]. While quantitative approaches dominate, scientific approaches with post-positivist theoretical perspectives sometimes include qualitative data collection and analyses, such as an RCT with interviews and focus groups in order to better understand causation, or participants' experiences of the intervention [24]. Qualitative methods here may be understood as exploratory, or as an adjunct to the quantitative methods. They may also be seen as a reflection of events/thoughts rather than socially constructed as in interpretivist approaches or critical enquiry. Consequently, data analyses within scientific approaches characteristically include descriptive, univariate, and multivariate statistics, for example, to establish statistically significant differences between groups (e.g., experimental and control groups) and/or determine statistically significant relationships between variables (e.g., causation or correlation). It is outside the scope of this book chapter on the foundations of scientific approaches to cover the wide-ranging scientific research methods in-depth, so instead we refer you to other sources [42]. Before moving on to the next section, pause and reflect on how you might apply scientific approaches to your HPER (see Box 5.5).

> **Box 5.5   Pause and reflect: Applying scientific methodologies/ methods to your research**
>
> - Think about a topic of enquiry in health professions education that you are especially interested in researching. This may relate to a challenge regarding your own teaching or learning, or it may link to previous research you have done, or could relate to key gaps in the literature.
> - What research question could you develop relating to this topic that would lend itself well to scientific approaches and why? What methodologies/ methods would be appropriate for this question and why?
> - Now think of a research question pertaining to your chosen topic that does not lend itself well to scientific approaches. What other methodologies/ methods are more appropriate for this question and why? What other chapters should you therefore read next?
> - Revisit this pause and reflect box once you have read the other chapters in Part II, and further developed your research ideas.

5.4 KEY QUALITY INDICATORS IN SCIENTIFIC APPROACHES

Quality indicators central to scientific approaches include generalisability, reproducibility, minimisation of bias, validity, reliability, and larger sample sizes [19, 21]. Although we briefly discuss each, it is worth noting that considerable interplay exists between these quality indicators. Generalisability involves claims about the extent to which study findings can be extrapolated to a broader population across various domains and contexts [1, 20, 43]. Also known as external validity, generalisability is typically assessed through the size and characteristics of the study sample, or the applicability of study findings to other settings [43]. Reproducibility can entail: 'replicability (i.e., the potential for replication) and replication (i.e., multiple instances of the same study)' [16 p. 696]. Minimisation of bias can be seen as attempts to minimise researcher practices or actions that could influence sampling, data collection, or interpretation, thereby threatening objectivity and neutrality [20]. In the context of trials, minimising biases can be seen as avoiding systematic errors [26]. This bias minimisation can be facilitated by paying close attention to issues of validity and reliability [35]. In the context of experimental methods, external validity equates to generalisability (as mentioned earlier in this section), whereas internal validity can be described as the ability to determine cause–effect relationships [19, 26, 27]. Assessment validity, in both experimental and non-experimental designs, can be seen as the extent to which a measurement construct assesses what it is supposed to measure [19, 35]. Cook and Hatala [44] provide a helpful primer on assessment validation in the context of simulation that includes popular frameworks by Messick [45] and Kane [46]. Reliability is seen as the extent to which a measurement instrument is dependable, stable, and consistent when repeated under identical conditions [43]. Larger sample sizes within scientific studies can serve to minimise bias, and enhance the generalisability of study findings, but can also help yield sufficient power to detect statistically significant changes in outcomes, thereby enabling inferences about studies to be made across other similar samples [43]. See Box 5.6 for a summary of the case studies' quality.

Box 5.6   Case studies: A summary of their quality

Systematic Review [3]: Our systematic review followed the Preferred Reporting of Items for Systematic Reviews and Meta-Analyses (PRISMA), to guide the quality of our reporting [47]. This approach helped ensure that our search strategy and data synthesis was reproducible. All screening and synthesis steps were conducted in duplicate to minimise bias. The individual quality of each study was appraised using a tool for reporting quality health simulations [40]. Using the STORIES (STructured apprOach to the Reporting In healthcare education of Evidence Synthesis) statement [48], we could have improved quality through clearly reporting a research question in our manuscript, as well as providing description/justification of our evidence synthesis method.

Randomised Controlled Trial [4]: Our findings demonstrated high external validity, replicating theoretical generalisability of cognitive integration in a novel context [7, 8]. Internal validity was high as our study design clarified the hypothesised causal relationships between integrated instruction, conceptual knowledge, and LP skill transfer. We minimised bias through highly controlled interventions and assessments with strong validity evidence. Although many CONSORT

(continued)

(continued)

(CONsolidated Standards Of Reporting Trials) criteria were met [49], we could have enhanced our study and reporting by registering the trial/protocol beforehand and including the randomised trial design in our paper's title.

<u>Non-experimental Observation</u> [5]: We employed the Consolidated Health Economic Evaluation Reporting Standards (CHEERS) statement [50] to guide our reporting of quality. The CHEERS statement incorporates items believed to be important to the reproducibility of economic studies, such as cost itemisation and currency conversion. To improve the study quality, we could have paid greater attention to our questionnaire's assessment validity. Furthermore, our reporting of the questionnaire could have been supported using the Checklist for Reporting Results of Internet E-Surveys (CHERRIES) [51], which pays particular attention to bias arising from participant sampling.

<u>Psychometrics</u> [6]: Although Guidelines for Reporting Reliability and Agreement Studies (GRRAS) exist [52], these were not relevant to our study because they exclude internal consistency (instead, focusing on inter-rater and test–retest reliability). While our reporting allowed for the reproducibility of the evaluation, our study participants (all volunteers) were self-selected (not random) and our sample size small, thereby potentially leading to bias and jeopardising the generalisability of our study findings.

Given these key quality indicators, multiple tools and checklists now exist for researchers working within scientific approaches to enhance the quality and reporting quality of research. For example, the Medical Education Research Study Quality Instrument (MERSQI) [53] was developed to appraise the quality of experimental and non-experimental observational studies in HPER (see Chapter 4). Furthermore, in the context of healthcare, reporting standards exist for different types of study design that can also be employed/adapted for HPER [38], including randomised trials (e.g., CONSORT) [49], observational studies (e.g., STROBE: STrengthening the Reporting of OBservation studies in Epidemiology) [54], systematic reviews (e.g., PRISMA: Preferred Reporting Items for Systematic Reviews and Meta-Analyses) [47], and economic evaluations (e.g., CHEERS) [50]. You can access many of these tools and further details about them on the EQUATOR Network: https://www.equator-network.org/reporting-guidelines. These tools either make explicit references to the quality indicators discussed earlier in this section (e.g., generalisability, validity, sample size, bias) or they imply these indicators through appraising other study features (e.g., minimising bias through the use of objective observer ratings, blinding or randomisation, enabling replication through sufficiently described interventions, or flagging potential conflicts of interest that could have affected the conduct or reporting of studies) [55].

While some elements of CONSORT are thought to be less relevant within HPER [38], a recent review of randomised studies in HPER has shown that most CONSORT elements were reported in less than 50% of studies [38]. This indicated problems in the completeness of reporting, plus most studies were assessed as having unclear or high risk for bias, especially for allocation concealment, participant blinding, personnel and outcome assessors [38]. Furthermore, Cook and Reed reviewed 26 HPER studies employing the MERSQI, finding that scores for the validity domain were suboptimal because validity evidence was infrequently reported (median score = 0.9/3) [53]. We would therefore encourage you to employ relevant tools to guide you on your HPER journey to: (a) determine the suitability of your study design for your research questions; (b) aid the rigorous design and conduct of your study; and (c) facilitate quality reporting of your study findings. Before moving on to the next section, we urge you to familiarise yourself with at least one of these tools, by critically appraising a paper (see Box 5.7).

Box 5.7   Stop and do: Critically appraise a scientific paper

- Read the abstract of the following open-access paper: Woolf et al. The attitudes, perceptions and experiences of medical school applicants following the closure of schools and cancellation of public examinations in 2020 due to the COVID-19 pandemic: a cross-sectional questionnaire study of UK medical applicants. *BMJ Open.* 2021;11(3):e044753. https://bmjopen.bmj.com/content/11/3/e044753 [56].

- Pick the most appropriate quality or quality reporting tool from those listed in section 5.4 and Box 5.6, and using your selected tool critically appraise this paper.

- How does this paper follow the reporting standards, and how does it not?

- What other scientific indicators of quality are apparent in this paper, and what could be better?

5.5   CHALLENGES AND STRENGTHS OF EMPLOYING SCIENTIFIC APPROACHES IN HPER

It is important to be aware of the challenges associated with scientific approaches, as well as their considerable strengths. Thinking first about the challenges, these can be articulated at the big-picture philosophical level, as well as the more fine-grained methodological/method level. Regarding the philosophical level, there are three key criticisms directed at scientific approaches. Firstly, published studies in HPER employing scientific approaches rarely make explicit their philosophical assumptions [11, 21]. This makes it hard to judge quality indicators like internal coherence; requiring the reader to guess the underlying philosophies. For example, if a study attempts to verify hypotheses, should we assume that it is underpinned by positivism? Or, if it attempts to falsify hypotheses, are we right to assume the study is underpinned by post-positivism? Secondly, the objectivist epistemology underpinning scientific approaches has been hotly contested. Many scholars have critiqued science's requirement for value-free research practices [22, 30], arguing that science serves to uphold only a 'pretence of dispassionate inquiry' [57 p. 254]. Many scholars are especially critical of positivism [2, 25, 30], believing that it is simply impossible for researchers to situate themselves outside of history, culture, and politics, and separate themselves off from their research participants. Such attempts at dualism have been criticised for dehumanising the research process, as well as research participants, and their subjectivities [22]. Finally, at this philosophical level, many regard education as a complex system, and consequently criticise its quasi-causal treatment for being unable to fully comprehend the multiple factors influencing education [1, 11, 38, 58–61].

At the methodological and method level, a key limitation of scientific approaches in HPER relates to small-scale explanatory experiments conducted in optimal conditions. While small RCTs examining the efficacy of interventions have been applauded for their internal validity [58, 62], their external validity have been criticised because of the nuanced conditions in which they take place, meaning that they can hold little practical consequence and value for educational decision-makers as the findings are context-dependent [2, 58, 62]. Context really does matter in education, and given its inherent complexities and uncertainties, scholars appreciate that interventions will produce different effects in different contexts (with different people and different circumstances) [24, 37]. These scholars suggest that experiments of social interventions could be better served by realist approaches underpinned by critical realism (rather than positivism) in order to unpack why interventions work or fail to work (mechanisms), and for whom and under what circumstances (contexts: see Chapter 6). Instead, what may be a more fruitful approach in HPER is employing scientific approaches in service of theory, that is, clarifying why an intervention works. Rather than comparing interventions and evaluating whether they worked or not, we should conduct studies that clarify the underlying principles, constructs, and mechanisms through which they operate. This distinction between studying interventions versus their underlying principles demonstrates that although on the surface two interventions in two different educational contexts may not necessarily look the same, they may nonetheless be implementing similar interventions at a conceptual level by stimulating the same underlying mechanisms [63]. Replication within educational studies, therefore, is not replication of an intervention at the level of its superficial packaging, but rather replication of its principles and philosophies [63–65]. See Box 5.8 for a summary of the case studies' strengths and challenges.

Box 5.8   Case studies: A summary of their strengths and challenges

Systematic Review [3]: Taking a scientific approach facilitated a defensible summary of the breadth of dietetics simulation employed before students' workplace learning. However, the scientific approach was limited to only measurable outcomes of preparedness for practice, thereby preventing more fulsome understandings of important narrative elements of dietetics practice (e.g., counselling patients). We struggled to define our scope, that is, just focusing on simulated activities involving simulated patients. We also debated including quality assessment of the individual studies, but instead chose a reporting standard related to simulation [40], which could better enable us to provide guidance to the profession on the need to enhance the educational design and quality of simulation-based learning using simulated patients.

Randomised Controlled Trial [4]: Our small, highly controlled experiment explicated mechanisms for how the intervention was thought to work building on previous clinical reasoning research [7, 8], thereby contributing generalisable knowledge. However, in balancing experimental control and external validity, developing knowledge and transfer test scenarios were challenging. Furthermore, we struggled to articulate the theoretical value of our findings to clinical educators, who were typically more interested in what worked rather than why. We addressed this by explaining that LP training was merely a specific instance of a general phenomenon (cognitive integration) that we sought to clarify to build understanding of instructional principles supporting psychomotor skills learning.

Non-experimental Observation [5]: Taking a scientific approach supported a reproducible calculation of cost of student failure, alongside clear causal pathways for how these costs were generated. However, economic studies such as ours are typically based on assumptions, and others may disagree with our assumptions (e.g., how to value student time). Furthermore, economic studies are context-dependent. Therefore, we strived to provide readers with sufficient information to understand what we did, why we did it, and create the opportunity to replicate our study using inputs from their own setting, thereby potentially reproducing our findings and enhancing our study's external validity.

Psychometrics [6]: Through our rigorous collection of multiple sources of quantitative data, plus our triangulation of those data (i.e., reliability and cost), we were able to identify the optimal number of OSCE stations to cover the assessment blueprint, enabling policymakers to make key decisions about the implementation of the OSCE going forward. Our biggest struggle related to the voluntary nature of participants' involvement in the OSCE, meaning that suboptimal numbers volunteered for the exam, plus several respondents simply failed to show on the day. However, we were able to run a second OSCE at a later stage, with different levels of learners, helping us to replicate our initial study findings.

There is no denying the considerable power of scientific approaches in HPER. Perhaps the most exciting strength associated with scientific approaches is that they offer the opportunity to discover generalisable facts to help us understand how the educational world works. Rigorous scientific studies clarifying how humans learn, as well as the factors supporting or inhibiting learning, hold much potential for educational practice [66, 67]. Randomised trials in HPER have, for example, confirmed the utility of pedagogical approaches [37]. Experimentation has particularly been advocated for comparative effectiveness studies [28, 37, 58], where researchers might compare an innovative educational intervention with a traditional one. The internal validity of small, well-controlled RCTs can be high [58],and through repeated well-controlled experiments in different settings and with diverse populations, external validity can be improved [28]. Larger pragmatic trials in real-world diverse settings evaluating the effectiveness of interventions have been applauded for enhancing generalisability, in addition to helping educators and policymakers make evidence-based decisions [26, 58]. Before moving on to the final section, stop and evaluate the strengths and challenges of an example scientific paper (see Box 5.9).

Box 5.9   Stop and do: Evaluating the strengths/challenges of an example scientific paper

- Read the following open-access paper: Monrouxe et al. Professional dilemmas, moral distress and the healthcare student: insights from two online UK-wide questionnaire studies. *BMJ Open*. 2015; 5(5):e007518. https://bmjopen.bmj.com/content/5/5/e007518 [68].

- Write down the strengths of the scientific approach employed in this study in terms of addressing its research questions.

- Note the challenges of the scientific approach for answering the study research questions.

- What alternative approaches may have addressed these research questions? You may need to revisit this query after reading other chapters in Part II.

- View the peer-review reports for this *BMJ Open* paper online to see peer-reviewer comments, and the author comments. How do these compare with your notes?

5.6   CHAPTER SUMMARY

In this chapter, we have discussed the philosophical underpinnings of scientific approaches to HPER – realist ontology, objectivist epistemology, and the values of empiricism, facts, objectivity, and dualism. We have provided a brief overview of common scientific methodologies used in HPER (i.e., systematic reviews, experimental and non-experimental approaches), and methods (i.e., random sampling, quantitative data collection, as well as statistical analyses). We have outlined key quality indicators (i.e., generalisability, reproducibility, minimisation of bias, validity, reliability, and larger sample sizes), and we have outlined key checklists relevant to HPER to appraise study quality (e.g., MERSQI) or reporting quality (e.g., CONSORT, STROBE, CHEERS, PRISMA). We have outlined numerous strengths of scientific approaches (e.g., creating generalisable facts about the utility of pedagogical approaches), as well as articulating well-worn criticisms of scientific approaches in educational research at both the philosophical level (e.g., treating a complex educational system in quasi-causal ways) and methodological levels (e.g., appreciating that interventions produce different effects in different contexts with different people). However, there is no denying the power of scientific approaches in HPER – perceiving the world as highly systematic and well-organised [18], and harnessing science's credibility, support, influence, and prestige, alongside what works in terms of influencing policy and policymakers [2, 22, 25, 57, 61]. However, like all the approaches outlined in Part II of this book, we urge you to be mindful of the ways in which you adopt scientific approaches – such approaches from basic and clinical sciences are not always transplantable to HPER. As suggested by Regehr: 'education research is not rocket science' [1 p. 38]. Therefore, we hope this chapter has clearly articulated the foundational terrain of HPER employing scientific approaches, to help you reflect critically on the applicability of scientific approaches for your own research. We invite you to continue your learning about scientific approaches through tackling the recommended reading in Box 5.10.

Box 5.10   Recommended reading for scientific approaches in HPER

Biesta GJJ, van Braak M. Beyond the medical model: thinking differently about medical education and medical education research. *Teach Learn Med.* 2020; 32(4):449–456 [60].

Cianciolo AT, Regehr G. Learning theory and educational intervention: producing meaningful evidence of impact through layered analysis. *Acad Med.* 2019; 94(6):789–794 [64].

Park YS, Konge L, Artino AR. The positivism paradigm of research. *Acad Med.* 2020;95(5):690–694 [19].

Regehr G. It's NOT rocket science: rethinking our metaphors for research in health professions education. *Med Educ.* 2010;44(1):31–39 [1].

Ringsted C, Hodges B, Scherpbier A. 'The research compass': an introduction to research in medical education: AMEE Guide no. 56. *Med Teach.* 2011;33 (9):695–709 [39].

Tolsgaard MG, Kulasegaram KM, Ringsted C. Practical trials in medical education: linking theory, practice and decision making. *Med Educ.* 2017;51(1): 22–30 [58].

Young ME, Ryan A. Postpositivism in health professions education scholarship. *Acad Med.* 2020;95(5):695–699 [16].

REFERENCES

1. Regehr G. It's NOT rocket science: rethinking our metaphors for research in health professions education. *Med Educ.* 2010;44(1):31–39.

2. Howe KR. Positivist dogma, rhetoric, and the education science question. *Educ Res.* 2009;38(6):428–440.

3. O'Shea M-C, Palermo C, Rogers GD, et al. Simulation-based learning experiences in dietetics programs: a systematic review. *J Nutr Educ Behav.* 2020;52(4):429–438.

4. Cheung JJH, Kulasegaram KM., Woods NN, et al. Knowing how and knowing why: testing the effect of instruction designed for cognitive integration on procedural skills transfer. *Adv Health Sci Educ.* 2018;23(1):61–74.

5. Foo J, Rivers G, Ilic D, et al. The economic cost of failure in clinical education: a multi-perspective analysis. *Med Educ.* 2017;51(7):740–754.

6. Brooks I, Dix S, Rees CE, et al. RN OSCE pilot and evaluation. Final confidential report to the funder; October 2019. Unpublished report.

7. Kulasegaram KM., Martimianakis MA, Mylopoulos M, et al. Cognition before curriculum: rethinking the integration of basic science and clinical learning. *Acad Med.* 2013;88(10):1578–1585.

8. Woods NN. Science is fundamental: the role of biomedical knowledge in clinical reasoning: clinical expertise. *Med Educ.* 2007;41(12):1173–1177.

9. Varpio L, MacLeod A. Philosophy of Science Series: harnessing the multidisciplinary edge effect by exploring paradigms, ontologies, epistemologies, axiologies, and methodologies. *Acad Med.* 2020;95(5):686–689.

10. Park YS, Zaidi Z, O'Brien BC. RIME foreword: what constitutes science in educational research? Applying rigor in our research approaches. *Acad Med.* 2020;95(11S):si–sv.

11. Bunniss S, Kelly DR. Research paradigms in medical education research. *Med Educ.* 2010;44(4):358–366.

12. Rees CE, Monrouxe LV. Theory in medical education research: how do we get there? *Med Educ.* 2010;44(4):334–339.

13. Carter SM, Little M. Justifying knowledge, justifying method, taking action: epistemologies, methodologies, and methods in qualitative research. *Qual Health Res.* 2007;17(10):1316–1328.

14. Veen M, Cianciolo AT. Problems no one looked for: philosophical expeditions into medical education. *Teach Learn Med.* 2020;32(3):337–344.

15. Gordon M. Are we talking the same paradigm? Considering methodological choices in health education systematic review. *Med Teach.* 2016;38(7):746–750.

16. Young ME, Ryan A. Postpositivism in health professions education scholarship. *Acad Med.* 2020;95(5):695–699.

17. O'Leary Z. Post-positivism. In *The Social Science Jargon Buster: The Key Terms You Need to Know.* London: SAGE; 2007:202–203.

18. Crotty M. *The Foundations of Social Research. Meaning and Perspective in the Research Process.* London: SAGE; 2003.

19. Park YS, Konge L, Artino AR. The positivism paradigm of research. *Acad Med.* 2020;95(5):690–694.

20. Varpio L, O'Brien B, Rees CE, et al. The applicability of generalisability and bias to health professions education's research. *Med Educ.* 2020;55(2):167–173.

21. Palermo C, Reidlinger DP, Rees CE. Internal coherence matters: lessons for nutrition and dietetics research. *Nutr Diet.* 2021;78(3):252–267.

22. Playle JF. Humanism and positivism in nursing: contradictions and conflicts. *J Adv Nurs.* 1995;22(5):979–984.

23. American Association for Anatomy. Anatomical Sciences Education author guidelines. 2021. https://ANATOMYPUBS.onlinelibrary.wiley.com/hub/journal/19359780/home page/forauthors.html(accessed 28 August 2021).

24. Bonell C, Moore G, Warren E, et al. Are randomised controlled trials positivist? Reviewing the social science and philosophy literature to assess positivist tendencies of trials of social interventions in public health and health services. *Trials.* 2018;19(1):238.

25. Saari A. Knowledge without contexts? A Foucauldian analysis of EL Thorndike's positivist educational research. *Stud Philos Educ.* 2016;35(6):589–603.

26. Patsopoulos NA. A pragmatic view on pragmatic trials. *Dialogues Clin Neurosci.* 2011;13(2):217–224.

27. Tonelli MR, Bluhm R. Teaching medical epistemology within an evidence-based medicine curriculum. *Teach Learn Med.* 2021;33(1):98–105.

28. Van Loon MH, Kok EM, Kamp RJA, et al. AM last page: avoiding five common pitfalls of experimental research in medical education. *Acad Med.* 2013;88(10):1588.

29. Loving CC. From the summit of truth to its slippery slopes: science education's journey through positivist-postmodern territory. *Am Educ Res J.* 1997;34(3):421–452.

30. Zyphur MJ, Pierides DC. Making quantitative research work: from positivist dogma to actual social scientific inquiry. *J Bus Ethics.* 2020;167(1):49–62.

31. Campbell DT, Stanley JC. *Experimental and Quasi-Experimental Designs for Research.* Chicago: Rand McNally; 1963.

32. Cook DA, Beckman TJ. Reflections on experimental research in medical education. *Adv Health Sci Educ.* 2010;15(3):455–464.

33. Higgins JPT, Thomas J, Chandler J, et al. Cochrane Handbook for Systematic Reviews of Interventions version 6.3 (updated February 2022). Cochrane; 2022. Available from https://www.training.cochrane.org/handbook (accessed 28 August 2021).

34. Gordon M, Daniel M, Patricio M. What do we mean by 'systematic' in health education systematic reviews and why it matters! *Med Teach.* 2019;41(8):956–957.

35. Cleland J, Durning SJ. *Researching Medical Education.* Chichester: Wiley Blackwell; 2015.

36. Greenhalgh T, Thorne S, Malterud K. Time to challenge the spurious hierarchy of systematic over narrative reviews? *Eur J Clin Invest.* 2018;48(6):e12931.

37. Cook DA. Randomized controlled trials and meta-analysis in medical education: what role do they play? *Med Teach.* 2012;34(6):468–473.

38. Horsley T, Galipeau J, Petkovic J, et al. Reporting quality and risk of bias in randomised trials in health professions education. *Med Educ.* 2017;51(1):61–71.

39. Ringsted C, Hodges B, Scherpbier A. 'The research compass': an introduction to research in medical education: AMEE Guide no. 56. *Med Teach.* 2011;33(9):695–709.

40. Cheng A, Kessler D, Mackinnon R, et al. Reporting guidelines for health care simulation research: extensions to CONSORT and STROBE statements. *Adv Simul.* 2016;1:25.

41. Bland M. *An Introduction to Medical Statistics,* 2nd ed. Oxford: Oxford Medical Publications; 1995.

42. Mukherjee SP. *A Guide to Research Methodology: An Overview of Research Problems, Tasks and Methods.* New York: Taylor and Francis; 2020.

43. Portney LG. *Foundations of Clinical Research: Applications to Evidence-based Practice.* 4th ed. Philadelphia, Pa.: FA Davis; 2020.

44. Cook DA, Hatala R. Validation of educational assessments: a primer for simulation and beyond. *Adv Simul.* 2016;1:31.

45. Messick S. Validity. In Linn L, ed. *Educational Measurement.* 3rd ed. New York: American Council on Education and Macmillan; 1989: 13–103.

46. Kane MT. Validation. In Brennan RL, ed. *Educational Measurement.* 4th ed. Westport: Praeger; 2006: 17–64.

47. Page MJ, McKenzie JE, Bossuyt PM, et al. The PRISMA 2020 statement: an updated guideline for reporting systematic reviews. *BMJ.* 2021;372:n71.

48. Gordon M, Gibbs T. STORIES statement: publication standards for healthcare education evidence synthesis. *BMC Med.* 2014;12:143.

49. Schulz KF, Altman DG, Moher D, for the CONSORT Group. CONSORT 2010 Statement: updated guidelines for reporting parallel group randomised trials. *BMJ.* 2010;340:698–702.

50. Husereau D, Drummond M, Petrou S, et al. CHEERS good reporting practices task force. consolidated health economic evaluation reporting standards (CHEERS)—explanation and elaboration: a report of the ISPOR health economic evaluation publication guidelines good reporting practices task force. *Value Health*. 2013;16(2):231–250.

51. Eysenbach G. Improving the quality of web surveys: the checklist for reporting results of internet e-surveys (CHERRIES). *J Med Internet Res*. 2004;6(3):e34.

52. Kottner J, Audige L, Brorson S, et al. Guidelines for Reporting Reliability and Agreement Studies (GRRAS) were proposed. *Int J Nurs Stud*. 2011;48(6):661–671.

53. Cook DA, Reed DA. Appraising the quality of medical education research methods: the Medical Education Research Study Quality Instrument and the Newcastle–Ottawa Scale-Education. *Acad Med*. 2015;90(8):1067–1076.

54. von Elm E, Altman DG, Egger M, et al. Strengthening the reporting of observational studies in epidemiology (STROBE) statement: guidelines for reporting observational studies. *BMJ*. 2007;335:806–808.

55. Young J, Solomon M. How to critically appraise an article. *Nat Clin Pract Gastroenterol Hepatol*. 2009;6(2):82–91.

56. Woolf K, Harrison D, McManus C. The attitudes, perceptions and experiences of medical school applicants following the closure of schools and cancellation of public examinations in 2020 due to the COVID-19 pandemic: a cross-sectional questionnaire study of UK medical applicants. *BMJ Open*. 2021;11(3):e044753.

57. Thomas G. Educational Research: an Unorthodox Introduction. *Educ Rev*. 2021;73(2):252–256.

58. Tolsgaard MG, Kulasegaram KM., Ringsted C. Practical trials in medical education: linking theory, practice and decision making. *Med Educ*. 2017;51(1):22–30.

59. Biesta G. Improving education through research? From effectiveness, causality and technology to purpose, complexity and culture. *Policy Futures Educ*. 2016;14(2):194–210.

60. Biesta GJJ, van Braak M. Beyond the medical model: thinking differently about medical education and medical education research. *Teach Learn Med*. 2020;32(4):449–456.

61. Biesta G, Filippakou O, Wainwright E, et al. Why educational research should not just solve problems, but should cause them as well. *Brit Educ Res J*. 2019;45(1):1–4.

62. Norman G. RCT = results confounded and trivial: the perils of grand educational experiments. *Med Educ*. 2003;37(7):582–584.

63. Leppink J, Pérez-Fuster P. What is science without replication? *Perspect Med Educ*. 2016;5(6):320–322.

64. Cianciolo AT, Regehr G. Learning theory and educational intervention: producing meaningful evidence of impact through layered analysis. *Acad Med*. 2019;94(6):789–794.

65. Horsley T, Regehr G. When are two interventions the same? Implications for reporting guidelines in education. *Med Educ*. 2018;52(2):141–143.

66. National Research Council. *Brain, Mind, Experience, and School*. Expanded ed. Washington DC: National Academies Press; 2000.

67. Hattie J, Yates G. *Visible Learning and the Science of How We Learn*. Thousand Oaks, Calif.: Routledge; 2014.

68. Monrouxe LV, Rees CE, Dennis I, et al. Professionalism dilemmas, moral distress and the healthcare student: insights from two online UK-wide questionnaire studies. *BMJ Open*. 2015;5(5):e007518.

Introducing Realist Approaches in Health Professions Education Research

Charlotte E. Rees[1,2], Paul E.S. Crampton[3], Van N.B. Nguyen[2], and Lynn V. Monrouxe[4]

[1] The University of Newcastle, Callaghan, New South Wales, Australia
[2] Monash University, Clayton, Victoria, Australia
[3] University of York, York, UK
[4] The University of Sydney, Camperdown, New South Wales, Australia

> **Box 6.1   Chapter 6 learning objectives: After reading this chapter you should be able to ...**
>
> - Describe the philosophical underpinnings (ontology, epistemology, and axiology) of realist approaches
> - Summarise common realist methodologies and methods in health professions education research (HPER), including key principles of sampling, data collection, and data analysis
> - Explain the main indicators of quality employed in realist approaches
> - Evaluate the strengths and challenges of realist approaches for HPER
> - Reflect critically on the applicability of realist approaches to your own HPER

6.1   INTRODUCING CHAPTER 6

... adoption of a realist ontology and ... the generative concept of causality, means that realist evaluation is able to provide, as it claims, a more realistic conception of the factors involved in the introduction and maintenance of complex ... interventions than experimental methods that confine themselves to artificial notions of unilinear causality. [1 p. 26]

Foundations of Health Professions Education Research: Principles, Perspectives and Practices,
First Edition. Edited by Charlotte E. Rees, Lynn V. Monrouxe, Bridget C. O'Brien, Lisi J. Gordon, and Claire Palermo.
© 2023 John Wiley & Sons Ltd. Published 2023 by John Wiley & Sons Ltd.

Increasingly popular in health professions education research (HPER) over recent years, realist approaches serve to unpack how programmes (interventions) work (or fail to work), for whom and under what circumstances, and why. For many educational researchers, realist approaches offer an alternative to the experimental methods discussed in Chapter 5, and the quote above illustrates why. Indeed, realist approaches recognise that educational interventions are complex and social, and therefore work differently for different people, in different settings, at different times, and so on. So, realist approaches privilege complexity, context, and a conception of causality foregrounding generative mechanisms (i.e., entities explaining why things occur). Realist approaches also privilege the building, testing, and refining of theory (see Chapter 2). This sixth chapter aims to provide you with a better understanding of realist approaches and consider their applicability to HPER questions that you are interested in (see Box 6.1). What we present in this chapter reflects the meeting point of our experiences – reading about, conducting, and reviewing realist approaches in HPER. Despite our diverse experiences to date, and disciplinary backgrounds, each of us lean towards critical realism, subjectivist, and qualitative accounts of realist approaches. In section 6.2, we outline the philosophical foundations (ontology, epistemology, and axiology) of realist approaches, and in section 6.3 we summarise common and emerging realist methodologies and methods in HPER. We discuss the key features of quality in realist approaches in section 6.4, and in section 6.5 we evaluate the strengths and challenges of realist approaches in HPER. Interwoven into each section are four recent and diverse cases employing different methodologies to bring realist approaches to life. These include realist reviews [2, 3], realist evaluations [3, 4], and a realist economic evaluation [5]. See Box 6.2. for a brief overview of these cases. Realist research is not for the faint-hearted, but for many of us who appreciate diverse research approaches addressing the real-world complexities of education, it really does feel like a practical way forward. While this chapter might take you longer to work through if you are new to realist approaches, we encourage you to persevere, especially with the realist terms employed; all of which are defined in our book glossary. We hope this chapter helps you to better understand the realist HPER work you will inevitably read throughout your HPER journey, as well as provides you with the basics to get started if you decide that realist approaches are for you.

Box 6.2   Case studies: An overview

Realist Synthesis [2]: We conducted a realist synthesis of selected papers focusing on research environments to understand their key features of success, for whom, how and in what circumstances. Although several reviews and commentaries had indicated the characteristics of successful research environments, our realist synthesis explored the contextual complexities, as well as the multiplicity of mechanisms involved to identify what really matters for successful medical education research environments and unpack successful research cultures.

Realist Evaluation I [3]: We embarked on a programme of realist studies primarily focusing on an intervention in New South Wales, Australia, whereby final-year medical students became assistants in medicine to support the COVID-19 pandemic hospital relief work. We began by undertaking a realist synthesis of the literature on similar types of interventions in hospitals (e.g., UK medical student Assistantships), as well as realist evaluation including interviewing programme designers to build programme theory, and then interviewing assistants in medicine and their supervisors to test and refine theory.

(continued)

(continued)

<u>Realist Evaluation II</u> [4]: We conducted a realist evaluation of a 12-week supervision training programme for nurses and allied health professionals involving one or two 3.5-hour face-to-face workshops followed by weekly reflexive longitudinal audio-diaries. Building on our previous realist synthesis [6], we aimed to test and refine programme theory to answer the question: to what extent does an extended-duration supervision training programme work, for whom, under what circumstances, and why?

<u>Realist Economic Evaluation</u> [5]: We conducted a preliminary realist economic evaluation of 3.5-hour online supervision training workshops for health and human services supervisors to evaluate how synchronous online training workshops and their cost-effectiveness works, and in what contexts. This realist economic analysis enabled us to develop a cost-optimised model based on identified costs and cost-sensitive mechanisms and contexts.

6.2   PHILOSOPHICAL UNDERPINNINGS OF REALIST APPROACHES

As previously discussed in Chapter 2, it is essential to understand the philosophical underpinnings of your research approach to enhance rigour through internal coherence – that is, the alignment in thinking and doing of ontology (nature of reality), epistemology (nature of knowing), methodology (how we come to know), and axiology (what we value) within a particular project as well as personal philosophies [7, 8]. In this section, we walk you through some fairly contested philosophical ground about realist approaches. We do this as simply as possible for an introductory text. However, we caution you that realist scholars are not unified in their thinking about realist philosophical foundations.

6.2.1   Realist Ontology: Scientific or Critical Realism?

> *Realism asserts that both the material and the social worlds are 'real', at least in the sense that anything that can have real effects is itself real* [9 p. 4]

Realist approaches have been described as underpinned by scientific [10], or critical realism [1, 11]. As suggested in Chapter 5, scientific realism sees the world and its structures and mechanisms as existing independent of our consciousness [12, 13]. Critical realism also imagines this objective, mind-independent reality but foregrounds the social, historical, and political features of scientific knowledge [12], so aligns with critical theory [1]. Critical realism suggests that objects are both products of scientific activity (so-called transitive) and objective laws independent of scientific activity (known as intransitive) [14]. This is stratified across three levels of reality: (1) the real (things existing independent of observation such as physical, social and psychological structures, powers, and mechanisms); (2) the actual (events occurring in space and time based on these real structures, powers, and mechanisms); and (3) the empirical (observable things) [12, 15–19]. Critical realists seek to understand mechanisms at the level of the real by examining the actual and empirical [15]. In science, scholars attempt to understand real and actual things through the empirical [12, 15–19]. Central to realism is the concept of emergence: new qualities emerging from interactions between entities at different stratified levels in open systems (e.g., individual, group, society) having causal impacts downward (e.g., groups impacting individuals), and/or upwards (e.g., individuals impacting groups) [9, 12, 16, 20, 21].

Some researchers consider scientific and critical realism to be closely related positions [13, 18, 19, 22, 23]. Whereas others suggest that they differ, primarily in their views about whether social science can appropriately create closed system investigations such as experiments [21]. Thus, scientific realism tends to argue pragmatically that closed systems are not a necessary precondition for investigation. Alternatively, critical realism tends to argue that closed systems are unachievable in social research and therefore substitutes, like moral or emancipatory lenses, should be employed instead (see Chapter 8). Furthermore, scientific and critical realism are thought to differ in terms of where the locus of change is situated. Within scientific realism, causal mechanisms are thought to sit primarily at the level of the individual (e.g., reasoning), whereas within critical realism, they are thought situated largely at the structural level (e.g., power and resources) [21].

6.2.2 Realist Epistemology: Objectivist or Subjectivist?

> Realism acknowledges that all enquiry and observation are shaped and filtered through the human brain and that there is, therefore, no such thing as 'final' truth or knowledge. [9 p. 4]

Scientific realism suggests that real entities can be articulated in theory, with mature, well-confirmed theories being approximately true [12]. Such truth-approximating theories can be true or false based on scientific methods, and if true, the entities proposed are deemed to exist, even if not observable [12]. Indeed, 'the [scientific realism] position is that our best science will be able to arrive at correct knowledge about the existence, structure, and functions of the self' [12 p. 25]. In this sense, scientific realism can be seen as underpinned by objectivist epistemology (as described earlier in Chapter 5). Critical realism, on the other hand, is seen as combining a realist ontology with a relativist/constructivist epistemology [16, 19, 20]. Such epistemological relativism means that theories are inherently subjective, as the above quotation implies, and thus only approximate reality [16, 19]. As with post-positivists, critical realists understand the fallibility of scientific observation, adopting a critical stance towards truth, while believing that reality exists outside of consciousness [19, 20]. While some argue that critical realism is compatible with post-positivism and constructivism [22], others suggest it was developed as a different scientific approach to positivism or constructivism [15]. Indeed, realism is often considered as an epistemological middle ground to the extremes of radical positivism and radical constructivism [24, 25].

6.2.3 Realist Methodology

> ... nothing works everywhere or for everyone, and that context really does make a difference to programme outcomes. [9 p. 4]

Realist methodologies seek to understand how things work in complex systems (that are open and social), offering a conceptualisation of causation different to the causality-as-constant-conjunction (i.e., A causes B) understanding inherent in scientific experimentation. Indeed, central to realist approaches are generative mechanisms. Furthermore, realist methodologies privilege context, unlike scientific experimentation that controls for, and thus neutralises, context. So, realist methodologies appreciate that causal mechanisms can be triggered by some contexts (e.g., medicine) but not others (e.g., nursing), as the quotation above implies [9]. Furthermore, at the heart of realist methodologies is the building, testing, and refining of programme theory (i.e., theories about how specific programmes work) and/or middle-range theory (i.e., theory that is testable yet sufficiently abstract to enable transferability beyond specific programmes). The realist methodologies most employed in HPER include realist review/synthesis [26–30], and realist evaluation [3, 4, 31–33]. However, more novel methodologies are emerging including realist economic evaluation [5, 34].

Many realist scholars employ, to some degree, mixed or multiple methods. However, scientific realism tends to advocate quantification and statistical modelling, whereas critical realism tends to reject such approaches [17]. Indeed, critical realists argue that, due to the importance of contextual conditions in the mediation of outcomes, qualitative approaches are optimal [20]. As such, scientific realist approaches have been criticised for replicating evidence-based practices inherent in randomised controlled trials, thereby promoting: 'technocratic interpretations of human problems' [1 p. 18], and abandoning emancipatory concerns often associated with critical enquiry. Further, statistical positivism within realist methodologies has been criticised for generating minimal new knowledge about programme outcomes. For example, critical realist research examining academic motivation identified a multiplicity of causal relationships among constructs employing qualitative case-based methodologies that were otherwise unattainable when employing statistical models [18, 23]. Thus, realist approaches are not bound by one particular methodology (despite many advocating mixed methods); but instead employ methodologies best aligned with chosen ontological and epistemological underpinnings.

6.2.4   Realist Axiology

Given that realist approaches seek to unpack the black box of how programmes work, for whom and under what circumstances, and why [35], it comes as no surprise that they value complexity, generative mechanisms, and contexts, alongside the building, testing, and refining of theory [9, 19]. Interestingly, while scientific and critical realism share some ontological understandings, there are differences in terms of their values. Differences include their approaches to individual agency versus social structures, and values versus facts [11, 17, 21]. For example, scientific realism regards social mechanisms as a conflation of agency (i.e., the capacity to act with free will) and structure (i.e., the role of social structures in constraining free will). Alternatively, critical realism privileges the (sometimes hidden) role of social structural influences in our world, pointing to the interplay between structure and agency (e.g., tensions, struggles, negotiations) but seeing structure and agency as distinct from each other [15]. Furthermore, scientific realism privileges the facts–values distinction discussed in Chapter 5, whereby empirical reality (i.e., what is and can be evidenced as objective facts) is seen as separate from value judgements (i.e., what ought to be and is debatable as subjective opinion) [36]. On the other hand, critical realism rejects the separation between facts and values, seeing reality as both objective and subjective. Furthermore, critical realism values emancipatory concerns (i.e., equality, empowerment, challenging the status quo: see Chapter 8) [37]. See Box 6.3 for a summary of the case studies' philosophical underpinnings.

Box 6.3   Case studies: A summary of their philosophical underpinnings

<u>Realist Synthesis</u> [2]: While our paper failed to state our philosophical approach, you could assume we employed a scientific realist ontology on surface reading of our methods. For example, we employed a systematic approach to our review including a PRISMA (Preferred Reporting Items for Systematic reviews and Meta-Analyses) flow chart. However, we explicitly stated that we adopted an 'interpretive approach' to our data synthesis [2 p. 941]. Therefore, our paper could best be described as underpinned by critical realism – combining a realist ontology with constructivist/relativist epistemology [16, 19, 20]. We believed that science is fallible, we rejected the facts–values distinction, and our synthesis foregrounded the structural elements of success factors – the social, environmental, and governance frameworks such as strategy, leadership, protected time, income, infrastructure, and facilities. We valued complexity, generative mechanisms, and the testing/refining of programme theory.

<u>Realist Evaluation I</u> [3]: We published our initial intentions, which heavily cited scientific realist literature: 'realist philosophy of science' [3 p. 3], thereby assuming scientific realist ontology and objectivist epistemology. However, during our data analysis, we acknowledge the existence of multiple truths aligned with interpretivist perspectives. Thus, while being relatively covert about this, we are approaching our analysis from a critical realist ontology and subjective constructivist epistemology. In terms of axiology, we value complexity, generative mechanisms, contexts, and testing/refining programme theory.

<u>Realist Evaluation II</u> [4]: Although we cite Pawson's 'scientific realism' in our paper's background [4 p. 2], our study is better described as underpinned by critical realist ontology with a subjective constructivist epistemology; firstly, because we believed in the fallibility of scientific observation, and secondly, because we privileged participants' diverse identifications of explanatory mechanisms. We rejected the facts–values distinction inherent in scientific realism, and foregrounded structural mechanisms and contexts (and the interplay between structures and agency) such as supervision-enabled or non-enabled workplace cultures. As with other realist approaches, we valued complexity, generative mechanisms, contexts, and testing/refining programme theory.

<u>Realist Economic Evaluation</u> [5]: Our realist economic evaluation is most appropriately described as underpinned by scientific realist ontology, and objectivist epistemology, but is post-positivist in nature, as we recognised the partiality of our findings and the imperfection of our methods. In this paper, we employed mixed methods with our quantitative cost data especially foregrounding facts, empiricism, and objectivity. However, this study was still realist in nature, so it integrated economic analysis within a realist framework, thereby valuing complexity, generative mechanisms, and contexts, as well as testing/refining economic programme theory.

6.3   COMMON AND EMERGING REALIST METHODOLOGIES AND METHODS IN HPER

As explained in section 6.2.1, realist approaches underpinned by scientific or critical realism have commonalities and divergences in how they approach methodologies and methods [1]. However, two common features are that they: (1) take a theory-driven approach based on generative mechanisms; and (2) are not bound by any singular methodological approach. While scholars vary in how they apply methodologies and methods to realist research across disciplines, we seek to illuminate how such approaches can be applied to HPER. We organise them here in the following ways: realist reviews/syntheses [2, 3]; realist evaluations [3, 4]; and realist economic evaluation [5]. Regardless of realist methodology and methods, publishing a peer-reviewed protocol ahead of undertaking work is increasingly common to ensure research accountability [3, 38, 39]. Publishing protocols might not always be practicable because you may have insufficient: (a) funds to publish protocols in fee-paying open-access journals; and/or (b) time to publish protocols ahead of conducting the work. However, it is good practice for a detailed protocol to be developed for internal team-based discussions. We discuss proposals in further detail in Chapter 10. See Box 6.4 for a summary of the case studies' methodologies and methods.

Box 6.4   Case studies: A summary of their methodologies and methods

Realist Synthesis [2]: Consistent with our critical realist ontology and constructivist epistemology, we gathered data (primary research articles) employing different methods (qualitative, quantitative, and mixed methods studies). By clarifying the scope of our review, conducting a systematic literature search, and then assessing study quality, we reviewed a final sample of 42 papers (none of which used realist approaches) to extract relevant data, that is, context–mechanism–outcome configurations (CMOCs) and recurring CMOCs – so called demi-regularities. An example of a CMOC includes: early career researchers (context) need protected time (mechanism) to increase their outputs (outcomes) [2 p. 942]. We then identified patterns as part of this synthesis to develop a modified realist programme theory to explain how research environments work under different circumstances.

Realist Evaluation I [3]: We began building programme theory through realist synthesis, identifying a variety of literature on interventions akin to the Australian assistants in medicine role. We examined their intended outcomes and identified associated contexts and mechanisms. We adopted an iterative approach to our synthesis to refine theory. We also interviewed programme developers through realist interviews. From both datasets, we developed CMOCs for subsequent testing with data from assistants in medicine, their team members, and supervisors (through group interviews and audio-diaries).

Realist Evaluation II [4]: Aligned with our critical realist ontology and constructivist epistemology, we employed qualitative realist evaluation methodology in this paper, with multiple methods commonly associated with interpretivist approaches. For example, employing maximum-variation sampling to amplify diversity, we collected data through semi-structured interviews and weekly longitudinal audio-diaries for three months; drawing on framework analysis as an organising framework for our realist analysis [47]. However, our data collection and analysis methods were realist in nature, with realist interviewing and realist analysis employed throughout to identify CMOCs, as well as test and refine programme theory. An example of a CMOC includes: health supervisors (context) with strong engagement (mechanism) increase supervision knowledge and practice (outcomes) [4 p. 6].

Realist Economic Evaluation [5]: Consistent with our scientific realist ontology and objectivist epistemology, we employed mixed methods realist economic evaluation methodology. We conducted 13 realist interviews with supervisors, employed the ingredients method to measure the costs associated with the online workshops [46], and conducted an analysis relevant to cost-sensitive mechanisms and contexts to propose an optimal cost-effective model for online faculty development workshops. Throughout this paper, we drew on a realist framework to integrate our realist and economic analyses, but we foregrounded costs to test and refine realist economic programme theory to determine how cost-effectiveness for online learning might work, and in what contexts.

6.3.1 Realist Review/Synthesis

Realist synthesis has become an increasingly popular approach to reviewing HPER literature over the last decade. Realist synthesis draws on secondary data sources relevant to building and testing programme theory to answer the question based on that literature: 'what works for whom under what circumstances, how and why?' [25 p. 2]. Realist synthesis can include both non-traditional outputs (e.g., grey materials, policy documents, commentaries), as well as traditional outputs such as peer-reviewed journal articles employing wide-ranging methods [40]. Many realist syntheses in HPER follow Pawson and colleagues' five stages [41]: (1) clarifying the scope of the review; (2) determining the search strategy; (3) study selection; (4) extracting data; and (5) synthesising the evidence and drawing conclusions [39]. Different from the scientific systematic reviews discussed in Chapter 5, realist syntheses focus on programme theory rather than interventions per se; meaning that they often include wide-ranging studies involving diverse programmes [40]. Furthermore, they employ an iterative approach to data inclusion, being less rigid than traditional systematic reviews. For example, Bansal et al. [27] used a realist review to unpack strategies to develop medical learners' person-centredness. They began by developing an initial programme theory to guide data collection by discussing the team's own perspectives, theories from grey literature, and drawing on learning theories more generally. Additional searches were then undertaken as their theory progressed with no restrictions on the type of study included, so long as studies contributed to theory building. They undertook multiple iterative cycles, moving between data and theory, developing realist causal explanations for the programme outcomes.

6.3.2 Realist Evaluation

Realist evaluation is a type of theory-based evaluation of programmes, interventions, initiatives, or policies that begins by elucidating programme theory explaining how mechanisms can generate outcomes and the contexts in which those mechanisms might be triggered [9, 42, 43]. Sometimes this programme theory is initially developed through a realist synthesis. Realist evaluation employs primary data sources (e.g., interviews, questionnaires), which can also be used to build programme theory (sometimes the first stage involving interviews with programme developers). Primary data sources are also used to test and refine programme theory [42]. Realist evaluation has become increasingly popular in HPER over the last five years given the complex and social nature of educational programmes. For example, Kerr et al. [32] examined how and why simulated patient role-play works for communication skills training for pharmacy students. They collected both quantitative (video recordings of interactions scored using a teaching/assessment scale for explanation/planning skills) and qualitative (focus groups) to test part of their programme theory (relating to videoed simulated patient role-play) previously developed through a realist synthesis [28]. They report mean score statistics for the communication skills assessment tool, plus qualitative data for the contexts, mechanisms, and outcomes from their realist analysis, along with students' perceptions of barriers to their learning.

6.3.3   Realist Economic Evaluation

While realist syntheses and realist evaluations are becoming increasingly popular in HPER, realist economic evaluations are only just beginning to emerge [5, 34]. Realist economic evaluations essentially integrate economic analyses and realist evaluations within a realist framework [38]. They are especially important in helping to inform programme design and implementation in resource-constrained environments, providing valuable insights for decision-makers [34]. They are theory-driven approaches to understanding causation explaining programme cost-effectiveness by focusing on cost-sensitive contexts, mechanisms, and/or outcomes [34]. Consequently, realist economic evaluation serves to unpack how programmes can optimise their cost-effectiveness for some people, in certain circumstances, and through what mechanisms [44, 45]. Therefore, realist economic evaluation builds and tests economic programme theory with theory explaining how programme costs and outcomes are produced in specific contexts and are causally linked [34]. A recent example of this includes our comparison of short versus extended-duration supervision training by developing and testing economic programme theory [34]. Starting with an initial economic programme theory based on our previous realist synthesis [6], we employed realist interviews with cost measurement (using the ingredients method) [46] to identify cost-sensitive mechanisms and contexts. From these cost-sensitive contexts and mechanisms, we developed cost-optimised models to maximise cost-effectiveness for short and extended-duration supervision training, as well as refining our economic programme theory.

6.3.4   Realist Sampling, Data Collection, and Analysis Methods

Realist approaches privilege context in terms of understanding how mechanisms are triggered (or not), leading to outcomes [35]. The application of realist research methods (sampling, data collection, and data analysis) may take flexible approaches; as long as they centre on eliciting data that informs programme theory building, testing, and refining. Indeed, programme theory and/or middle-range theory lies at the heart of realist approaches; and its testability is linked to research methods [48–50]. It is outside the scope of this foundations book to cover the practicalities of how to undertake realist approaches in depth, but we highlight key considerations below, and refer you to other sources for detailed guidance [25, 43, 51, 52].

In terms of sampling, realist approaches typically draw on purposive rather than random sampling because intra-programme, and intergroup comparisons are prioritised. This differs from comparisons between participants completing the intervention or not, as in experimental designs employing random sampling [9, 51]. So, purposive sampling can serve to maximise the diversity of your realist sample relevant to the building/testing of programme theory, especially the testing of contexts, such as questions about who the intervention is for and which subgroups the intervention works for (or not) [9, 51].

Regarding data collection, HPER realist approaches typically involve qualitative methods such as individual and/or group interviews, observations, or case studies, and to lesser extents quantitative approaches such as performance data, questionnaires, or validated scales [25, 43, 51, 53]. Like pragmatism, mixed methods within realist approaches are seen as complementing each other to answer research questions. However, different from pragmatism, mixed methods in realist approaches serve to answer realist research questions, as well as build/test/refine programme theory. Interestingly, while quantitative approaches may yield valuable insights into contextual and outcomes data, qualitative methods can illuminate more detailed understandings of mechanisms, plus the nuances of how programme theories may operate in practice. Importantly, realist data collection methods (e.g., realist interviews) differ from their non-realist counterparts because they focus on building, testing, and refining programme theory rather than simply eliciting exploratory subjective accounts of participants' lived experiences [51, 54]. Therefore, the realist researcher asks questions specifically about outcomes (e.g., what positive outcomes resulted from the intervention?), mechanisms (e.g., what generated those positive outcomes?), and contexts (in what circumstances were those mechanisms triggered?), and developing causal configurations [51, 55].

In terms of realist data analysis, this also contrasts with other non-realist approaches such as qualitative interviews identifying themes, or quantitative questionnaires providing descriptive and inferential data to test hypotheses [35]. Realist analysis focuses on the identification of contexts, mechanisms, outcomes, and CMOCs to build, test, and refine programme theory and middle-range theory across cases [52]. Before moving on to the next section, pause and reflect on how you might apply realist approaches to your own HPER (see Box 6.5).

Box 6.5 Pause and reflect: Applying realist methodologies/methods to your research

- Think about an HPER topic that you are interested in researching, either relating to a gap in existing literature and/or relating to a problem you are experiencing with an educational programme.

- What research questions could you develop relating to this topic that would optimally be answered through realist approaches and why? What methodologies/methods would be appropriate for this question and why?

- Think of a research question relating to your topic of interest, and think of research questions that would not lend themselves to a realist approach and why? What other chapters should you read next?

- Revisit this pause and reflect box once you have read other Part II chapters, and further developed your research ideas.

6.4   KEY QUALITY INDICATORS IN REALIST APPROACHES

While quality indicators for critical realism and scientific realism may differ slightly due to different philosophical underpinnings, some quality indicators apply to both approaches. These indicators include but are not limited to: (1) centrality of theory; (2) trustworthiness; (3) coherence; (4) respect for configurational analysis; and (5) adherence to RAMESES (Realist And Meta-narrative Evidence Syntheses: Evolving Standards) reporting standards [25, 43].

First, while theory is at the centre of all realist approaches [48–50], a common question asked by novice realist researchers is: how do I find initial programme theories for my realist study? Marchal et al. [49] suggested three possible options: (a) exploring the assumptions of those who designed, developed, and/or implemented the intervention; (b) conducting exploratory research; and (c) conducting realist synthesis. In thinking about what theories to select, scholars suggest that your chosen theory should [56]: (a) be at the appropriate level of abstraction (not too specific, not too general); (b) best fit with your topic; (c) be relatively simple, and with the potential to inspire theory development in a straightforward manner; and (d) be compatible with realist approaches.

Second, placing theories at the centre of realist research means that they will dictate the methods used to collect relevant data to achieve realist rigour – trustworthiness [57]. For example, according to Manzano [51], interviewing is mostly used to collect qualitative data in realist evaluations, despite this constructivism-informed method not being traditionally developed for theory-testing purposes. It is therefore important to highlight the integral features of realist interviewing, which make it methodologically different from qualitative interviewing. Realist interviewing includes using the interviewer–interviewee cycle with suitable/knowledgeable interviewees, with its three phases to glean, refine, and consolidate theories, while still maintaining conversational flow [51, 54, 58]. To enhance trustworthiness, realist researchers are recommended to: (a) use credible realist data collection methods; (b) collect realist data from multiple sources; (c) collect as much realist data as possible; and (d) treat realist data with scepticism, especially where data sources are unknown, as in realist syntheses [57].

Third, this data trustworthiness is crucial in allowing the conceptualisation of contexts, mechanisms, and outcomes, which subsequently informs the development of coherent arguments to support theory building, testing, and refining [57]. Coherence is helped enormously if a realist approach is adopted from start to finish, rather than adopted part-way through a study such as applying realist analysis to data collected through non-realist means and/or without a programme theory in mind [59]. According to Wong [57], such coherence can be judged by the explanatory breadth of theory to cover most data, and its simplicity. As such, the most coherent theory is the: 'inference to the best explanation' [57 p. 10].

Fourth, configurational analysis is a key quality marker for realist approaches. These privilege CMOCs to explain realist causality (based on generative mechanisms) rather than reporting contexts, mechanisms, and outcomes separately [60]. Such configurational analysis is an iterative case-by-case process, whereby researchers are required to articulate, test, and refine conjectured CMOCs to arrive at explanatory accounts of what outcomes are generated, through which mechanisms, and triggered in what contexts [49]. Here, applying retroductive thinking (i.e., shuttling back and forth between theory and data) can help researchers, especially those using scientific realism, to connect the dots by identifying outcomes and examining the necessary conditions required to achieve them [61].

Finally, high-quality realist research is that which follows latest reporting standards [25, 43]. Two reporting standards currently exist to guide realist research reporting: (a) realist syntheses [25] and (b) realist evaluations [43], although the authors concede that standards will continue to evolve over time. It is noted that reporting standards do not yet exist for realist economic evaluations [5, 34]. Using these standards will not only assist reviewers, editors, and publishers in the peer-review process, but should also assist researchers in designing their realist research, as well as providing sufficient information to make their realist findings more accessible and digestible to a broader range of end-users such as educators and policymakers [25, 43]. See Box 6.6 for a summary of the case studies' quality. Before moving on to the next section, critically appraise a realist paper (see Box 6.7).

Box 6.6   Case studies: A summary of their quality

Realist Synthesis [2]: We employed a rigorous team-based realist approach from start to finish, with a clear initial programme theory based on exploratory research, which we refined through the analytic process. We included quality checks and realist relevance throughout the literature selection processes and included a large sample of papers in the synthesis including qualitative, quantitative, and mixed methods studies. However, an element of incoherence existed in our synthesis because none of the included papers employed realist approaches, meaning that it was hard for us to tease out contexts that triggered outcome-generating mechanisms. While we presented CMOCs in our paper, we presented three cross-cutting mechanisms separately for clarity, which served to lose the centrality of configurational analyses presented in our paper. However, we followed the RAMESES reporting guidelines for realist syntheses [25].

Realist Evaluation I [3]: Despite currently analysing our data, we have used a realist approach throughout (coherence). Regarding theory building, we undertook exploratory data collection via realist synthesis, as well as exploring programme designer assumptions. These two datasets kick-started our team-based realist analysis employing computer-assisted qualitative data analysis software (CAQDAS), enabling analytical comparisons between the two datasets. We began developing individual CMOCs and their descriptions (privileging configurational analyses), then merging codes to identify a smaller number of demi-regularities. We will report our findings following RAMESES I and II reporting standards [25, 43].

Realist Evaluation II [4]: We collected large amounts of qualitative data (over sixty hours) from a diverse sample, conducted a rigorous analytical approach involving multiple analysts and CAQDAS, and our study was realist from start to finish – with the building, testing, and refining of programme theory central to all stages of data collection and analysis. Our study could be criticised from a *scientific* realist perspective for not employing mixed methods, and for not including objective outcome measures such as knowledge tests [54]. However, we followed the RAMESES II reporting standards for realist evaluations [43].

Realist Economic Evaluation [5]: We conducted rigorous team-based realist analysis employing CAQDAS, and the testing, building, and refining of realist economic programme theory was omnipresent across the study. However, we collected a relatively small amount of qualitative realist data, making it difficult to determine

(continued)

(continued)

robust patterns. Although reporting standards for realist economic evaluations do not yet exist, wherever possible, we followed both the RAMESES II reporting standards for realist evaluations [43], and the Consolidated Health Economic Evaluation Reporting Standards (CHEERS) [62].

Box 6.7   Stop and do: Critically appraise a realist paper

- Read the abstract of one of the following open-access papers: Carrieri et al. Optimising strategies to address mental ill-health in doctors and medical students: 'Care Under Pressure' realist review and implementation guidance. *BMC Med.* 2020;18(1):76. https://bmcmedicine.biomedcentral.com/articles/10.1186/s12916-020-01532-x or Lefroy et al. Can learning from workplace feedback be enhanced by reflective writing? A realist evaluation in UK undergraduate medical education. *Educ Prim Care.* 2021;32(6):3 26–335. https://www.tandfonline.com/doi/full/10.1080/14739879.2021.19 20472.

- Pick the most appropriate quality or quality reporting tool from those listed in Box 6.6, and using your selected tool critically appraise your chosen paper.

- How does your chosen paper follow the reporting standards, and how does it not?

- What other realist indicators of quality are apparent in your chosen paper, and what could be better?

- Improve your critical appraisal skills further by doing the same exercise with the other paper, or choose another realist paper relevant to your research questions.

6.5   CHALLENGES AND STRENGTHS OF EMPLOYING REALIST APPROACHES IN HPER

It is important to understand the challenges and strengths of realist approaches within HPER. In terms of challenges, it is worth noting that realist approaches can be difficult for novice researchers, so team-based approaches including senior researchers with more advanced realist understandings is beneficial. Moreover, due to the emergent and iterative nature of realist approaches, it can be difficult to develop and follow rigid protocol formats; meaning that sampling, data collection, and data analysis can be hard to plan at the outset of your project [42, 56]. Additionally, as a realist researcher you might find it difficult to develop initial programme theories at the start of your research; either because of an over-abundance of potential candidate theories, or because the theories you identify are not terribly novel [56]. Although central to providing realist causal explanations, teasing out contexts, mechanisms, and outcomes in data (especially voluminous qualitative data) can also be challenging [63]. Mechanisms are not directly observable and thus need to be inferred through, for example, theories [56]. Be mindful that it can be easy to erroneously conflate mechanisms with programme activities [49, 64]. Additionally, although scholars suggest that teasing out mechanisms into resources and reasoning can help distinguish between mechanisms and contexts [20], it is often difficult to identify whether something is operating as a mechanism or context in any given explanation [49, 65, 66]. Moreover, it can be challenging to identify configurations (i.e., CMOCs) and recurring patterns (so-called demi-regularities) in your data, and then communicate those rich and complex configurations to other researchers and end-users in a clear, parsimonious, and transparent manner. Often, researchers do not explicitly articulate their configuration types to end-users [63, 67], especially given that configuration types can be flexible – for example, researchers might include extra explanatory factors and/or vary the order of CMO presentation, such as IOMC [intervention-outcome-mechanism-context] configurations. Finally, realist researchers can often experience significant problems communicating their study findings to researchers and end-users. This is especially so for recipients who are more comfortable with (and knowledgeable of) scientific approaches. For example, they might understand causality as constant conjunctions, rather than generative causality, and want (or expect) clear-cut findings about whether an intervention works (or not), or whether it is cost-effective or not. Indeed, Westhorp [9] suggested that realist approaches are suboptimal if end-users do not need/want to know how, where, and why programmes work, but instead want to know the average net effect of a programme, or whether a simple programme works.

Despite these challenges, realist approaches possess considerable strengths at philosophical, methodological, and pragmatic levels. First, realist approaches fundamentally appreciate educational programmes as complex interventions in that they: (a) are influenced by things outside the programme (open); (b) are based on interactions influenced by meaning (semiotic); and (c) include system elements that influence each other (recursive) [68]. Indeed, 'education works as a result of the intentional activities of reflexive agents [such as teachers and learners]. This means that an important avenue for educational change towards improvement is to be found in the ways in which the agents in the situation make sense of it and the activities going on inside it' [68 p. 206]. In simple terms, this suggests that a programme does not work universally for everyone at all times and in all contexts. With this nod to complexity [50], and how realist approaches serve to unpack the black box of how and why programmes work [35], Westhorp [9] suggests that realist approaches are best-suited to evaluating interventions that: (1) are new and/or pilot; (2) seem to work but how and for whom is unknown; (3) have mixed outcomes to understand why and how differences occur; and (4) require scaling up to other contexts (so might not work in new contexts). Second, scholars have applauded critical realism for being methodologically pluralist and inclusive, thereby overcoming epistemological objectivist–subjectivist dichotomies and methodological qualitative–quantitative dichotomies [16]. Third, realist evaluation enables you to critically consider an educational programme but to generalise to wider contexts through programme and middle-range theory. For example, Tilley suggests that: 'one of the roles of the realist, applied social scientist is to formulate and test the theory at a middle-range level of abstraction that speaks neither universally to all cases nor specifically only to one particular case' [69 p. 22]. Indeed, such realist research aligns itself well with the research impact agenda in HPER, appealing to various research end-users including practitioners, policymakers, regulators, and funders [9]. Before moving on to the chapter summary, read the summary of the case studies' strengths and challenges in Box 6.8. Also, stop and evaluate the strengths and challenges of an example realist paper (see Box 6.9).

Box 6.8   Case studies: A summary of their challenges and strengths

Realist Synthesis [2]: We experienced difficulties identifying contexts, mechanisms, and outcomes in such a large dataset of non-realist primary articles focusing on multiple interventions for successful research environments. For example, time could operate as an outcome, a mechanism, or context across or within the interventions. Consequently, we found it challenging to present our findings using an explicit articulation of CMOCs [63]. Instead, we presented three key cross-cutting mechanisms and their interactions. While this presentation downplayed our configurational analysis, it highlighted novel findings of interest to researchers and end-users (e.g., between protected time and researcher identities), highlighting the complexity of how interventions work (or not) and for whom, and thereby explaining mixed findings in the literature. For example, why protected time could work for the researcher with a strong researcher identity but not for the researcher without a strong researcher identity.

Realist Evaluation I [3]: Our team comprises researchers with varying levels of realist expertise; necessitating the upskilling of novice team members. Team-based analysis is time-consuming, leading to much debate about analytic steps and decisions, and conversations about CMO descriptions and levels of abstraction. This elongated duration led to changes in team members and the onboarding of new members, further extending our study duration. However, our realist approach is helping us to unpack the 'black box' of this assistants in medicine programme, with the findings of interest to researchers and end-users.

Realist Evaluation II [4]: Although we privileged context-triggering mechanisms in this study (unlike our earlier realist synthesis) [6], we found it challenging and highly time-consuming to identify demi-regularities from voluminous CMOCs identified in the vast qualitative dataset (over sixty hours of transcribed data). Because of the volume of data/codes, it was laborious keeping track of the extent to which programme theories were unsupported, supported, or completely new; requiring us to extend the timelines of our project. It was also sometimes difficult to tease out whether something was a mechanism or context, as well as guarding against conflating mechanisms with programme activities. We also found it challenging to present our nine demi-regularities parsimoniously, especially regarding our findings relating to the contexts likely to trigger outcome-generating mechanisms. However, our realist approach served to privilege (and better understand) the training programme as a complex intervention, thereby providing practical recommendations to end-users about future training.

Realist Economic Evaluation [5]: Our biggest struggle was working out how to integrate our realist and economic data analyses, to make realist-informed decisions (about cost-sensitive mechanisms and contexts) to develop our cost-optimised model, especially because realist economic evaluation is relatively new and guidelines do not yet exist. Also challenging was our having to defend the paper against positivist accusations that it: (a) lacked clear findings about whether online learning really worked; and (b) failed to properly examine causality (substitute here constant conjunctions). As with previous published realist papers [5], we needed to add a glossary of realist terms to our paper to help explain the approach to readers. However, through our rigorous analysis of multiple data sources and our novel integration of economic and realist analyses, we were able to develop a cost-optimised model for online workshops, thereby enabling multiple end-users (e.g., educators, funders, policymakers) to make decisions about how to balance effectiveness and cost in online learning.

Box 6.9   Stop and do: Evaluating the strengths/challenges of an example realist paper

- Read the following open-access realist paper: Kerr et al. A realist evaluation exploring simulated patient role-play in pharmacist undergraduate communication training. *BMC Med Educ.* 2021;21(1). https://bmcmededuc.biomed central.com/articles/10.1186/s12909-021-02776-8.
- Write down the strengths of the realist approach employed in this study in terms of addressing its research questions.
- Note the challenges of the realist approach for conveying the study research questions.
- What alternative approaches may have addressed these research questions? You may need to revisit this query after reviewing other chapters in Part II.
- View the peer-review reports for this *BMC Medical Education* paper online to see peer-reviewer comments, and the author comments. How do these compare with your notes?

6.6   CHAPTER SUMMARY

In this chapter, we have outlined the somewhat contested philosophical terrain associated with realist approaches to HPER – realist ontology (either scientific or critical realism), objectivist or subjectivist epistemology respectively, and the realist values of complexity, generative mechanisms, contexts, and the building, testing, and refining of theory. As you read this chapter, the debates may have moved on, with more and more realist papers being published in HPER. We have provided a short summary of common and emerging realist methodologies in HPER (realist synthesis, realist evaluation, and realist economic evaluation), and methods (i.e., purposive sampling, mixed methods realist data collection, as well as realist configurational analyses). We have outlined the key quality indicators for realist approaches (common to both scientific and critical realism) including theory, trustworthiness, coherence, and configurational analyses, as well as reporting standards for realist synthesis [25] and realist evaluation [43]. We have articulated the challenges associated with realist approaches including their iterative nature, difficulties developing initial programme theories, challenges identifying CMOCs and recurring patterns, and communicating those to researchers and end-users unfamiliar with realist approaches. However, realist approaches have compelling strengths – they respect educational interventions as social and complex, privilege methodological pluralism and inclusivity, and enable theory-driven evaluators to generalise from one programme to others through programme and middle-range theory. Realist approaches offer a solution to unpack complex educational interventions in HPE, and therefore we encourage you to build your understanding of (and capabilities in) realist approaches in HPER. As a start, make sure you work your way through the cases presented in this chapter, including the examples suggested in the stop and do boxes (Boxes 6.7 and 6.9), and engage with the recommended reading in Box 6.10. As with all the approaches to HPER covered in Part II of this book, we urge you to carefully consider the suitability of your approach in relation to your own epistemological beliefs and the research question(s) you seek to answer.

It is high time for an end to the domination of the quasi-experimental (or OXO) model of evaluation. Such an approach is a fine strategy for evaluating the relative performances of washing powders ... but is a lousy means of expressing the nature of causality and change going on within social programmes. [70 p. 292]

Box 6.10   Recommended reading for realist approaches in HPER

Ellaway RH, Kehoe A, Illing J. Critical realism and realist inquiry in medical education. *Acad Med.* 2020;95(7):984–988 [19].

Emmel N, Greenhalgh J, Manzano A, et al. eds. *Doing Realist Research*. London: SAGE; 2018 [50].

Manzano A. The craft of interviewing in realist evaluation. *Evaluation*. 2016; 22(3):342–360 [51].

Westhorp G. *Realist Impact Evaluation: An Introduction*. London: Overseas Development Institute; 2014 [9].

Wong G, Greenhalgh T, Westhorp G, et al. RAMESES publication standards: Realist syntheses. *BMC Med.* 2013;11:21 [25].

Wong G, Westhorp G, Manzano A, et al. RAMESES II reporting standards for realist evaluations. *BMC Med.* 2016;14(1):96 [43].

Wong G, Greenhalgh T, Westhorp G, et al. Realist methods in medical education research: what are they and what can they contribute? *Med Educ.* 2012; 46(1);89–96 [35].

REFERENCES

1. Porter S, O'Halloran P. The use and limitation of realistic evaluation as a tool for evidence-based practice: A critical realist perspective. *Nurs Inq.* 2011;19(1):18–28.

2. Ajjawi R, Crampton PES, Rees CE. What really matters for successful research environments? a realist synthesis. *Med Educ.* 2018;52(9):936–950.

3. Monrouxe LV, Hockey P, Khanna P, et al. Senior medical students as assistants in medicine in COVID-19 crisis: a realist evaluation protocol. *BMJ Open.* 2021;11(9):e045822.

4. Rees CE, Nguyen VNB, Ottrey E, et al. The effectiveness of extended-duration supervision training for nurses and allied health professionals: a realist evaluation. *Nurs Educ Today.* 2022;110:105225.

5. Rees CE, Nguyen VNB, Foo J, et al. Balancing the effectiveness and cost of online education: a preliminary realist economic evaluation. *Med Teach.* 2022;44(9):977–985.

6. Rees CE, Lee SL, Huang E, et al. Supervision training in healthcare: a realist synthesis. *Adv Health Sci Educ.* 2020;25(3):523–561.

7. Carter SM, Little M. Justifying knowledge, justifying method, taking action: epistemologies, methodologies, and methods in qualitative research. *Qual Health Res.* 2007;17(10):1316–1328.

8. Palermo C, Reidlinger DP, Rees CE. Internal coherence matters: lessons for nutrition and dietetics research. *Nutr Diet.* 2021;78(3):252–267.

9. Westhorp G. *Realist Impact Evaluation: An Introduction*. London: Overseas Development Institute; 2014.

10. Pawson R. *The Science of Evaluation: A Realist Manifesto*. London: SAGE; 2013.

11. Porter S. The uncritical realism of realist evaluation. *Evaluation*. 2015;21(1):65–82.

12. Brekke J, Anastas J, Floersch J, et al. The realist frame: scientific realism and critical realism. In Brekke J, Anastas J, eds. *Shaping a Science of Social Work: Professional Knowledge and Identity*, Online ed. New York: Oxford Academic; 2019: 22–40.

13. Niiniluoto I. *Critical Scientific Realism*. New York: Oxford University Press; 2002.

14. Bhaskar R. *A Realist Theory of Science*. London: Routledge; 1979.

15. Fletcher AJ. Applying critical realism in qualitative research: methodology meets method. *Int J Soc Res Methodol*. 2017;20(2):181–194.

16. Vincent S, O'Mahoney J. Critical realism and qualitative research: an introductory overview. In Cassell C, Cunliffe AL, Grandy G, eds. *The SAGE Handbook of Qualitative Business and Management Research Methods*. London: SAGE; 2018: 201–216.

17. Nash R. Explanation and quantification in educational research: the arguments of critical and scientific realism. *Br Educ Res J*. 2005;31(2):185–204.

18. Chirkov V, Anderson A. Statistical positivism versus critical scientific realism. A comparison of two paradigms for motivation research: part I. A philosophical and empirical analysis of statistical positivism. *Theory Psychol*. 2018;28(6):712–736.

19. Ellaway RH, Kehoe A, Illing J. Critical realism and realist inquiry in medical education. *Acad Med*. 2020;95(7):984–988.

20. McEvoy P, Richards D. Critical realism: a way forward for evaluation research in nursing? *J Adv Nurs*. 2003;43(4):411–420.

21. Dalkin SM, Greenhalgh J, Jones D, et al. What's in a mechanism? Development of a key concept in realist evaluation. *Implement Sci*. 2015;10:49.

22. Chernoff F. Critical realism, scientific realism, and international relations theory. *Millennium: J Int Stud*. 2007;35(2):399–407.

23. Chirkov V, Anderson J. Statistical positivism versus critical scientific realism. A comparison of two paradigms for motivation research: part 2. A philosophical and empirical analysis of critical scientific realism. *Theory Psychol*. 2018;28(6):737–756.

24. Astbury B. Some reflections on Pawson's Science of Evaluation: A Realist Manifesto. *Evaluation*. 2013;19(4):383–401.

25. Wong G, Greenhalgh T, Westhorp G, et al. RAMESES publication standards: realist syntheses. *BMC Med*. 2013;11:21.

26. Gorchs-Font N, Ramon-Aribau A, Yildirim M, et al. Nursing students' first experience of death: identifying mechanisms for practice learning. A realist review. *Nurs Educ Today*. 2021;96:104637.

27. Bansal A, Greenley S, Mitchell C, et al. Optimising planned medical education strategies to develop learners' person-centredness: a realist review. *Med Educ*. 2022;56(5):489–503.

28. Kerr A, Kelleher C, Pawlikowska T, et al. How can pharmacists develop patient-pharmacist communication skills? A realist synthesis. *Patient Educ Couns*. 2021;104(10):2467–2479.

29. Carrieri D, Mattick K, Pearson M, et al. Optimising strategies to address mental ill-health in doctors and medical students: 'Care Under Pressure' realist review and implementation guidance. *BMC Med*. 2020;18:76.

30. Pierce C, Corral J, Aagaard E, et al. A BEME realist synthesis review of the effectiveness of teaching strategies used in the clinical setting on the development of clinical skills among health professionals: BEME Guide no. 61. *Med Teach*. 2020;42(6):604–615.

31. Browne F, Hannigan B, Harden J. A realist evaluation of a safe medication administration education programme. *Nurs Educ Today*. 2021;97:104685.

32. Kerr A, Strawbridge J, Kelleher C, et al. A realist evaluation exploring simulated patient role-play in pharmacist undergraduate communication training. *BMC Med Educ*. 2021;21:325.

33. Lefroy J, Walters B, Molyneux A, et al. Can learning from workplace feedback be enhanced by reflective writing? A realist evaluation in UK undergraduate medical education. *Educ Prim Care*. 2021;32(6):326–335.

34. Rees CE, Foo J, Nguyen VNB, et al. Unpacking economic program theory for super-vision training: preliminary steps towards realist economic evaluation. *Med Educ.* 2022;56(4):407–417.

35. Wong G, Greenhalgh T, Westhorp G, et al. Realist methods in medical education research: what are they and what can they contribute? *Med Educ.* 2012;46(1):89–96.

36. Davydova I, Sharrock W. The rise and fall of the fact/value distinction. *Sociol Rev.* 2003;51(3):357–375.

37. Wilson M, Greenhill A. Theory and action for emancipation: elements of a critical realist approach. In Kaplan B, Truex DP, Wastell D, et al., eds. *Information Systems Research: Relevant Theory and Informed Practice.* IFIP International Federation for Information Processing. vol. 143. London: Springer; 2004: 667–674.

38. Brown S, Dalkin SM, Bate A, et al. Exploring and understanding the scope and value of the Parkinson's nurse in the UK (The USP project): a realist economic evaluation protocol. *BMJ Open.* 2020;10(10):e037224.

39. Lee S, Denniston C, Edouard V, et al. Supervision training interventions in the health and human services: realist synthesis protocol. *BMJ Open.* 2019;9(5):e025777.

40. Greenhalgh T, Pawson R, Wong G, et al. Realist evaluation, realist synthesis, realist research – what's in a name. The RAMESES II Project. National Institute for Health Research; 2017. https://www.ramesesproject.org/media/RAMESES_II_RE_RS_RR_whats_in_a_name.pdf (accessed 9 July 2022).

41. Pawson R, Greenhalgh T, Harvey G, et al. Realist review – a new method of systematic review designed for complex policy interventions. *J Health Serv Res Policy.* 2005;10(S1):21–34.

42. Greenhalgh T, Pawson R, Wong G, et al. Realist evaluation and ethical considerations. The RAMESES II Project; National Institute for Health Research; 2017. https://www.ramesesproject.org/media/RAMESES_II_Realist_evaluation_and_ethical_consid-erations.pdf (accessed 9 July 2022).

43. Wong G, Westhorp G, Manzano A, et al. RAMESES II reporting standards for realist evaluations. *BMC Med.* 2016;14(1):96.

44. Anderson R, Hardwick R, Pearson M, et al. Using realist approaches to explain the costs and cost-effectiveness of programs. In Emmel N, Greenhalgh J, Manzano A, et al., eds. *Doing Realist Research.* London: SAGE; 2018: 107–130.

45. Anderson R, Hardwick R. Realism and resources: towards more explanatory economic evaluation. *Evaluation.* 2016;22(3):323–341.

46. Foo J, Cook DA, Tolsgaard M, et al. How to conduct cost and value analyses in health professions education: AMEE Guide no. 139. *Med Teach.* 2021;43(9): 984–998.

47. Ritchie J, Spencer L. Qualitative data analysis for applied policy research. In Bryman A, Burgess R, eds. *Analyzing Qualitative Data.* London: Routledge; 1994: 173–194.

48. Williams M. Making up mechanisms in realist research. In Emmel N, Greenhalgh J, Manzano A, et al., eds. *Doing Realist Research.* London: SAGE; 2018: 25–40.

49. Marchal B, Kegels G, Van Belle S. Theory and realist methods. In Emmel N, Greenhalgh J, Manzano A, et al., eds. *Doing Realist Research.* London: SAGE; 2018: 79–89.

50. Emmel N, Greenhalgh J, Manzano A, et al. Introduction: doing realist evaluation, synthesis and research. In Emmel N, Greenhalgh J, Manzano A, et al., eds. *Doing Realist Research.* London: SAGE; 2018: 1–13.

51. Manzano A. The craft of interviewing in realist evaluation. *Evaluation.* 2016; 22(3):342–360.

52. Gilmore B, McAuliffe E, Power J, et al. Data analysis and synthesis within a realist evaluation: towards more transparent methodological approaches. *Int J Qual Methods.* 2019;18:1–11.

53. Crampton P, Mehdizadeh L, Page M, et al. Realist evaluation of UK medical education quality assurance. *BMJ Open.* 2019;9(12):e033614.

54. Pawson R, Tilley N. *Realistic Evaluation.* London: SAGE; 1997.

55. Westhorp G, Manzano A. Realist evaluation interviewing – a 'starter set' of questions. The RAMESES II Project; National Institute for Health Research; 2017. https://www.ramesesproject.org/media/RAMESES_II_Realist_interviewing_starter_questions.pdf (accessed 9 July 2022).

56. Shearn K, Allmark P, Percy H, et al. Building realist program theory for large complex and messy interventions. *Int J Qual Methods.* 2017;16:1–11.

57. Wong G. Data gathering in realist reviews – looking for needles in haystacks. In Emmel N, Greenhalgh J, Manzano A, et al., eds. *Doing Realist Research.* London: SAGE; 2018: 131–145.

58. Greenhalgh T, Pawson R, Wong G, et al. The realist interview. The RAMESES II Project; National Institute for Health Research; 2017. http://www.ramesesproject.org/media/RAMESES_II_Realist_interviewing.pdf (accessed 9 July 2022).

59. Ogrinc G, Ercolano E, Cohen ES, et al. Educational systems factors that engage resident physicians in an integrated quality improvement curriculum at a VA hospital: a realist evaluation. *Acad Med.* 2014;89(10):1380–1385.

60. Pawson R, Manzano-Santaella A. A realist diagnostic workshop. *Evaluation.* 2012;18(2):176–191.

61. Jagosh J. Retroductive theorizing in Pawson and Tilley's applied scientific realism. *J Crit Realism.* 2020;19(2):121–130.

62. Husereau D, Drummond M, Petrou S, et al. Consolidated Health Economic Evaluation Reporting Standards (CHEERS) statement. *BMJ.* 2013;346:f1049–f1049.

63. De Weger E, Van Vooren NJE, Wong G, et al. What's in a realist configuration? Deciding which causal configuration to use, how, and why? *Int J Qual Methods.* 2020;19:1–8.

64. Astbury B, Leeuw F. Unpacking black boxes: mechanisms and theory building in evaluation. *Am J Eval.* 2010;31(3):363–381.

65. Greenhalgh J, Manzano A. Understanding 'context' in realist evaluation and synthesis. *Int J Soc Res Methodol.* 2022;25(5):583–595.

66. Jolly H, Jolly L. Telling context from mechanism in realist evaluation: the role for theory. *Learning Communities: Int J Learn in Soc Contexts.* 2014;14:28–45.

67. Nguyen VNB, Rees CE, Ottrey E, et al. What really matters for supervision training workshops? A realist evaluation. *Acad Med.* 2022;97(8):1203–1212.

68. Biesta G. Improving education through research? From effectiveness, causality and technology to purpose, complexity and culture. *Policy Futures Educ.* 2016;14(2):194–210.

69. Tilley N. The middle-range methodology of realist evaluation. In Emmel N, Greenhalgh J, Manzano A, et al., eds. *Doing Realist Research.* London: SAGE; 2018: 15–24.

70. Pawson R, Tilley N. What works in evaluation research? *Br J Criminol.* 1994;34(3):291–306.

Introducing Interpretivist Approaches in Health Professions Education Research

Lynn V. Monrouxe[1], Megan E.L. Brown[2], Ella Ottrey[3], and Lisi J. Gordon[4]

[1] The University of Sydney, Camperdown, New South Wales, Australia
[2] Imperial College London, London, UK
[3] Monash University, Clayton, Victoria, Australia
[4] University of Dundee, Dundee, Scotland, UK

> **Box 7.1 Chapter 7 learning objectives: After reading this chapter you should be able to ...**
>
> - Describe the philosophical underpinnings (ontology, epistemology, and axiology) of interpretivist approaches
> - Summarise the common interpretivist methodologies in health professions education research (HPER)
> - Identify key principles of interpretivist methods in HPER (sampling, data collection, and data analysis)
> - Explain the main indicators of quality employed in interpretivist approaches
> - Evaluate the strengths and challenges of interpretivist approaches for HPER
> - Reflect on the applicability of interpretivist approaches to your own HPER

7.1 INTRODUCING CHAPTER 7

[some] educational researchers believe that scientific inquiry must focus on the study of multiple social realities, that is, the different realities created by different individuals as they interact in a social environment. They also believe that these realities cannot be studied by the analytic methods of positivist research. [1 p. 19]

Foundations of Health Professions Education Research: Principles, Perspectives and Practices,
First Edition. Edited by Charlotte E. Rees, Lynn V. Monrouxe, Bridget C. O'Brien, Lisi J. Gordon, and Claire Palermo.
© 2023 John Wiley & Sons Ltd. Published 2023 by John Wiley & Sons Ltd.

Historically, interpretivist approaches and their assertion that the world comprises a set of socially constructed meanings, was a perspective brought about as: 'a reaction to the positivist approach to social science inquiry' [1 p. 19], with positivist approaches preferring quantitative methods and interpretivist approaches qualitative. In this chapter we aim to help you think through the hows and whys of applying interpretivist approaches to HPER (see Box 7.1). Those new to research sometimes struggle with understanding the differences between interpretivist, constructivist, social constructivist, and social constructionist approaches. See our book glossary for definitions of these terms, as well as other complex terms employed across this chapter. We therefore begin with an outline of key differences in Box 7.2, while acknowledging there are weak and strong versions of all philosophies, and many overlaps between them [2]. This chapter, however, focuses on interpretivist approaches. We hope that this helps you see that this dichotomous 'either–or' argument is no longer relevant in health professions education research (HPER) and that your choice of taking an interpretivist approach is based on the well-established concepts we introduce to you in this chapter. The broad premise behind interpretivist approaches is that what we say, do, and have hold meaning and shape our understanding of the world. For example, we use words (spoken and written) to construct our world and give it meaning. Furthermore, what we say, do, and have will mean something to others. However, these meanings might be different and will depend on what you and others choose to identify and magnify as important. This is called social sense-making and is an ongoing process that is central to interpretivist research [3]. For an interpretivist researcher, social interaction, the context, and the researcher's position in relation to the research are important [4]. Interpretivist approaches encompass diverse perspectives, which are 'not always in harmony'[5 p. 6], reflecting the different disciplines from which interpretivist approaches have originated [6]. Indeed, you may have already delved into the literature around these approaches, only to become confused by this discord. We hope this chapter helps clarify the interpretivist approach in HPER and your thinking about why and how you might choose this path.

Box 7.2 Interpretivism, constructivism, social constructivism, and social constructionism

Interpretivism rejects positivist approaches that seek to examine the social world in the same way we examine the physical world: arguing that we can only know the world from within the social system itself. This approach asserts it is possible for a researcher to identify subjective meanings (e.g., participants' beliefs and intentions) through interpretation [2].

Constructivism asserts that a person: 'selects information, constructs hypotheses, and makes decisions, with the aim of integrating new experiences into his [*sic*.] existing knowledge and experience' [7 p. 11]. Constructivists often make claims around knowledge being stored in our cognition (as mental models) and how this develops in stages over time (cognition precedes knowledge) [7].

Social constructivism adopts an: 'anti-realist position and states that the process of knowing is affected by other people and is mediated by community and culture' [7 p. 10], with knowledge preceding cognition [7].

Social constructionism focuses on interactions between individuals and how we socially construct meaning through language and action (typically with no claim to cognitive representations) [8]. This position is agnostic to ontological matters around whether things exist, but is interested in how language and action work as social and rhetorical practices in everyday life [2].

What we present in this chapter reflects our reading of the interpretivist literature, as well as our own experiences of conducting and reviewing interpretivist approaches in HPER. In section 7.2, we describe the philosophical underpinnings of interpretivist approaches including historical origins. Section 7.3 then outlines common interpretivist methodologies and methods used in HPER. We introduce and discuss key indicators of quality in interpretivist research in section 7.4 and we then consider the challenges and strengths associated with interpretivist approaches to HPER in section 7.5. Throughout this chapter, we provide real-world examples of research using different interpretivist approaches, including a narrative review, a longitudinal qualitative research (LQR) study, a phenomenology study, and a study conducted within an ethnomethodological framework (see Box 7.3 for a brief overview). We hope this chapter helps you decide if an interpretivist approach is appropriate for your research, plus prepares you for any challenges you may encounter along the way.

Box 7.3   Case studies: An overview

<u>Narrative Review</u> [9]: We conducted a narrative review on developing and implementing longitudinal methods of clinical education within the UK. This involved conducting a systematic search of international literature, and synthesising findings to create a practical guide for UK implementation.

<u>Longitudinal Qualitative Research</u> [10, 11]: In this Australian study, we explored preparedness for practice journeys of graduates from multiple healthcare professions (dietetics, medicine, nursing, pharmacy) over their final-year student to new graduate transition. Our aims were to explore understandings and experiences of preparedness for practice and transition.

<u>Phenomenology</u>: [12] We explored new doctors' experiences of the transition from medical student to clinical practice in the UK. We were interested in a thick description of how doctors live through this transition and, particularly, the influence of new doctors' experiences on whether and how they discussed distress.

<u>Ethnomethodology</u>: [13, 14] Using audio and video recordings in naturalistic settings, we explored doctor–student–patient triadic teaching/patient care interactions across UK healthcare settings. Following data immersion with participant representatives we examined how patients are included (and excluded) in the teaching of medical students, interactional student feedback practices, and how trust is enacted within these triadic encounters.

7.2   PHILOSOPHICAL UNDERPINNINGS OF INTERPRETIVIST APPROACHES

As described in Chapter 2, an appreciation of the underpinning philosophies of specific research approaches is key to achieving research rigour. Articulating the alignment of ontology (nature of reality), epistemology (nature of knowing), methodology (how we come to know), and axiology (what we value) within a particular project, as well as personal philosophies, is important. It is also an important part of developing your research design, from inception through to data analyses. In this section, we outline the philosophical foundations of interpretivist approaches with the aim of developing your thinking around the appropriateness of these for your own work, and also to guide your research design in a way that ensures internal coherence between ontological, epistemological, methodological, and axiological considerations [15].

7.2.1 Relativist Ontology

Interpretivist approaches are underpinned by a relativist ontological perspective [16]. From a relativist perspective, reality is socially constructed as we interact with each other: influenced by our own backgrounds and past experiences, and the world around us [16]. Thus, as an interpretivist researcher, you are not looking to discover an objective, single, pre-existing reality of the world (as discussed in Chapter 5). Rather, you will accept that there can be many truths coexisting. Accordingly, you are seeking to understand these truths through your interpretation: identifying particular patterns within the data and attempting to understand their meaning within the context that they were collected [17]. Furthermore, while a relativist ontology asserts that our worlds are socially constructed, this is not a free-for-all: our worlds also sit within wider (and often shared) social structures and contexts (e.g., cultures, hierarchies, professions, education systems, national and international contexts). Part of our social construction of reality through interaction serves to reinforce, resist, or develop these social structures and contexts [18, 19]. Some interpretivists, therefore, adopt a critical realist ontological perspective, whereby there is an acceptance that some knowledge is dependent on an external reality but it is merely an approximation of that reality (see Chapter 6 for an introduction to critical realism) [8].

7.2.2 Subjectivist Epistemology

Building on the notion that knowledge is constructed, interpretivist research is underpinned by a subjectivist epistemology, recognising that you, the researcher, are integral to the process. Thus, as social reality is embedded within social settings, our interpretation of this social reality is more of a sense-making process (rather than hypothesis testing: as described in Chapter 5). Your focus is processes rather than objects; and meanings rather than causality [20]. Thus, at the very heart of a subjectivist epistemology is a consideration of how you as the researcher influence this process and the interpretation of data: you will layer your own meanings onto data. Furthermore, accepting that knowledge is constructed means that you might use first-person language to report on your research, which emphasises the subjectivity and openness of the processes you have undertaken [21]. This acceptance that knowledge is inherently subjective means that as an interpretivist researcher you should be mindful of your influence. This mindfulness is referred to as reflexivity. We will revisit reflexivity in more depth later in section 7.4.

7.2.3 Interpretivist Methodology

Because your aim as an interpretivist researcher is to understand the intricacies of our social world by identifying and understanding social phenomena within context, interpretivist research methodologies are typically qualitative [20]. Qualitative methodologies facilitate the generation of new understandings through research that is 'interactive and iterative' [3, 22 p. 168]. This means that while you will sometimes generate research questions a priori based on previous work in the field, you may also generate them from other places including your own experiences (direct experience and listening to others' stories) and from the research data itself during or after collection (as in post hoc research questions) [3]. When you work from the data, formulating questions that generate new understandings, you will use either induction or abduction [23]. Induction uses a stepwise process of identifying new understandings and theories from the data alone [3]. Abductive methodology is different in that it advocates moving back and forth between the data and multiple existing theories and research to identify what is 'surprising', generating new insights [22]. Common interpretivist methodologies used in HPER include ethnography, LQR, narrative review, narrative enquiry, and ethnomethodology.

7.2.4   Interpretivist Axiology

Connected with the ontological and epistemological viewpoints described in sections 7.2.1 and 7.2.2, interpretivist axiology aligns with the notion that knowledge can never be value-free [24]. As interpretivist researchers, we see research and practice as intertwined, each guiding and influencing the other [6]. Thus, your research is influenced by your personal interest in the topic and beliefs about the most appropriate way to approach data collection, analysis, and dissemination. Other influences include institutional, economic, and political values [25]. These influences impact on the research process, irrespective of the research approach you have adopted. However, due to the acceptance of subjectivity in interpretivist approaches, you go beyond merely acknowledging specific biases (e.g., researcher or funding biases) by considering the systemic nature of biases as inherent to your research processes [25]. As an interpretivist researcher, you will openly discuss values embedded in your research. The language you use as an interpretivist researcher also differs from other approaches [26]. For example, the term participant is preferred over subject. See Box 7.4 for a summary of the case studies' philosophical underpinnings.

Box 7.4   Case studies: A summary of their philosophical underpinnings

Narrative Review [9]: While we did not discuss the philosophical foundation of our review at the time, we implicitly assumed that reality was subjective, multiple, and context-dependent (relativist ontology), and that knowledge formation involved researcher perspectives (subjectivist epistemology). In considering international literature through a local lens, we contemplated the influence of context, holding regular team meetings to discuss how our own perspectives and values might deepen our interpretation (axiology). We selected a narrative review (methodology) to critically consider the impact of context.

Longitudinal Qualitative Research [10, 11]: We adopted a relativist ontology and subjectivist epistemology based on social constructionism: recognising multiple views and experiences of reality, construction of knowledge through social interaction, and researcher involvement in knowledge production [27]. We sought to uncover the different ways that participants articulated 'preparedness for practice' and 'transition' by asking them what these terms meant to them. In terms of axiology, we valued diverse perspectives, complexity, and fluidity in transition experiences, and sense-making in the moment.

Phenomenology [12]: We considered reality and knowledge to be subjective, with many realities existing (relativist ontology). We recognised ourselves as part of the research process: acknowledging and embracing our own experiences, considering how they might add depth to our interpretations (axiology). We focused on individuals who shared an experience (new doctors), but acknowledged that each participants' experiences would be influenced by social, cultural, and political contexts.

Thus, we also embraced a subjectivist epistemology. To explore commonalities and differences in lived experience, we adopted a hermeneutic phenomenological approach (methodology).

Ethnomethodology [13, 14]: Our ontological underpinning was relativist, understanding that social groups share the same collective understanding of the world, but these may differ according to who and where we are. Our epistemological position was associated with constructionism: understanding our social world is in continual flux, being constituted in and through social means. We valued an approach to studying behaviour (axiology) that privileged studying it from within the system: both from participants' perspectives, as well as within specific linguistic sequential social interactions, rather than using existing social theory. Ethnomethodology was our methodology, using: 'video-recorded data as a preferred method with detailed attention to talk-in-interaction and gestures as interaction' [28 p. 270].

7.3 COMMON INTERPRETIVIST METHODOLOGIES AND METHODS IN HPER

In this section we outline a selection of common methodological approaches used within interpretivist research in HPER. We present these alphabetically and they are not exhaustive. Our aim is to provide you with a few possibilities to help you with your research design decision-making. Using our research examples, we bring some of these to life, providing a rationale for our choices around the specific methodological approach we adopted (see Box 7.5). Note that grounded theory methodology is considered in Chapters 2 and 9 (see sections 2.3.3 and 9.3.3).

7.3.1 Phenomenology

Phenomenology is concerned with how we imbue meaning within our lived experiences [29]. Whilst there are many approaches to phenomenology, they do not all sit within an interpretivist framework. Therefore, we focus on hermeneutic (interpretative) phenomenological research [30]. This approach centres on analysing the meaning of a person's lived experience of a phenomena (i.e., how something was experienced), rather than describing the structure and content of that experience (i.e., what was experienced) [30]. Experience and sense-making considers our world of meaning, shaped by social, cultural, and political contexts. In-depth qualitative interviews are typically used. Unstructured or semi-structured interviews offer the time, space, and freedom to explore how participants experience common meanings and practices [31]. There are many ways to analyse data phenomenologically. Common to most interpretivist approaches, phenomenology recognises the impossibility of bracketing off previous experiences, thus conceptualises researchers as reflexive in the social world in which research occurs. Moving between data (such as interview transcripts) and interpretations (known as the hermeneutic cycle [32]) can help us develop an understanding of how something was experienced. This can happen within one text (researchers moving between sections of a transcript, developing or challenging interpretations), across texts, or across an entire project. In HPER, interpretative phenomenology has been applied to many topics including transitions [12].

7.3.2 Ethnography

Ethnography has grounding in social anthropology [33]: seeking to live, understand, and embody culture and society (i.e., whatever connects a group together) through an ethnographer's immersion in that culture and society. Hammersley identifies seven key dimensions of an ethnographic approach: (1) time spent in a context; (2) occurring in natural settings; (3) researcher observation and participant engagement; (4) multiple (mostly qualitative) methods (e.g., observation, interviews, documentary analysis); (5) documenting experiences as they are lived; (6) emphasising culture; and (7) having a holistic focus. The range of topics using ethnographic approaches for HPER includes professional identities [34], peer-assisted learning [35], interprofessional education [36], and leadership [37].

7.3.3 Longitudinal Qualitative Research (LQR)

LQR is typified by a sequence of qualitative data collection points (e.g., observation, interviews, diaries) with the same participant group, to explore the complexity of experiences as they shift, evolve, or even remain stable over time [38–41]. LQR facilitates access to repeated accounts of sense-making around experiences close to the time they are lived, especially when data are collected ethnographically or via diary methods [39]. Criticised for lacking philosophical and theoretical articulation [42], researchers tend to use longitudinal approaches in conjunction with other methodologies, for example narrative enquiry or interpretative phenomenology [10, 11, 38, 43]. LQR is characterised by an increasingly familiar relationship between participants and the researcher, and the opportunity to return to experiences and explore change, which can lead to new insights and understandings about a phenomenon [44, 45]. LQR is an increasingly popular methodology in HPER, being used to explore transitions across career trajectories [41, 46], preparedness for practice [10, 11], and professional identity construction [38, 39].

7.3.4 Narrative Enquiry

Narrative enquiry collects and analyses stories of events: these can be written, spoken, or even visually represented [47]. Some theorists argue that as we recount events, there is an element of sense-making that can lead to new understandings for researchers and participants [48]. Thus, when a story is told, the narrator (often the research participant) will construct and present theirs and others' identities, interactions, and relationships. As an interpretivist researcher, there are multiple ways in which you can explore narratives including individual biographies focusing on the inner world of the narrator, with phenomenology being a common strand [49, 50]. Some focus on how people construct their identities in relation to others: ethnomethodology and ethnographic approaches featuring strongly [51–53]. Finally, some consider the broader narratives of an organisation. Indeed, even within an interpretivist approach, there is no agreement as to what comprises a narrative nor how they should be analysed. Furthermore, as we demonstrate in our case study examples, narrative enquiry is often undertaken alongside other methodologies, for example LQR or ethnography. In HPER, narrative enquiry has been applied to topics such as feedback dialogues [11], leadership and followership [54, 55], preparedness for practice [39], professionalism dilemmas [56], and identities [38].

7.3.5 Narrative Literature Review

Narrative literature reviews are a form of literature synthesis focused on the impact of context, and with the ability to answer multiple questions on contemporary topics simultaneously [57, 58]. Narrative reviews offer scope for the critical interpretation of literature on a topic through a particular lens (that might be to do with role, geographical location, etc.). As they are interpretivist, they can also integrate expert opinion, whereby narrative review authors draw on their own experiences and perspectives in shaping review findings [58]. They differ from systematic reviews in that literature searches are not always systematic; they may focus solely on known critical papers within a field. However, narrative review searches are increasingly systematic, with many now searching widely, and providing clear search strategies and inclusion criteria to enhance transparency [59]. Another difference is that quality assessment of the evidence is not necessary [60]. This is because the philosophical foundation of narrative reviews is different: while literature quality is a key concern for post-positivist approaches asserting the existence of one reality and one truth, narrative reviews adopt an interpretivist approach, recognising and embracing ontological and epistemological plurality [61]. Indeed, narrative reviews acknowledge that there are multiple realities and truths. They aim to consider how context and experience helps us to understand key questions within our subjectively experienced practice, rather than an objective way to definitively answer questions [59]. Narrative reviews have been used extensively in HPER, examining wide-ranging topics such as student burnout [62], recruitment of ethnic minorities and Indigenous peoples into medical and surgical training [63], teaching clinical reasoning [64], perceptions of rural medicine [65], emotional intelligence [66], and psychological safety [67].

Box 7.5   Case studies: A summary of their methodologies and methods

---

Narrative Review [9]: We searched four databases using keywords for Longitudinal Integrated Clerkships (LICs). Setting inclusion and exclusion criteria, we identified 164 publications for inclusion. We proposed an initial form to collate data, based on our research question, which included study demographic detail, and information on barriers and enabling factors to development of LICs. Other categories of the form (e.g., questions arising from included studies) were added iteratively as it became apparent that there were common questions within the community we hoped would help structure our practical development guide. Data collected using this form were analysed thematically: grouping comments regarding similar enablers together (like the LIC environment) and considering how they might relate. We generated a practical application guide: 10 questions to consider when introducing a LIC into a medical curriculum based on both the review and our experience as educators.

Longitudinal Qualitative Research [10, 11]: We used maximum variation sampling (i.e. selecting four professions to represent diversity in degrees, registration requirements, and employment certainty) and snowballing (i.e., recruiting participants through other participants). We collected qualitative data across three phases: entrance interviews, longitudinal audio-diaries (LADs), and exit interviews. We asked participants about their understandings of transition to and preparedness for practice, eliciting personal stories that explored factors that impacted

(continued)

(continued)

their preparedness. We also delved into the emotional and psychosocial impacts of their experiences. We analysed data using a team-based approach to framework analysis [68]. Using NVivo software we explored patterns within our data, across the whole cohort (e.g., cross-sectional similarities and differences between professions) and individual participants (e.g., longitudinal changes over time).

Phenomenology [12]: Being interested in a thick description of transition to practice experiences, we purposively recruited a small sample with at least six months' experience of this transition (seven recently qualified UK doctors). We undertook in-depth, one-to-one interviews, prompting them to reflect on their recent experiences. We initially analysed our data inductively using Ajjawi and Higgs'[69] six stages of hermeneutic analysis to ground interpretations of our participants' lived experiences in their accounts. We then moved abductively between data, background literature, and reflections on our own experiences to inform interpretations. We used Poetic Inquiry to dive deeply into the meaning of participants' experiences [70], enhancing researcher reflexivity, and exploring the relationship between language and meaning [12]. To do so, we constructed 'participant-voiced poems', using words and stories from interview transcripts to communicate core themes. We moved between interview audio, text, and our poems in a hermeneutic cycle to create and communicate a richer understanding of new doctors' transitions to practice.

Ethnomethodology [13, 14]: Focusing primarily on 43 video recordings of naturally occurring interactional data during bedside teaching encounters (BTEs: totalling 937 minutes videoed from two angles) we examined 'the socially constructed, ongoing and reflexive (rather than causative) activities within the encounter' [13 p. 126]. Participants comprised a convenience sample of clinicians, students and patients who were engaging in hospital bedside teaching locally. We interpreted data through Conversation Analysis (CA) or CA-informed data interrogation. Primarily using an inductive approach, we stumbled across research questions by watching the data (sometimes with participants), developing topics of interest. We extracted data sections relating to the topic, looking for recurring patterns (e.g., linguistically and bodily) [28]. Through this method we explored how students and patients negotiate trust, how supervisors provided feedback to students, and how patients are included/excluded during teaching moments using verbal/non-verbal interactions [13, 14, 71]. All research questions arose through participant engagement and/or data familiarisation (see Chapter 8 for more on co-design).

7.3.6 Interpretivist Sampling, Data Collection, and Analysis Methods

Interpretivist research explores and constructs meaning through interaction, often with subjectivity as a core value. Thus, sampling strategies target groups who might understand and/or have experience of the phenomenon being researched [72]. As an interpretivist researcher, you will make several choices when deciding who to invite to participate in your research. The sampling strategy you use will help you achieve research efficiency and credibility. Purposive sampling is the most common approach, facilitating the collection of information-rich participants for your research. There is a range of purposive approaches, depending on your requirement. For example, do you want diversity within your sample (maximum variation), or are you looking for specific expert groups/individuals to inform certain constructs (theory-based), or even looking to reduce variation by looking at a particular subgroup (homogeneity). However, convenience sampling can also be appropriate (e.g., asking those who happen to be present). Additionally, you may ask current participants to bring along other potential participants, as in snowballing (see Box 7.5).

Data collection methods within interpretivist HPER can include interviews, focus groups, diaries, documentary analysis, and observation [73]. Using these types of methods, you will gather rich data often in multiple formats including (but not exhaustively): textual (e.g., transcripts, documents, field notes); audio (e.g., interview recordings, audio-diaries); or visual data (e.g., video-recordings, photographs, drawings) [74].

Perhaps unsurprisingly, data analysis methods within interpretivist HPER are wide ranging: from thematic analysis [75], to complex types of discourse analysis (e.g., emotional talk) [76], and everything in between. Although the development of research questions can include participant involvement, data analysis is researcher-led. This contrasts with critical approaches discussed in Chapter 8 that also include participants in the analytical process. Typically, qualitative data comprises large documents and files that require storage, management, and systematic interrogation. As such, computer assisted qualitative data analysis software (CAQDAS), such as NVivo and ATLAS.ti, are often used to facilitate the process. Before moving on to the next section, pause and reflect on how you might apply interpretivist approaches to your HPER (see Box 7.6).

> ### Box 7.6 Pause and reflect: Applying interpretivist methodologies/ methods to your research
>
> - Think about a topic of enquiry in health professions education that you are especially interested in researching. This may relate to a challenge regarding your own teaching or learning, or it may link to previous research you have done, or could relate to key gaps in the literature.
>
> - What research question could you develop relating to this topic that would lend itself well to an interpretivist approach and why? What methodologies/ methods would be appropriate for this question and why?
>
> - Now think of a research question pertaining to your chosen topic that does not lend itself well to an interpretivist approach. What other methodologies/ methods are more appropriate for this question and why? What other chapters in this book should you therefore read next?
>
> - Revisit this pause and reflect box once you have read the other chapters in Part II, and further developed your research ideas.

7.4 KEY QUALITY INDICATORS IN INTERPRETIVIST APPROACHES

As we have discussed in this chapter, an interpretivist approach to HPER does not search for a single truth but accepts multiple constructed realities affected by time and context. Thus, your interpretivist research will be bound by your values as a researcher, the research choices you make, your theoretical perspectives, and the context in which you undertake the research [77]. It is important therefore that you attend to and articulate how you have ensured research quality through a rigorous approach to your research from beginning to end. This rigour also entails that we engage in a continuous decision-making process as we conduct our research ethically. Indeed, it has been argued that interpretivist approaches are ethically mandated for the promotion of an equitable forum in which every voice has an opportunity to be heard and valued [78]. This valuing includes ownership and intellectual property, issues around harm and exploitation, and power relations. These are discussed further in Chapter 3. The key take-home message in terms of research quality is that serious considerations regarding how we will conduct our work respectfully reflects the credibility of our research. Some researchers have highlighted various procedural ways of ensuring research rigour, mainly under the broad construct of trustworthiness [77, 79, 80]. Thus, from the very inception of your research, key foundational considerations around quality include ensuring an internal coherence between ontology, epistemology, methodology, and methods [15, 81]. The issues around credibility and authenticity (referring to the plausibility of findings) are also key. Scholars have argued that these can be achieved through things like triangulation, member checking, peer-debriefing, auditing, continuous fully informed consent, prolonged engagement, and data saturation, although several of these concepts have been problematised more recently in HPER [82]. Confirmability and dependability are also related to trustworthiness and can be addressed by demonstrating how the findings clearly link to the data (rather than just researcher opinion) and the articulation of rigorous data collection and analysis processes, respectively. This detail of reporting relates to the issue of transparency in terms of how you tell your story, including what you have chosen to report, whose voices you have represented, and the meta-story (e.g., the background, methods, interpretation, limitations, and implications of the work) [83]. Finally, trustworthiness also includes transferability. This refers to the extent to which the findings are relevant to different contexts and can be addressed via thick description and/or the judicious use of theory.

In addition to procedural ways to enhance quality, we suggest that your goal should be to embody research quality, which can be achieved through engaging deeply in the process of researcher and team reflexivity [84]. Reflexivity serves to emphasise your presence within the research process with the aim of improving research quality through critical consideration of your influence on the research process, researcher–participant relationships, and how you report the research [85]. Embodying reflexivity intertwines with the trustworthiness constructs discussed above and can comprise critically considering a number of factors, including: how we might influence data generation (via our selection of tools, processes of data collection), the interpretive process (personal, a priori perspectives or expectations), potential ideological and power relationships that may impact on the research process (e.g., how data are reported and potentially used), alongside what is reported and how (e.g., claims to authority, which voices are represented) [83]. In practical terms, this can mean: keeping and maintaining a research diary; recording personal reflections; regular meetings as a research team; and regular presentation and discussion of research with peers in both formal (e.g., conferences) and informal settings (e.g., team meetings).

It is beyond the scope of this chapter to delve into all these constructs, but we encourage you to critically evaluate the utility of each for your interpretivist approach. Indeed, researchers change their minds over time as to how to assess quality in interpretivist research [76]. Further, due to the range of approaches within interpretivist research, constructs recommended as a quality indicator for one perspective might highlight a lack of rigour for another. As indicated above, the constructs of triangulation, member checking, and data saturation have come from a particular version of grounded theory methodology but can be problematic when undertaking a different interpretivist approach such as narrative enquiry using positioning analysis [82]. Therefore, other studies instead draw on related concepts of crystallisation, reflexivity, and information power respectively [82]. See Box 7.7 for a summary of our case studies' quality.

Box 7.7   Case studies: A summary of their quality

Narrative Review [9]: We considered our own perspectives and experiences in team discussions as we synthesised our findings. All authors were involved with LIC design and/or implementation, actively examining our experiences alongside insights from the literature for correspondences and divergences. Drawing on our experiences to practically ground the review, our discussions allowed us to acknowledge our own thoughts and opinions (we engaged with the data reflexively), considering whether our data were dependable: whether insights from included papers were consistent with our experiences. We attended to credibility by auditing our review process, though we could have presented this audit trail in a more well-recognised format (e.g., by using a PRISMA diagram).

Longitudinal Qualitative Research [10, 11]: We completed a team reflexivity exercise at the start of the study to encourage individual and collective self-reflection, and support understandings of one another's perspectives and differences in our understandings [85]. We audio-recorded the interviews and LADs, transcribing them verbatim, to promote credibility and dependability. In terms of transferability, we described the degrees that our participants were undertaking, including the different degree types and lengths, and workplace learning requirements.

Phenomenology[12] : Early within the design of our research, we held team discussions where we reflected on internal coherence within our project design. We paid particular attention to reflexivity. Spending an extended period considering participant language through Poetic Inquiry led us to realise that representing others' experiences requires interpretation that inevitably invokes one's own experiences. As we poetically recreated participants' experiences, we were able to reflect on our own similar experiences, and stories we had heard, facilitating reflection on how we had interpreted and presented the data. Confirmability and dependability were enhanced as we challenged our data interpretation, questioning whether our findings fairly represented our data.

Ethnomethodology [13, 14]: Initially, we were concerned that our analysis focused on what and how things were said, being mindful not to categorise participants as particular types of people, to infer intentions, and to claim causality. In terms of authenticity, we often included key stakeholders to drive topic development (e.g., tactical authenticity: patients, students, and educators repeatedly watched videos with us). While patients noted being excluded in the teaching activity, this led us to interrogate the data for interactional patterns exploring this rather than co-analysing the data with participants, as in critical enquiry discussed in Chapter 8 [13]. Students noticed different feedback practices [71]. Internal coherence and dependability was achieved by having an expert conversation analyst on the team, and a reflexive process for assuring we stayed within the boundaries of our data (reporting what we saw in the data, not what we thought we knew from experience).

By now you will have developed an appreciation of the wide range of research undertaken within an interpretivist approach. Given this appreciation, it will be unsurprising that what comprises research quality will vary accordingly. There are ongoing debates and discussions about what comprises markers of quality [82, 86]. It is important to remember that research quality is intimately entwined with research ethics, which varies contextually. As such, it is impossible to create a completely satisfactory checklist of things for you to do (or not). Despite this, scholars have developed sets of reporting standards with quality at the fore such as the Standards for Reporting Qualitative Research (SRQR) and the COnsolidated criteria for REporting Qualitative research (COREQ) [87–91] However, in doing so they tend to focus on listing the constructs with little concern for their contested nature across the different approaches to interpretivist research. Furthermore, it has been argued that when ticking a checklist, researchers are simplifying their responses [17]. For example, techniques for trustworthiness might be ticked and referenced in the article but dealt with as an afterthought or at a superficial level. Before moving on to the next section, we encourage you to familiarise yourself with one set of reporting standards, by critically appraising a paper (see Box 7.8).

> ### Box 7.8   Stop and do: Critically appraise an interpretivist paper
>
> - Read the following open-access paper: Offiah, et al. Gender matters: understanding transitions in surgical education. *Front Med.* 2022;9:884452. https://www.frontiersin.org/articles/10.3389/fmed.2022.884452/full
> - Use the SRQR and the quality indicators discussed in section 7.4 to critically appraise this paper.
> - How does this paper follow the reporting standards, and how does it not?
> - What interpretivist indicators of quality are apparent in this paper, and what are missing or could be better?

7.5   CHALLENGES AND STRENGTHS OF EMPLOYING INTERPRETIVIST APPROACHES IN HPER

entrenched in the positivist paradigm of scientific values and objectivity ... Extricating me was ... slow and painful ... after 20 years on a well-trodden and familiar road and yet emancipatory because it opened so many previously unknown lanes to explore. Every decision I made concerning the most suitable research paradigm, ontology, epistemology and methodology involved long periods of confusion and uncertainty. [92 p. 206]

We now turn to consider relative challenges and strengths of adopting an interpretivist approach for your HPER. We do so with one caveat: this is not an exhaustive list of negatives and positives, but a few select issues identified by us as we have engaged in our interpretivist endeavours (see Box 7.9). In line with an interpretivist perspective, we accept that it is entirely possible that there are numerous aspects of employing this approach, many of which are context-specific. As you read through this section, therefore, we urge you to consider your own thoughts on the matter: what aspects of this perspective feel uneasy for you and where is your own particular comfort zone?

Considering the challenges first, when thinking about the process of undertaking research, for those of you coming from a background rooted within a positivist/post-positivist tradition discussed in Chapter 5 (as most healthcare professions are), as seen from the excerpt above, shifting perspectives to an interpretivist approach can be challenging [92]. Ensuring coherence as you make this transition requires continual checking: what assumptions are you making? What of the notions of truth and reality in your knowledge claims? For example, while interpretivist researchers have the explicit ideology of a relativist ontological perspective, it has been noted that it is all too easy for researchers to inadvertently slip into a (neo)realist ontology [5]. To clarify using an example from our own work, Monrouxe and Sweeney [93] report data from medical students' LADs analysing them within an interpretivist approach. However, in doing so we classify the narratives (looking onto, living alongside, and living with illness, dying, and death) and focus on the interior tensions for each narrator: 'between two aspects of the self: the student as clinician-to-be and the student as myself' [93 p. 61]. As a consequence, we slip into this (neo)realist ontology by claiming to know the tensions, understand them, and posit they are familiar to all medical students as they develop their professional identities. Furthermore, living with uncertainty (e.g., without clear patterns being identified, concerns about our interpretations being 'right') can be difficult, even for those not initially versed in a positivist framework. There is a tangible tension felt between the general messiness of storytelling (in all its forms) and the tidiness required in our reporting. Others who share the same socially constructed understandings of what research comprises are more likely to understand and accept your interpretivist research. Those from outside (i.e., positivists) may find this hard as they have their own socially constructed understanding of research. Therefore, peer reviews from those who are unfamiliar with interpretivist approaches, or those who do not share the same epistemological understanding, can cause tension around beliefs of fairness in the peer-review process [94]. Moreover, responding to these reviews, politely challenging requests for revisions that would threaten internal coherence, can be problematic.

Another challenge is that data collection can be time-consuming. For example, a traditional ethnography can be problematic in HPER where there is increasing pressure to publish and a paucity of funding sources [95]. This has led a movement towards shorter, more intensive fieldwork methods [96]. However, these have come under criticism as to whether they are within the ethnographic tradition of prolonged engagement with the field [95, 97]. Further challenges include: establishing, maintaining, and ending relationships with participants especially during longitudinal research [44]; issues around transcription content (should we transcribe, and if so how, paralinguistic elements of talk such as laughter, pauses, tone of voice, and cross-talk?); and whether we note visual as well as audio information [98]. All of these concerns around what information is relevant and what is omitted reflect on our wider epistemological and axiological values and impact on how we might analyse our data [98]. Indeed, in terms of axiology, some have argued that interpretivist perspectives largely neglect issues of power and agency [99], a stance taken on by critical approaches (as discussed in Chapter 8).

Finally, data analysis can be challenging, with further questions around whether to use data management software and decisions around how the coding might be developed and actualised. It is beyond the scope of this chapter to delve into all these challenges in depth, but we encourage you to critically evaluate the utility and quality of each interpretivist methodological approach. Indeed, researchers change their minds over time as to how to assess quality in interpretivist research [77], and many accepted (and now expected) practices arise from specific theoretical approaches. This can result in an aspect being recommended as a quality indicator for one interpretivist perspective but highlights a lack of rigour for another.

Box 7.9   Case studies: A summary of their challenges and strengths

Narrative Review: [9] In selecting a narrative approach, we were able to consider our own experiences of implementing LICs, which sparked the idea for this review. Our narrative approach facilitated a focus on the influence of context, considering how international literature applies to UK healthcare and higher education. This focus allowed us to produce a practical application guide in the hope of informing practice. Limiting our scope when mapping review findings to a UK context was challenging. We had a lot to say but the paper needed to be an acceptable length for readers. While we wanted to generate insights for UK institutions, we also hoped the guide would be of interest to international educators: making the judgement on how much detail is required for transferability to this audience was difficult. We addressed this by responding to informal feedback from peers unfamiliar with this review, and with our specific context.

Longitudinal Qualitative Research [10, 11]: Through developing strong researcher–participant relationships, we captured rich data and promoted study engagement. Building trust and developing rapport with participants helped facilitate their sharing of stories. However, at times the LAD process resulted in brief accounts. We addressed this by encouraging them to identify memorable experiences in depth, and providing an LAD prompt sheet with points to consider in their narratives. We struggled during data analysis with the volume of data collected and complexities associated with analysing data cross-sectionally and longitudinally. We addressed this by making decisions around our approach to coding, such as whether to prioritise coding by phase across the whole sample, by participant across all phases, or a combination of both [100].

Phenomenology [12]: This was our first time using Poetic Inquiry. We saw Poetic Inquiry's strengths as facilitating rich enquiry, providing us with space to comprehensively consider the meaning of participants' experiences. One of our greatest challenges however was coherently communicating our philosophical perspective and demonstrating how this informed our Poetic Inquiry approach. In our paper, we describe reality and knowledge as subjective and multiple. On reflection, this is incomplete. While each participant is an embodied being, our experiences in the world (like transitions) are situated and shaped by context. We could have further emphasised our understandings of how participants are influenced by common meanings and practices within transition periods, which enables us to present common interpretations (including the poems we created) as findings.

Ethnomethodology [13, 14]: We faced many challenges over our research, but these intertwined with the strengths of our approach. Our interdisciplinary team comprised researchers with different methodological backgrounds in interpretivist approaches: narrative enquiry, conversation analysis, and thematic analysis. We also had different professional backgrounds: cognitive linguistics, sociology, and medicine. Thus, we had different experiences in how to approach the analysis, and the degree to which prior research and personal opinions should be used.

These challenges required reflexive practice and patience, ensuring the team had clarity of purpose. We collected a great deal of video interactional data. This was time-consuming: embedding ourselves in hospital wards, gaining consent, recording interactions, reviewing data, data storage, and transcribing dilemmas (e.g., if and how to transcribe overlapping talk, micro pauses, longer pauses, laughter, hesitation, emphasis, reported talk). Through these challenges of how to transcribe, the strengths of our approach became apparent, enabling us to answer our novel research questions, grounding our interpretations in authentic interactions, and providing strong recommendations for practice.

Interpretivist approaches have numerous strengths in the context of HPER. When selecting a specific interpretivist perspective (rather than adopting a generic qualitative approach), a key strength is that you have multiple resources to draw upon to help guide your research decisions, ensuring you develop a coherent approach [101]. Furthermore, as interpretivist researchers, we tend to write more openly about our philosophical assumptions: clarifying for ourselves and consumers of our research the status of our findings and claims therein [102]. Indeed, our attention to researcher reflexivity across the entire research process not only facilitates quality in the work we produce, but also supports successful teamworking [85]. Moreover, shining a spotlight on interactions within our social world can illuminate interesting facets and cast new light onto old issues [103]. Furthermore, the interpretivist approach affords space for you to develop questions based on your own experiences, facilitating understanding of important issues that might otherwise not be active topics of conversation in the community, particularly when you are embedded in clinical environments. Interpretivist approaches also go beyond an explanation of observable, measurable, and generalisable facts (i.e., the whats), towards a deep understanding and explanation of the hows and whys of phenomena within social contexts. Before moving on to the final section, stop and evaluate the strengths and challenges of an example interpretivist paper (see Box 7.10).

> **Box 7.10   Stop and do: Evaluating the strengths and challenges of an example interpretivist paper**
>
> - Read the following open-access paper: Gordon, et al. Leadership and followership in the healthcare workplace: exploring medical trainees' experiences through narrative inquiry. *BMJ Open*. 2015;5(12):e008898. https://bmjopen.bmj.com/content/5/12/e008898.
> - Write down the strengths of the interpretivist approach employed in this study in terms of addressing its research questions.
> - Note the challenges of the interpretivist approach for answering the study research questions.
> - What alternative approaches may have addressed these research questions? You may need to revisit this query after reading other chapters in Part II.
> - View the peer-review reports for this *BMJ Open* paper online to see peer-reviewer comments, and the authors' comments. How do these compare with your notes?

7.6   CHAPTER SUMMARY

In this chapter, we highlighted key constructs of interpretivist perspectives, acknowledging the complexity and confusion that exists in the literature. We began by explaining the main philosophical underpinnings of relativist ontology and subjectivist epistemology, before discussing core aspects of interpretivist methodology and the values of subjectivity, researcher involvement, and multiple meanings gained from language, actions, and objects. We mentioned how interpretivist approaches were developed to counteract positivist thinking around social research [1]. We discussed how this ascription of meaning is both an individual and a social practice, thereby avoiding the notion that our own understanding is the only one we can know [103]. These foundations of interpretivist perspectives entail us engaging reflexively across all research processes: from inception through data collection and analyses. We then highlighted five common interpretivist methodologies and methods used across HPER: phenomenology, ethnography, longitudinal qualitative research, narrative enquiry, and narrative review, each bringing its own way of recognising knowledge and knowing, data collection techniques, and analytical approaches. Following this we considered the issues of quality when engaging with interpretivist perspectives including: credibility and authenticity; transferability; dependability; confirmability; reflexivity; transparency; and internal coherence. Throughout our chapter, we shared with you our own experiences through case studies, drawing on work undertaken within this framework. We concluded by highlighting some of the challenges (e.g., reporting messy data in a tidy fashion) and strengths of interpretivist perspectives (e.g., their openness about philosophical underpinnings). As with other approaches to HPER covered in Part II of this book, we urge you to carefully consider the suitability of the approach you employ in relation to your own epistemological beliefs and the research question(s) you seek to answer, alongside judicious use of reflexivity. It has been asserted that: 'Self-understanding (in so far as this is possible) lies at the heart of this new epistemology of qualitative education research' [104 p. 155]. We invite you to consider the merits of this approach and to learn more about interpretivist approaches by pursuing the recommended readings in Box 7.11.

> **Box 7.11   Recommended reading for interpretivist approaches in HPER**
>
> Atkinson P, Pugsley L. Making sense of ethnography and medical education. *Med Educ.* 2005;39(2):228–234 [33].
>
> Barry CA, Britten N, Barber N, et al. Using reflexivity to optimize teamwork in qualitative research. *Qual Health Res.* 1999;9(1):26–44 [85].
>
> Bressers G, Brydges M, Paradis E. Ethnography in health professions education: slowing down and thinking deeply. *Med Educ.* 2020;54(3):225–233 [95].
>
> Cleland J, MacLeod A, Ellaway RH. The curious case of case study research. *Med Educ.* 2021;55(10):1131–1141 [105].
>
> Gordon L. Making space for relational reflexivity in longitudinal qualitative research. *Med Educ.* 2021;55(11):1223–1224 [45].
>
> Monrouxe LV. Solicited audio diaries in longitudinal narrative research: a view from inside. *Qual Res.* 2009;9(1):81–103 [39].
>
> Rees CE, Crampton PES, Monrouxe LV. Re-visioning academic medicine through a constructionist lens. *Acad Med.* 2020;95(6):846–850 [8].

Varpio L, Ajjawi R, Monrouxe LV, et al. Shedding the cobra effect: problematising thematic emergence, triangulation, saturation and member checking. *Med Educ.* 2017;51(1):40–50 [82].

REFERENCES

1. Gall M, Borg W, Gall J. *Educational Research: An Introduction.* White Plains, NY: Longman; 1996.

2. Schwandt T. Three epistemological stances for qualitative inquiry: interpretivism, hermeneutics and social constructionism. In Denzin NK, Lincoln YS, eds. *Handbook of Qualitative Research,* 2nd ed. Thousand Oaks, Calif.: SAGE; 2000: 189–214.

3. Schwartz-Shea P, Yanow D. *Interpretive Research Design: Concepts and Processes.* Armonk, NY: Taylor & Francis Group; 2011.

4. Ryan G. Introduction to positivism, interpretivism and critical theory. *Nurse Res.* 2018;25(4):14–20.

5. Smith B, Sparkes AC. Contrasting perspectives on narrating selves and identities: an invitation to dialogue. *Qual Res.* 2008;8(1):5–35.

6. Willis JW. *Foundations of Qualitative Research: Interpretive and Critical Approaches.* Thousand Oaks, Calif.: SAGE; 2007: 95–146.

7. Amineh RJ, Asl HD. Review of constructivism and social constructivism. *J Soc Sci Lt Lang.* 2015;1(1):9–16.

8. Rees CE, Crampton PES, Monrouxe LV. Re-visioning academic medicine through a constructionist lens. *Acad Med.* 2020;95(6):846–850.

9. Brown ME, Anderson K, Finn GM. A narrative literature review considering the development and implementation of longitudinal integrated clerkships, including a practical guide for application. *J Med Educ Curric Dev.* 2019;6:2382120519849409.

10. Ottrey E, Rees CE, Kemp C, et al. Exploring health care graduates' conceptualisations of preparedness for practice: a longitudinal qualitative research study. *Med Educ.* 2021;55(9):1078–1090.

11. Rees CE, Ottrey E, Kemp C, et al. Understanding health care graduates' conceptualizations of transitions: a longitudinal qualitative research study. *Acad Med.* 2022;97(7):1049–1056.

12. Brown MEL, Proudfoot A, Mayat NY, et al. A phenomenological study of new doctors' transition to practice, utilising participant-voiced poetry. *Adv Health Sci Educ.* 2021;26(4):1229–1253.

13. Elsey C, Challinor A, Monrouxe LV. Patients embodied and as-a-body within bedside teaching encounters: a video ethnographic study. *Adv Health Sci Educ.* 2017;22(1):123–146.

14. Elsey C, Monrouxe LV, Grant A. The reciprocal nature of trust in bedside teaching encounters. In Pelsmaekers K, Jacobs G, Rollo C, eds. *Trust and Discourse: Organizational Perspectives.* Amsterdam: John Benjamins Publishing Company; 2014: 45–70.

15. Palermo C, Reidlinger DP, Rees CE. Internal coherence matters: lessons for nutrition and dietetics research. *Nutr Diet.* 2021;78(3):252–267.

16. Berger PL, Luckmann T. *The Social Construction of Reality: A Treatise in the Sociology of Knowledge.* New York: Anchor Books; 1966.

17. Carter SM. Enacting internal coherence as a path to quality in qualitative inquiry. In Higgs J, Cherry N, Macklin R, et al., eds. *Researching Practice: A Discourse on Qualitative Methodologies*. Practice, Education, Work and Society Series, Vol. 2. Rotterdam: Sense Publishers; 2010: 143–152.

18. Denzin NK, Lincoln YS. *Handbook of Qualitative Research*. 3rd ed. Thousand Oaks, Calif.: SAGE; 2005.

19. Pring R. *Philosophy of Educational Research*. London and New York: Continuum; 2000.

20. Ismaeel M. Philosophical paradigms underlying discourse analysis: methodological implications. In Crossman J, Bordia S, eds. *Handbook of Qualitative Research Methodologies in Workplace Contexts*. Cheltenham: Edward Elgar; 2021: 47–66

21. Webb C. The use of the first person in academic writing: objectivity, language and gatekeeping. *J Adv Nurs*. 1992;17(6):747–752.

22. Timmermans S, Tavory I. Theory construction in qualitative research: from grounded theory to abductive analysis. *Sociol Theory*. 2012;30(3):167–186.

23. Philipsen K. Theory building: using abductive search strategies. In Freytag PV, Young L, eds. *Collaborative Research Design: Working with Business for Meaningful Findings*. Singapore: Springer Singapore; 2018: 45–71.

24. Littlejohn SW, Foss KA. *Encyclopedia of Communication Theory [Internet]*. Thousand Oaks, Calif.: SAGE; 2009: https://sk.sagepub.com/reference/communicationtheory (accessed 23 January 2022).

25. Biedenbach T, Jacobsson M. The open secret of values: the roles of values and axiology in project research. *Proj Manag J*. 2016;47(3):139–155.

26. Kivunja C, Kuyini AB. Understanding and applying research paradigms in educational contexts. *Int J High Educ*. 2017;6(5):26.

27. Burr V. *Social Constructionism*. 3rd ed. London and New York: Routledge; 2015.

28. Pillay R. Ethnomethodology. In Liamputtong P, ed. *Handbook of Research Methods in Health Social Sciences*. Singapore: Springer Singapore; 2019: 269–283.

29. van Manen M. *Researching Lived Experience: Human Science for an Action Sensitive Pedagogy*. 2nd ed. London and New York: Routledge; 2016.

30. Neubauer BE, Witkop CT, Varpio L. How phenomenology can help us learn from the experiences of others. *Perspect Med Educ*. 2019;8(2):90–97.

31. Wimpenny P, Gass J. Interviewing in phenomenology and grounded theory: is there a difference? *J Adv Nurs*. 2000;31(6):1485–1492.

32. McAuley J. Hermeneutic understanding. In Cassell C, Symon G, eds. *Essential Guide to Qualitative Methods in Organizational Research*. London: SAGE; 2004: https://sk.sagepub.com/books/essential-guide-to-qualitative-methods-in-organizational-research (accessed 4 July 2022).

33. Atkinson P, Pugsley L. Making sense of ethnography and medical education. *Med Educ*. 2005;39(2):228–234.

34. Arreciado Marañón A, Isla Pera MP. Theory and practice in the construction of professional identity in nursing students: a qualitative study. *Nurse Educ Today*. 2015;35(7):859–863.

35. Carey MC, Chick A, Kent B, et al. An exploration of peer-assisted learning in undergraduate nursing students in paediatric clinical settings: an ethnographic study. *Nurse Educ Today*. 2018;65:212–217.

36. Bridges SM, Chan LK, Chen JY, et al. Learning environments for interprofessional education: a micro-ethnography of sociomaterial assemblages in team-based learning. *Nurse Educ Today*. 2020;94:104569.

37. Gordon L, Rees CE, Ker J, et al. Using video-reflexive ethnography to capture the complexity of leadership enactment in the healthcare workplace. *Adv Health Sci Educ.* 2017;22(5):1101–1121.

38. Monrouxe LV. Negotiating professional identities: dominant and contesting narratives in medical students' longitudinal audio diaries. *Current Narratives.* 2009;1(1):41–59.

39. Monrouxe LV. Solicited audio diaries in longitudinal narrative research: a view from inside. *Qual Res.* 2009;9(1):81–103.

40. Gordon L, Rees CE, Jindal-Snape D. Doctors' identity transitions: choosing to occupy a state of 'betwixt and between'. *Med Educ.* 2020;54(11):1006–1018.

41. Balmer DF, Teunissen PW, Devlin MJ, et al. Stability and change in the journeys of medical trainees: a 9-year, longitudinal qualitative study. *Acad Med.* 2021;96(6):906–912.

42. Hermanowicz JC. The longitudinal qualitative interview. *Qual Sociol.* 2013;36(2):189–208.

43. McCoy LK. Longitudinal qualitative research and interpretative phenomenological analysis: philosophical connections and practical considerations. *Qual Res Psychol.* 2017;14(4):442–458.

44. Balmer DF, Varpio L, Bennett D, et al. Longitudinal qualitative research in medical education: time to conceptualise time. *Med Educ.* 2021;55(11):1253–1260.

45. Gordon L. Making space for relational reflexivity in longitudinal qualitative research. *Med Educ.* 2021;55(11):1223–1224.

46. Gordon L, Jindal-Snape D, Morrison J, et al. Multiple and multidimensional transitions from trainee to trained doctor: a qualitative longitudinal study in the UK. *BMJ Open.* 2017;7(11):e018583.

47. Squire C, Davis M, Esin C, et al. *What Is Narrative Research?* The 'What is?' Research Methods Series. New York: Bloomsbury Academic; 2014: 1–22.

48. Bruner J. The narrative construction of reality. *Crit Inq.* 1991;18(1):1–21.

49. Crossley M. *Introducing Narrative Psychology.* Buckingham: Open University Press; 2000.

50. McAdams D. Identity and the life story. In Fivush R, Haden C, eds. *Autobiographical Memory and the Construction of a Narrative Self: Development and Cultural Perspectives.* Mahwah, NJ: Lawrence Erlbaum Associates; 2003: 187–208

51. Bamberg M. Positioning between structure and performance. *J Narrat Life Hist.* 1997;7(1–4):335–342.

52. De Fina A, Georgakopoulou A. *Analyzing Narrative. Discourse and Sociolinguistic Perspectives.* Cambridge, UK: Cambridge University Press; 2012.

53. De Fina A, Georgakopoulou A. *The Handbook of Narrative Analysis.* Hoboken, NJ: John Wiley & Sons, Inc; 2015.

54. Gordon L, Rees CE, Ker JS, et al. Leadership and followership in the healthcare workplace: exploring medical trainees' experiences through narrative inquiry. *BMJ Open.* 2015;5(12):e008898.

55. Samuriwo R, Bullock A, Webb K, et al. 'Nurses whisper.' Identities in nurses' patient safety narratives of nurse–trainee doctors' interactions. *Med Educ.* 2021;55(12):1394–1406.

56. Monrouxe LV, Rees CE. "It's just a clash of cultures": emotional talk within medical students' narratives of professionalism dilemmas. *Adv Health Sci Educ.* 2012;17(5):671–701.

57. Ferrari R. Writing narrative style literature reviews. *Medical Writing*. 2015;24(4): 230–235.

58. Green BN, Johnson CD, Adams A. Writing narrative literature reviews for peer-reviewed journals: secrets of the trade. *J Chiropr Med*. 2006;5(3):101–117.

59. Greenhalgh T, Thorne S, Malterud K. Time to challenge the spurious hierarchy of systematic over narrative reviews? *Eur J Clin Invest*. 2018;48(6):e12931.

60. Grant MJ, Booth A. A typology of reviews: an analysis of 14 review types and associated methodologies. *Health Info Libr J*. 2009;26(2):91–108.

61. Gough D, Thomas J, Oliver S. Clarifying differences between review designs and methods. *Syst Rev*. 2012;1:28.

62. Dyrbye L, Shanafelt T. A narrative review on burnout experienced by medical students and residents. *Med Educ*. 2016;50(1):132–149.

63. Koea J, Rahiri J-L, Ronald M. Affirmative action programs in postgraduate medical and surgical training—a narrative review. *Med Educ*. 2021;55(3):309–316.

64. Schmidt HG, Mamede S. How to improve the teaching of clinical reasoning: a narrative review and a proposal. *Med Educ*. 2015;49(10):961–973.

65. Somporn P, Ash J, Walters L. Stakeholder views of rural community-based medical education: a narrative review of the international literature. *Med Educ*. 2018;52(8):791–802.

66. Lewis GM, Neville C, Ashkanasy NM. Emotional intelligence and affective events in nurse education: a narrative review. *Nurse Educ Today*. 2017;53:34–40.

67. Daniels AL, Morse C, Breman R. Psychological safety in simulation-based prelicensure nursing education: a narrative review. *Nurse Educ*. 2021;46(5):E99–E102.

68. Ritchie J, Spencer L. Qualitative data analysis for applied policy research. In Bryman A, Burgess R, eds. *Analysing Qualitative Data*. London and New York: Routledge; 1994: 173–194.

69. Ajjawi R, Higgs J. Using hermeneutic phenomenology to investigate how experienced practitioners learn to communicate clinical reasoning. *Qual Rep*. 2007;12(4):612–638.

70. Bynum W, Varpio L. When I say … hermeneutic phenomenology. *Med Educ*. 2018;52(3):252–253.

71. Rizan C, Elsey C, Lemon T, et al. Feedback in action within bedside teaching encounters: a video ethnographic study. *Med Educ*. 2014;48(9):902–920.

72. Marshall C, Rossman GB. *Designing Qualitative Research*, 5th ed. Thousand Oaks, Calif.: SAGE; 2011.

73. Monrouxe L, Ajjawi R, Verma AK. Observing, interviewing, diarising: understanding personal and professional identities in health professions education. *Med Educ*. 2010;44:40–49.

74. Rees C. Drawing on drawings: moving beyond text in health professions education research. *Perspect Med Educ*. 2018;7(3):166–173.

75. Ritchie J, Spencer L. Qualitative data analysis for applied policy research. In Huberman AM, Miles MB, eds. *The Qualitative Researcher's Companion: Classic and Contemporary Readings*. Thousand Oaks, Calif.: SAGE; 2002:305–330.

76. Rees CE, Monrouxe LV. "I should be lucky ha ha ha ha": the construction of power, identity and gender through laughter within medical workplace learning encounters. *J Pragmat*. 2010;42(12):3384–3399.

77. Guba EG, Lincoln YS. Paradigmatic controversies, contradictions, and emerging confluences. In Denzin NK, Lincoln YS, eds. *The SAGE Handbook of Qualitative Research*, 3rd ed. Thousand Oaks, Calif.: SAGE; 2005: 191–215.

78. Haraway D. Situated knowledges: the science question in feminism and the privilege of partial perspective. *Fem Stud*. 1988;14(3):575–599.

79. Lincoln YS, Guba EG. *Naturalistic Inquiry*. Newbury Park, Calif.: SAGE; 1985.

80. Amin MEK, Nørgaard LS, Cavaco AM, et al. Establishing trustworthiness and authenticity in qualitative pharmacy research. *Res Social Adm Pharm*. 2020; 16(10):1472–1482.

81. Rees CE, Monrouxe LV. Theory in medical education research: how do we get there? *Med Educ*. 2010;44(4):334–339.

82. Varpio L, Ajjawi R, Monrouxe LV, et al. Shedding the cobra effect: problematising thematic emergence, triangulation, saturation and member checking. *Med Educ*. 2017;51(1):40–50.

83. Alvesson M, Sköldberg K. *Reflexive Methodology: New Vistas for Qualitative Research*, 3rd ed. Thousand Oaks, Calif.: SAGE; 2018.

84. Vettraino E, Linds W, Downie H. Embodied reflexivity: discerning ethical practice through the Six-Part Story Method. *Reflective Practice*. 2019;20(2):218–233.

85. Barry CA, Britten N, Barber N, et al. Using reflexivity to optimize teamwork in qualitative research. *Qual Health Res*. 1999;9(1):26–44.

86. Varpio L, O'Brien BC, Rees CE, et al. The applicability of generalisability and bias to health professions education's research. *Med Educ*. 2021;55(2):167–173.

87. O'Brien BC, Harris IB, Beckman TJ, et al. Standards for reporting qualitative research: a synthesis of recommendations. *Acad Med*. 2014;89(9):1245–1251.

88. Tong A, Sainsbury P, Craig J. Consolidated criteria for reporting qualitative research (COREQ): a 32-item checklist for interviews and focus groups. *Int J Qual Health Care*. 2007;19(6):349–357.

89. D'Souza DM, Sade RM, Moffatt-Bruce SD. The many facets of research integrity: what can we do to ensure it? *J Thorac Cardiovasc Surg*. 2020;160(3):730–733.

90. Stewart Jr CN. *Research Ethics for Scientists: A Companion for Students* Chichester: John Wiley & Sons, Ltd; 2011.

91. Poff DC, Ginley DS. Publication ethics. In Iphofen R, ed. *Handbook of Research Ethics and Scientific Integrity*. Cham: Springer International Publishing; 2020: 107–126.

92. Lacey AJ. Novice researchers' nightmare journey of paradigms and methodologies: 'It's hard to know what is right or wrong'. In Costa A, Reis L, Souz F, et al. eds. *Computer Supported Qualitative Research: Second International Symposium in Qualitative Research (ISQR 2017)*. Advances in Intelligent Systems and Computing, Vol. 621. Cham: Springer; 2018.: 204–212

93. Monrouxe LV, Sweeney K. Between two worlds: medical students narrating tensions. In Figley C, Huggard P, Rees C, eds. *First Do No Self-Harm: Understanding and Promoting Physician Stress Resilience*. New York: Oxford University Press; 2013: 44–66.

94. Mallard G, Lamont M, Guetzkow J. Fairness as appropriateness: negotiating epistemological differences in peer review. *Sci Technol Human Values*. 2009;34(5):573–606.

95. Bressers G, Brydges M, Paradis E. Ethnography in health professions education: slowing down and thinking deeply. *Med Educ*. 2020;54(3):225–233.

96. Andreassen P, Christensen MK, Møller JE. Focused ethnography as an approach in medical education research. *Med Educ*. 2020;54(4):296–302.

97. Monrouxe LV, Ajjawi R. Ethnography, methodology: striving for clarity. *Med Educ*. 2020;54(4):284–286.

98. McMullin C. Transcription and qualitative methods: implications for third sector research. *Voluntas*; 2021;34(1):140–153. https://doi.org/10.1007/s11266-021-00400-3 (accessed 20 November 2022).

99. Mack L. The philosophical underpinnings of educational research. *Polyglossia.* 2010;19:5–11.

100. Vogl S, Zartler U, Schmidt E-M, et al. Developing an analytical framework for multiple perspective, qualitative longitudinal interviews (MPQLI). *Int J Soc Res Methodol.* 2018;21(2):177–190.

101. Hunt MR. Strengths and challenges in the use of interpretive description: reflections arising from a study of the moral experience of health professionals in humanitarian work. *Qual Health Res.* 2009;19(9):1284–1292.

102. Ataro G. Methods, methodological challenges and lesson learned from phenomenological study about OSCE experience: overview of paradigm-driven qualitative approach in medical education. *Ann Med Surg.* 2020;49:19–23.

103. Olave-Encina K, Moni K, Renshaw P. Exploring the emotions of international students about their feedback experiences. *Higher Educ Res Dev.* 2021;40(4):810–824.

104. Garrick J. Doubting the philosophical assumptions of interpretive research. *Int J Qual Stud Educ.* 1999;12(2):147–156.

105. Cleland J, MacLeod A, Ellaway RH. The curious case of case study research. *Med Educ.* 2021;55(10):1131–1141.

CHAPTER 8

Introducing Critical Approaches in Health Professions Education Research

Claire Palermo[1], Nicole Redvers[2], Gabrielle Brand[1], and Lisi J. Gordon[3]

[1] Monash University, Clayton, Victoria, Australia
[2] University of Western Ontario, London, Ontario, Canada
[3] University of Dundee, Dundee, Scotland, UK

> **Box 8.1 Chapter 8 learning objectives: After reading this chapter you should be able to ...**
>
> - Explore the multiple philosophical underpinnings (ontology, epistemology, and axiology) of critical approaches to health professions education research (HPER), including Western and Indigenous philosophies
> - Summarise common critical methodologies and methods in HPER (including key principles of sampling, data collection, and analysis)
> - Explain the main indicators of quality employed in critical approaches
> - Evaluate the strengths and challenges of critical approaches for HPER
> - Reflect on the applicability of critical approaches to your own HPER

8.1 INTRODUCING CHAPTER 8

> Today, we are called to change the world and to change it in ways that resist injustice while celebrating freedom and full, inclusive, participatory democracy. [1 p. 8]

Collectively, critical approaches aim to: 'understand and to disrupt notions of truth and the structures of power that come to be taken for granted' [2 p. 1043]. We use the term critical approaches to describe a range of different research methodologies such as critical enquiry, critical pedagogy, co-design, critical discourse analysis,

Foundations of Health Professions Education Research: Principles, Perspectives and Practices,
First Edition. Edited by Charlotte E. Rees, Lynn V. Monrouxe, Bridget C. O'Brien, Lisi J. Gordon, and Claire Palermo.
© 2023 John Wiley & Sons Ltd. Published 2023 by John Wiley & Sons Ltd.

decolonising methodologies, and critical action research. Common critical theories that inform critical approaches include critical theory, critical realism, race, class or cultural theory, gender and queer theory, and feminism theory. See our book glossary for definitions of key terms employed throughout this chapter. Critical approaches enquire about a phenomenon in a way that disrupts existing knowledges by asking questions that confront prevailing and often unexamined assumptions, illuminating them and encouraging reflexive awareness of the status quo. Critical analysis leads to the uncovering and dismantling of omissions and invisibilities, paying increased attention to power, privilege, and hierarchy [3]. Taking a critical approach allows researchers to emphasise the perspectives of those who may be in less powerful positions, for the purposes of empowerment, equality, emancipation, social justice, and enacting change. In doing so, critical approaches examine broad contexts and structures along with individual agency, and use questions that challenge existing ways of knowing and the conditions giving rise to the ways things are [3].

Critical approaches are described as having four key elements. First, *values* whereby enquiry is driven by and with the people for whom the phenomenon of interest exists. Second, an assumption of *quality*, in that the research process should produce more profound insights or generate depth of knowledge because those participating or impacted by the research are engaged in, or indeed co-designing the process. Third, the *reciprocity* premise, in that *both* researchers and research participants benefit from the research. This contrasts with other approaches that privilege knowledge developed by the researcher, including scientific and interpretivist approaches. Fourth is *utility*, whereby knowledge is exchanged for the benefit of all participants as they themselves are part of the process of gathering data and acting on or translating findings [4].

This chapter will help you consider the applicability of critical approaches to your health professions education research (HPER). For example, what methods may be used to explore the roles of individual educators and education systems in maintaining existing power structures and privilege in healthcare education? What are decolonising methodologies? How might we engage with healthcare consumers in HPER and education itself? In this chapter, we aim to help you think through the hows and whys of applying critical approaches to HPER (see Box 8.1). In section 8.2, we explore the philosophical underpinnings of critical approaches and why you should choose a critical approach in HPER, and in section 8.3, we summarise common critical methodologies and methods used in HPER. We explain and critique the key indicators of quality in critical approaches in section 8.4, and in section 8.5, we reflect on the challenges and strengths of critical approaches for HPER, before summarising the chapter in section 8.6. We bring these issues to life throughout this chapter by illustrating details associated with three case studies based on our own research employing different critical methodologies (see Box 8.2). What we present in this chapter reflects our reading of the critical literature, as well as our own experiences conducting and reviewing critical approaches in HPER. Given the limited studies using critical approaches in HPER, we have chosen methodology-focused papers highlighting what it means to take a critical approach and the processes of undertaking a critical approach. One paper focuses on a research approach for co-designing health professions education [5], and a second paper on decolonising methodologies to highlight how this philosophical positioning offers a different lens [6]. In addition, we have showcased one of our studies that took a critical approach to explore cultural and historical factors influencing recognition of excellence in dietetics [7]. We hope this chapter helps you decide if a critical approach is appropriate for your research, and prepares you for any challenges you may encounter along the way.

Box 8.2   Case studies: An overview

Co-design [5]: We describe how HPER and practice is predominantly underpinned by Western, biomedical framing of health and illness that negates the authentic and experiential knowledges derived from healthcare consumers' lived experiences. This paternalistic approach positions health professionals as the experts in health reinforcing the status quo. This is challenged through describing a research approach to partnering and legitimising healthcare consumers' lived experience knowledge and expertise in health professions education using innovative, arts and humanities-based teaching methodologies.

Decolonising Methodology [6]: We challenge the status quo of health professions education through the lens of education for sustainable healthcare. Critical global dialogues are engaged: 'on the significance of Indigenous knowledge systems in educating health professionals for a sustainable future' [6 p. 1085]. The current state of affairs is examined through a lens of decolonisation while platforming underrepresented Indigenous voices and their knowledge systems within health profession educational spaces. Attention is focused on critically examining the epistemological underpinning of current education delivery methods and its connection to research and leadership.

Critical Qualitative Study [7]: We conducted a qualitative action research study that aimed to describe the characteristics of dietetics excellence and critically review factors relevant to the recognition and promotion of excellence within the profession. We conducted focus groups to give a voice to those in the profession who had previously not been heard. After thematic analysis of the data we sought further meaning from the results using cultural–historical activity theory.

8.2 PHILOSOPHICAL UNDERPINNINGS OF CRITICAL APPROACHES

As discussed in Chapters 2 and 4, understanding the philosophical underpinnings of your research is important to enhance quality. Describing ontology (nature of reality), epistemology (nature of knowing), methodology (how we come to know) and axiology (what we value) within a particular project is important. A key part of this understanding is our personal philosophies and their influence on our research. Together this supports ensuring the internal coherence or lens of the research undertaken. That is, the alignment in thinking and doing of ontology, epistemology, methodology, and axiology within a particular project [8]. Critical approaches can be examined through a Western or decolonial lens. Section 8.2 describes a critical approach from both a Western and decolonised perspective. For the philosophical underpinnings of our case studies see Box 8.3.

8.2.1   Historical Realism Ontology

As described in Chapter 2, ontology relates to the nature of reality. Historical and critical realism typically underpins Western approaches to critical research. Historical realism attests that reality is shaped by social structures and language [9]. Critical realism suggests there is an objective reality but acknowledges the social, historical, and political features of knowledge [10]. Critical ontology acknowledges that our understanding of the world or reality is shaped by underlying social (including gender), political, cultural, economic, environmental, and ethical structures [9, 11]. Further, historical realism recognises that these structures are inherently unequal leading to a constant interaction between privilege and oppression [12]. From a decolonising perspective, reality is shaped by the lived experience of Indigenous Peoples as first peoples of the land on which the research is being conducted and through their languages and world views that inform structures and practices [13]. Decolonising ontology privileges history and lived experience pre- and postcolonisation and recognises that research is fundamentally political [13].

8.2.2 Collectivist and Subjectivist Epistemology

Western-based critical approaches are underpinned by a collectivist and subjectivist epistemology whereby knowledge is socially constructed, influenced by social structures and privileges participants' voices [9, 11]. Straddling both poststructuralism and post-positivism (also discussed in Chapter 5), critical epistemologies are seen to be reciprocal through planning and conducting research alongside participants, assuming that knowledge is subjective and dynamic in nature. Unlike other approaches, critical approaches assume that what is seen to be knowledge and knowing is continually contested by competing groups. Thus, understandings of experiences are thought to be unequal, and differ across groups because of power, position, and values associated with these collective ways of knowing [1, 12]. From a decolonising perspective, the generation of new knowledge is led by Indigenous Peoples that recognise the power of Indigenous knowledges and ways of being [14]. A decolonising philosophy to research must meaningfully contribute to the generation of knowledge that can lead to change – not just knowledge for the sake of knowledge [13]. Traditional research approaches can aim to objectify or examine struggles, whereas decolonising scholars may aim to use this knowledge for activism [13].

8.2.3 Critical Methodology

Aiming to understand and challenge existing structures, both Western and decolonising critical methodologies draw on participatory approaches that place research participants at the centre of research. Critical methodologies focus on challenging values and assumptions, and exposing structures or systems that can reinforce power differentials and keep certain groups oppressed [1]. The process of engaging in critical methodologies is transformative for both participants and researchers alike as it fosters critical consciousness and what educationist Paulo Freire describes as a re-reading of the world [15]. Thus, methodologies used in critical approaches tend to be more organic, iterative, and emergent as the researchers and participants engage in a relationally reflexive dialogue with questions and answers about the nature of the reality of phenomena being explored [16]. In this way, researchers facilitate change with participants, not of (or for) them. Examples of critical methodologies include co-production [17], participatory action research [18], visual methods (e.g., photovoice [19, 20], video-reflexive ethnography [21]), critical discourse analysis [22], critical review [23], critical ethnography [24], and decolonising methodologies [25].

8.2.4 Emancipatory Axiology

Central to critical approaches is valuing a commitment to raising awareness of, and exposing and changing what already exists. In other words: 'the critical paradigm … considers how things ought to be' [9 p. 13]. These approaches value democracy, egalitarianism, emancipation (liberation or to set free), and change [11]. At its core is building and upholding mutually respectful researcher–participant relationships, whereby participants are often co-researchers. For example: 'critical scholars in medical education study the socioeconomic, gender, racial, sexual, cultural, and linguistic correlates of persistent or growing inequities. They shed light on how medical schools and organisations function as social actors that can either foster diversity or further privilege an elite group through practice of admission' [2 p. 1044]. Critical approaches in HPER should be used when education researchers wish to challenge the status quo or deeply understand how power and privilege play out in health professions education, research, and practice. Decolonising approaches value Indigenous ways of knowing, being, and doing, respecting these ways over the dominant population where researchers learn by thinking, listening, and operating in ways that are grounded in community [13]. Decolonising approaches go beyond emancipation, to transform and develop consciousness. If your HPER questions involve issues of inequity, injustice or control, power imbalance, or focus on ideas that go against mainstream thought, critical approaches may be for you.

Box 8.3   Case studies: A summary of their philosophical underpinnings

---

Co-design [5]: Our methodology paper adopted a critical approach to co-designing education as we sought to question whose knowledge is of value in HPER? Although not specifically stated in our paper, our approach was underpinned by critical realism as we recognised that the reality (ontology) of healthcare education and related practice has been dominated by the knowledge of a single group (health and scientific experts). We aimed to shed light on the inherent power imbalance and hierarchy that exists across health professions education, research, and practice. We held the position that by partnering with healthcare consumers in the research process (collectivist epistemology) of co-designing education will: 'rebalance traditional pedagogical power relationships towards more active and collaborative consumer roles in education' [5 p. 5].

Decolonising Methodology [6]: As Indigenous Peoples, our ontological positioning for this paper was based on the concept of interconnectedness, which sees all reality from a relational lens. This interconnected worldview means that ourselves as community members, the scholarships we carry out, and the greater planet become the basis of our reality without hierarchy or imposition. We carried a Land-based epistemology with the Land and Country being an active host and originator of the learning process through traditional protocols relevant to the participants present in the dialogue.

Critical Qualitative Study [7]: We adopted a critical approach in this research whereby we sought to shed light on the structural, cultural, historical, and power issues shaping behaviour and through uncovering these issues facilitating change. Using historical realism, we recognised that the reality (ontology) was influenced

(continued)

(continued)

by structural and cultural factors. As researchers with the experience of achieving excellence or being eligible for this recognition, we worked alongside others with similar lived experiences (collectivist epistemology) to develop knowledge. We valued shedding light on issues that had previously not been uncovered in attempts to create change.

8.3 COMMON CRITICAL METHODOLOGIES AND METHODS IN HPER

There are a variety of different methodologies and methods used in critical approaches. In this section, we focus on some common and emerging critical methodologies used in HPER and provide examples of these. These include do-design, decolonising methodologies, visual methodologies, and autoethnography. Common to critical approaches is an iterative, co-design, and co-production process of continual redefinition of problems and cooperative interaction [16]. Therefore, core to these methodologies (except autoethnography) is the multidirectional, often longitudinal, dialogue and engagement between researchers and participants (both individuals and collectives). Using our case study examples, we provide examples of these methodologies and methods (see Box 8.4).

8.3.1 Co-design

Co-design methodologies align with the principles of participatory action research: partnering with key stakeholders (consumers/end-users of research) in understanding a phenomenon and using these new understandings to inform and ultimately change policies, services, and programmes as part of practice [18]. See Chapter 9 for more details on action research. Stakeholder participation in research is essential for knowledge co-creation that benefits health professionals, health professions educators, researchers, and produces impactful research outcomes [26]. Perhaps most importantly, co-design should be meaningful, relevant, and reflect the needs and expectations of the people who participate in, and will be affected by, the outcomes. This movement towards consumer involvement in health was further extended in the 2015 Vancouver Statement to ensure the patient voice is embedded across health and social care education [27]. Co-design and co-production methods are gaining momentum in HPER and can involve health professions students, faculty, or health service users, at varying levels of participation across the education continuum, including informing discipline content, curriculum design and pedagogy, and research [17]. The data collection methods that can be used to co-design education are limitless but must align with co-design aims that situate consumers/end-users at the centre of the participatory research process.

8.3.2 Decolonising Methodologies and Methods

Decolonising research methodologies are a set of approaches used to challenge Eurocentric or Western research processes that have often served to undermine the local knowledge and experiences of marginalised and oppressed populations [13, 28, 29]. More importantly, decolonising research methodologies prioritise strengths-based narratives and approaches that platform a unique way of knowing (i.e., epistemology)

> *Yarning*
> '... a conversational process that involves the sharing of stories and the development of knowledge. It prioritizes Indigenous ways of communicating, in that it is culturally prescribed, cooperative, and respectful' [36 p. 1216]. 'Yarning is a fluid ongoing process, a moving dialogue interspersed with interjections, interpretations, and additions.' [31 p. 15]
>
> *Deep listening*
> 'The Indigenous concept of Deep Listening describes a way of learning, working, and togetherness that is informed by the concepts of community and reciprocity. Deep Listening involves listening respectfully, which can help build community. It draws on every sense and every part of our being.' [37 p. 91]
>
> *Indigenous consensus processes*
> The decisions that are made through extensive collective discussion and consultation with Indigenous Peoples and communities, where ideas are legitimately shared and result in strong relations and actions [33].
>
> *Narratives*
> Stories told by communities that reflect shared aspects of experiences that help to make sense of the world [34, 35].

FIGURE 8.1   Description of examples of decolonising methods.

grounded within local community knowledge. This research approach most often has a specific intent to have positive effects and does not seek to conform to standard research structures inherent within standard Western academic processes [30]. Inherent throughout most decolonising research approaches are: a sense of responsibility to those served through the research process; a focus on relationship to the research and to the community; and the need for actioned reciprocity with the community involved or directing the research process. The methods used in a decolonised approach may vary depending on the community context, cultural protocols, and purpose of the research. Some examples of potential methods used in decolonising approaches are yarning [31], deep listening [32], Indigenous consensus processes [33], and community-based narratives (or storytelling) [34, 35]. See Figure 8.1 for more on these methods.

8.3.3   Participatory Visual Methodologies

Visual methods are emerging as a useful method in the social sciences [38, 39]. From a critical perspective, visual methods can help manage typical power relations between researchers and participants as more often than not, participants themselves manage what will, and will not, be recorded or collected [21, 40, 41]. Examples of using visual methodologies for critical approaches in HPER are photovoice and video-reflexive ethnography (VRE). Photovoice is a method whereby participants are given a camera and invited to take pictures of the phenomenon that represents their experiences [19, 20]. Through discussions of the pictures, participants can expose structural factors impacting their lives [19]. VRE is a participatory methodology that uses video methods to capture participants in their naturalistic working environment (ethnographic) before playing this footage back to participants, so they can explore the footage as a group and discuss opportunities for change (in reflexivity sessions) [21, 42]. Through watching the videos back, everyday practices are made visible and can reveal, and open up conversations about, in-the-moment unseen habits of power and practice often filtered through memory when using other methodologies [21, 41, 42]. In these approaches, these multiple realities and understandings are co-constructed with researchers who have spent time in the context, thus the researcher position is 'alongside' participants [43, 44]. This differs from the use of visual methods within interpretivist approaches, whereby researchers conduct research from the inside, serving to understand rather than change things (as discussed in Chapters 2 and 7).

8.3.4 Autoethnography

Autoethnography is a methodology used for documenting and making sense of personal experiences from the individual's own and wider sociological and cultural perspective [45]. Autoethnographers document significant and meaningful lived experiences that are grounded in personal experience to raise awareness around identity politics and silenced voices, and in doing so develop new knowledge [45]. In comparison to ethnography (see Chapter 7), autoethnography focuses on the individual participant's experience rather than a group of participants. Autoethnographers not only use their own narratives, but may also consult texts or other artefacts (for example, photographs, illustrations, or other art) and gather perspectives from others to assist in the analysis process [45]. In this approach, research is considered a: 'political, socially-just and socially conscious act' [45 p. 1], as researchers engage in a continual process of self-reflexivity to question the interplay between themselves and social life [46].

Box 8.4   Case studies: A summary of their methodologies and methods

Co-design [5]: Drawing on the five core principles of co-design (inclusive, respectful, participative, iterative, outcomes-focused) we describe an example of how you can use research co-design to reframe health professions education and practice. Genuine and trusting partnerships were developed with key industry and consumer stakeholders prior to a series of individual, in-depth, narrative-based conversations with consumers (including collecting narrative artefacts) over a two-year period. Grounded in an open, reciprocal, narrative analysis approach and rich with healthcare consumers' lived experience knowledge and understandings, we co-designed a series of humanities-based learning activities to support learners to bridge clinical and lived experience knowledges. This critical approach was chosen to deconstruct and reposition traditional, paternalistic relations in health professions education (i.e., limited consumer involvement) towards more humanised models of healthcare. Traditionally in co-design, consumers are only brought in to consult and are not involved in the co-planning, co-design, co-delivery, and co-evaluation of education. Our work describes a research approach that encompasses consumer participation throughout the whole process.

Decolonising Methodology [6]: We took an Indigenous decolonial critical approach that platformed Indigenous community voices. A narrative and reflective practice was utilised to elicit shared understandings at the community level of what needed to be amplified on the topic within health professions education spaces. The narrative and reflective practice was operationalised through the method of deep listening which is a way of learning through a state of togetherness [32], as well as through a sharing circle method focused on gathering and sharing from an interdependent perspective [47].

Critical Qualitative Study [7]: We used action research to conduct focus groups with 30 participants. Discussion explored descriptions of expertise, and perceptions of (and barriers to) recognition of excellence in the profession. Data were examined using a thematic analysis approach and participants further engaged with our interpretation of the data. Additional meaning of the initial themes was explored through cultural historical activity theory (CHAT: see Chapter 2, Box 2.3 for a further description of CHAT) [48]. The findings were shared with those in positions of influence to change the way excellence is recognised and rewarded in the profession with the aim of facilitating change.

8.3.5 Critical Sampling, Data Collection, and Analysis Methods

Critical research aims to explain and disrupt existing knowledges and uncover structures of power and privilege. Purposive sampling, also used in realist and interpretivist approaches, is a common sampling approach employed in critical research to obtain a sample that can provide a rich and lived experience of the phenomenon of interest [49]. Critical sampling approaches aim to explore an issue in depth and uncover meaning. Therefore, sample sizes are often smaller than in scientific or some interpretivist approaches. In participatory approaches, for example, visual methods or decolonising methodologies, the sample involves those who are best placed to co-design the research. Similar to interpretivist approaches, data collection methods in critical approaches are typically qualitative. Interviews, conversations with or without artefacts (e.g., photographs), focus groups, observations, and other visual methods (e.g., VRE or photovoice) are common. In addition, secondary analysis of documents, literature, or artefacts (e.g., reports, policies, paintings, photographs, drawings) with a critical lens is possible. Data collection methods draw on gathering narratives from participants themselves. Therefore, data analysis often uses narrative or thematic analysis techniques in the first instance, whereby reflexivity is central to the data analysis process, and emancipation is the goal. In addition, data collection and analysis techniques used in critical approaches must facilitate mutual trust between researchers and participants, and build participants' capacity and empower them through the process. In this co-analysis, participants and researchers work together to analyse the data, which contrasts to an interpretivist approach where the analysis is led by the research team. It is outside the scope of this book chapter on the foundations of critical approaches to cover the wide-ranging critical research methods in depth, so instead, we refer you to other sources [3, 22, 50]. Before moving on to the next section, pause and reflect on how you might apply critical approaches to your own HPER (see Box 8.5).

Box 8.5 Pause and reflect: Applying critical methodologies/methods to your research

- Think about a topic of enquiry in health professions education that you are especially interested in researching. This may relate to a challenge regarding your own teaching or learning, or a taken-for-granted assumption on your own education, or it may link to previous research you have done, or could relate to key gaps in the literature.

(continued)

(continued)

- How might you involve the affected community in co-designing, co-developing, refining, and operationalising your research questions and methodologies/methods?
- Now think of a research question pertaining to your chosen topic that does not align well with critical approaches. What other methodologies/methods are more appropriate for this question and why? What other chapters should you therefore read next?
- Revisit this pause and reflect box once you have read the other chapters in Part II, and further developed your research ideas.

8.4   KEY QUALITY INDICATORS IN CRITICAL APPROACHES

Given that critical approaches typically draw on qualitative data collection methods, similar indicators of quality central to interpretivist approaches can also be recommended for critical approaches. Authenticity or the credibility of the research is a key marker of quality [49]. Research is credible when it exposes the multiple realities of participants and the researchers, and the findings are eloquent [49, 51]. In critical approaches, credibility also relates to whether the research process and outcomes have empowered participants and led to change for marginalised groups [51]. Transferability or applicability refers to whether the findings of the research can be transferred to other participant groups or contexts, and the usefulness of the findings [49, 51]. Dependability is the qualitative equivalent to objectivity that relates to the trustworthiness of the data [49]. Confirmability is about whether the findings and their interpretation clearly match the data from which they are drawn [49]. Confirmability can be maintained through reflexivity whereby researcher experience is acknowledged as part of the research and it is made visible how this experience will add to the multiple understandings embraced by these research approaches [51, 52].

As part of reflexivity in all approaches, researchers are encouraged to actively engage in a personal reflexive process. This is often undertaken through diarising and discussion with other research team members, and acknowledgement of these influences [49]. Reflexivity serves to emphasise both the researcher and the team's presence in the research [53]. In critical approaches, reflexivity requires researchers to be aware of their position in the research, which is often evolving alongside co-researchers (the participants) through the research journey together [54, 55]. In critical approaches, researchers need to examine their own values and beliefs, including personal and professional privileges. For example, researchers supporting decolonising approaches within communities must engage in self-reflection and reflexive relational practice of their experiences, ideas, and preconceptions [56]. As a researcher this can make you feel quite exposed as your relationships, influences, and understandings are mutually explored by participants as much as you will be exploring theirs [45]. These research encounters provide a potent space to co-produce new knowledge that neither researcher nor participants previously considered – highlighting the importance of relational reflexivity [57]. Through engaging in research itself, relational reflexivity becomes a process of co-production and a central tenet of critical research [58]. In Box 8.6, we provide brief reflexive commentaries from the researchers about their experiences of undertaking each of the case studies.

Transparency is also a useful marker of quality in critical approaches ensuring that both participants and researchers are clearly involved in data collection and interpretation [4]. Another key marker of quality in critical approaches is ethics. Given the participatory involvement of those engaged in the research, the role participants play needs careful consideration in terms of ethical principles with a particular focus on justice, beneficence, and respect (see Chapter 3 for more details on ethics).

Box 8.6   Case studies: Reflections on experiences as critical researchers

Co-design [5]: Working with co-design methodologies in HPER presents both opportunities and challenges. The inclusive, collaborative, and participatory nature of this approach, which most often occurs over a prolonged period of time, requires researchers to be open, reflexive, and adaptable. For example, in this paper, we share our experience of co-designing education with mental health consumers and how it reframed how we work with people, as health professionals, educators, and researchers. The relational experience stimulated deep, critical reflection on how Western reductionist framing of illness pathologises the problem of mental illness, and thus extends to how we educate health professionals. This uncomfortable realisation highlights the need to shift this deficit discourse towards more inclusive, strengths-based, recovery-oriented language and practice.

Decolonising Methodology [6]: In decolonising methodologies, positionality is foundational to the research process [25]. Who you are, your lived experience, your family connections, and your Land and environmental connections all position you as a researcher within the relationship of the research and the communities served through the research process. HPER has not been historically attuned to positionality due to the needs of reducing bias, as per scientific approaches discussed previously in Chapter 5. Due to this, we were required in this paper to push critical boundaries by stating clearly our positionality in the context of the work, placing us as members of Indigenous communities of practice to ensure our decolonising premise of the paper was not lost in the presentation and Western format of delivery. For critical dialogues to occur, we recognised the importance of not compromising on the established Indigenous community norms inherent within decolonised methodologies.

Critical Qualitative Approach [7]: Using critical approaches in a profession whose roots lie in scientific approaches challenged us as authors, as well as the audience for which our manuscript was intended. We were challenged in our position in the research, feeling uncomfortable being both the researchers and the participants. Through our writing, we wanted to disrupt current practice and change the way the profession recognises excellence. As such, we were challenged in our writing to prepare a manuscript that provided an outcome, that is, description of excellence, together with a critical lens on why so few in the profession achieved this recognition. This may have resulted in some misalignment of internal coherence in our reporting [11].

For scientific and realist approaches, quality indicators translate neatly into multiple tools and checklists for researchers that enhance the quality conduct and reporting of research. As with interpretivist approaches, in critical approaches, we may challenge the use of quality tools and checklists due to the wide range of research undertaken [59]. While there is no specific tool recommended for use in critical approaches, the Standards for QUality Improvement Reporting Excellence (SQUIRE) [60] and Standards for QUality Improvement Reporting Excellence in Education (SQUIRE-EDU) [61] are recommended for: 'the reporting of qualitative and quantitative evaluations of the nature and impact of interventions intended to improve healthcare, with the understanding that the guidelines may be adapted as needed for specific situations' [60 p. e7]. In addition, the Public and Patient Engagement Evaluation Tool [62], GRIPP2 [63] or the National Health and Medical Research Council's Statement on Consumer and Community Involvement in Health and Medical Research [64] can assist researchers when planning and conducting their studies, to consider how and when consumers or participants are engaged in the research process. Used together they may support quality checking and reporting for critical approaches. Box 8.7 provides some guidance on how to achieve key quality markers for a critical approach. Before moving on to the next section test your knowledge of quality indicators in critical approaches by completing the activity in Box 8.8.

Box 8.7   Case studies: A summary of their quality

Co-design [5]: Despite prioritising the active participation of consumers in healthcare improvement [65], research [64], and accreditation standards for health professional degrees, to date there is a lack of clarity on what constitutes quality in co-design across both healthcare and HPER. Therefore, to ensure the credibility of our work we demonstrated transparency through clearly describing five core principles for undertaking successful co-design, including co-authoring the paper with both academic and lived experience researchers and educators (authenticity). Reflexivity was demonstrated through the authors sharing their evolving health professional or personal reflexive accounts of power disparities during the co-design process. Finally, the ongoing participative nature of co-design requires attention to ethics, and a heightened awareness of consumers shifting recovery processes that require regular check-ins, so that ethical principles of justice, beneficence, and respect are upheld throughout the research.

Decolonising Methodology [6]: We did not utilise any Western quality metrics or frameworks in our research process. Within many Indigenous research methodologies, it can be cultural incongruent and inappropriate to judge or assess the quality of others' work. As quality frameworks are primarily rooted within Western ways of knowing, using a Western paradigm for quality assessment can be seen as an extension of colonial processes. For example, traditional Indigenous medicine is considered very sacred and it would therefore be culturally unacceptable in many instances to critique the application or method of another Indigenous communities' traditional medicine protocols from one's own. The appropriateness of using Western quality frameworks within Indigenous research contexts should be explored with Indigenous communities directly ensuring community cultural protocols are followed. As Indigenous Nations around the globe are incredibly diverse, how a community decides what is relevant for them will be contextual to the place of the work.

Critical Qualitative Approach [7]: The credibility of our work was evident in that it led to change in how the process of awarding excellence in the profession was administered. Engaging research participants in data collection and data interpretation supported the transparency and dependability of the findings. Being clear about our position as researchers in the reporting of the work and how we managed this positioning during data collection and analysis provided evidence of our reflexivity.

Box 8.8   Stop and do: Critically appraise a critical paper

- Read the following open access paper: Lepre et al. Nutrition competencies for medicine: an integrative review and critical synthesis. *BMJ Open.* 2021;11(3):e043066. https://bmjopen.bmj.com/content/11/3/e043066

- Pick the most appropriate quality reporting tool from those listed in section 8.4, and using your selected tool, critically appraise this paper.

- What critical indicators of quality are apparent in this paper, and what is missing or could be improved?

- Reflect on the limitations of the quality reporting tool and why quality checklists may not be appropriate for critical approaches? What could be better?

8.5   CHALLENGES AND STRENGTHS OF EMPLOYING CRITICAL APPROACHES IN HPER

Embarking on critical approaches in HPER is not without its challenges. A key challenge is that of reflexivity, which goes beyond the reflexivity used in interpretivist approaches (as discussed in Chapter 7), whereby researchers need to examine their own values and beliefs, including personal and professional privileges. As described above, critical approaches are not common in HPER so researchers in this area may experience mainstream resistance to their approach as they depart from traditional ways of knowing and doing HPER [16]. Another key challenge is the vulnerability of the researcher during the research process [58]. This includes relinquishing control and truly partnering with participants as co-researchers and being an agent of change through speaking out about hidden issues, structures, and systems that challenge the status quo [66]. Participatory research approaches take time and can be intensive because they are led by the participants themselves as co-researchers who may have competing priorities (i.e., not solely focused on research) [67]. In addition, many participatory and co-design projects do not have a natural end and require a long-term commitment by researchers, which may be challenging for time-limited research grants or funded research positions [17].

While opportunities exist to examine health professions education phenomena from critical perspectives, researchers still typically opt for more traditional approaches. For example, traditional systematic review approaches have been used for reviewing clinical placements in underserved areas [68], and interpretivist philosophies have been used for participatory research to guide education for those living in poverty [69], and examine culture and power in a profession [70].

However, there have been recent calls to use more critical theory such as feminist theory in HPER [71], and we hope this chapter provides guidance to support more researchers to undertake HPER using critical approaches.

Key strengths of critical approaches include the potential for reciprocal benefits for researchers and participants in that there is two-way learning through this dual process of trust and reciprocity. Another key strength is capacity building with participant groups who may be under-represented or misrepresented in HPER [72]. Critical approaches also align with health professions educators' philosophy to work with (instead of on) those at the centre of the research. This positions the consumer at the heart of the research process to work towards making a difference to individual and community health outcomes. This is in contrast to other, more positivist philosophies that generate new knowledge for the research community. Most importantly perhaps, critical approaches aim to raise awareness of hidden phenomena that often disrupt existing knowledges and hierarchical or power structures in education systems. Critical approaches have the potential to challenge the status quo regarding health professions education practice that could lead to positive changes. See Box 8.9 for reflections on the strengths and challenges in our case studies.

Box 8.9   Case studies: A summary of their strengths and challenges

Co-design [5]: A key strength of our study was the rich potential of participatory, co-design research to rebalance pedagogical power relations towards more equal, collaborative consumer roles in education that enhance health professional learning and practice. However, challenges included the time it took for collaborative data collection and analysis cycles, which contrasted with unrealistic time frames set by funding bodies. In addition, the diversity of our research team (academics and consumers) disrupted usual ways of knowing and doing in HPER, challenging our team's personal and professional values and belief systems. This was overcome by deliberate checking in around sharing power and decision-making that demanded all researchers remain open, adaptive, responsive, and reflexive during the entire research process.

Decolonising Methodology [6]: Through global Indigenous representation, we were able to transcend traditional geographic health professions educational boundaries and critique overarching notions of knowledge application within developing sustainability spaces in healthcare. Our largest struggle using a decolonial approach was fitting the narrative into a Westernised journal structure. Due to established norms in academic processes, Indigenous research methodologies often have to conform their narratives to Western structures to even get the ability to be heard. As participants in this work came from Indigenous communities across the world, we had to be very mindful and respectful of the different traditional protocols and processes that can exist in different Indigenous communities. Although there are many synergies across Indigenous communities in terms of the structures of power and processes that they face, due to geographic differences, and different Land and cultural histories, consensus was a really important process to embody to ensure all participants were speaking from one heart.

Critical Qualitative Approach [7]: The key challenge was how we managed reflexivity as key people experiencing the phenomenon of recognition of excellence in the profession. We overcame this challenge by regularly reminding ourselves of our own experiences and position, and how, throughout data collection and analysis, this may be contributing to and shaping the research. The strengths of our work were in uncovering novel findings about our profession and its identity, which helped shape understandings and how excellence in the profession was rewarded in the future. The work has led to changes in the way excellence is recognised and the process for which leaders in the profession apply to be rewarded.

8.6 CHAPTER SUMMARY

In this chapter, we have explored and discussed the philosophical underpinnings of critical approaches to HPER – historical realism ontology, collectivist and subjectivist epistemology, and the emancipatory axiology or values underpinning this approach. We have provided a brief overview of common critical methodologies used in HPER (i.e., co-design, decolonising and visual methodologies, autoethnography), data collection methods (e.g., interview, photovoice, VRE), and data analysis (e.g., narrative, thematic). We have also outlined key quality indicators (i.e., confirmability, relational reflexivity, and ethics), including guidelines that may support the appraisal of critical research (e.g., SQUIRE guidelines, Public and Patient Engagement Evaluation Tool). We have outlined strengths (e.g., reciprocal benefits, facilitating change, challenging existing assumptions and structures) and have articulated key challenges (e.g., relational reflexivity, long-term commitment) of critical approaches in HPER. There is, however, no denying the potential value of critical approaches in HPER – raising awareness of issues, disrupting existing knowledges and facilitating change – albeit that these are still underutilised in HPER currently [73, 74]. However, like all approaches outlined in Part II of this book, we urge you to be mindful of the ways in which you adopt critical approaches, which may not always transfer appropriately to HPER. We encourage you to think critically about the use of critical approaches in HPER. We hope this chapter has clearly articulated the basics of critical approaches, while also encouraging you to see how you may use critical approaches in your own research. We invite you to continue your learning about critical approaches through completing the reflexive activity outlined in Box 8.10. We also encourage you to consider the merits of critical approaches and to learn more about this approach by pursuing the recommended readings in Box 8.11. As with all approaches to HPER covered in Part II of this book, we urge you to consider the suitability of the approach you employ in relation to your own epistemological beliefs and the research question(s) you seek to answer.

It is time to turn the mirror towards ourselves so we can unpack some uncomfortable truths and tackle the role of the profession in reproducing inequalities. [75 p. 1348]

> **Box 8.10   Stop and do: What are your positions in critical research approaches?**
>
> Practise having an honest conversation with someone from a different gender, sex, cultural or educational background, or discipline from your own. Consider:
>
> - What assumptions did you make before commencing the conversation? Where did these assumptions come from?
> - Who does the person remind you of? Is this positive or negative?
> - What influences your impression?
> - Whose knowledge is of value? Do you value objective or subjective knowledges, and why?
> - Are these influences grounded in evidence or your unexplored assumptions?

> **Box 8.11   Recommended reading for critical approaches in HPER**
>
> Hodges BD. When I say ... critical theory. *Med Educ.* 2014;48(11):1043–1044 [2].
> Cleland J, Razack S. When I say ... privilege. *Med Educ.* 2021;55(12):1347–1349 [75].
> Brand G, Sheers C, Wise S, et al. A research approach for co-designing education with healthcare consumers. *Med Educ.* 2021;55(5):574–581 [5].
> Matias, CE. *The Handbook of Critical Theoretical Research Methods in Education.* London and New York: Routledge; 2021 [73].
> Paradis EL, Nimmon L, Wondimagegn D, et al. Critical theory: broadening our thinking to explore the structural factors at play in health professions education. *Acad Med.* 2020;95(6):842–845 [74].
> Redvers N, Schultz C, Vera Prince M, et al. Indigenous perspectives on education for sustainable healthcare. *Med Teach.* 2020;42(10):1085–1090 [6].
> Tuhiwai Smith L. *Decolonizing Methodologies: Research and Indigenous Peoples.* London: Bloomsbury Publishing; 2021 [13].

REFERENCES

1. Denzin N. Critical qualitative inquiry. *Qual Inq.* 2017;23(1):8–16.

2. Hodges B. When I say ... critical theory. *Med Educ.* 2014;48(11):1043–1044.

3. Swaminathan R, Mulvihill T. *Critical Approaches to Questions in Qualitative Research.* New York and London: Routledge; 2017.

4. Patton MQ. *Qualitative Research and Evaluation Methods: Integrating Theory and Practice.* 4th ed. Thousand Oaks, Calif.: SAGE; 2014.

5. Brand G, Sheers C, Wise S, et al. A research approach for co-designing education with healthcare consumers. *Med Educ.* 2021;55(5):574–581.

6. Redvers N, Schultz C, Vera Prince M, et al. Indigenous perspectives on education for sustainable healthcare. *Med Teach.* 2020;42(10):1085–1090.

7. Palermo C, Allen L, Dart J, et al. Hidden Jedi: a critical qualitative exploration of the fellow credential and advanced expertise. *Nutr Diet.* 2020;77(1):167–176.

8. Rees CE, Monrouxe LV. Theory in medical education research: how do we get there? *Med Educ.* 2010;44(4):334–339.

9. Scotland J. Exploring the philosophical underpinning of research: relating ontology and epistemology to the methodology and methods of the scientific, interpretive and critical research paradigms. *English Language Teaching*. 2012;5(9):9–16.

10. Brekke J, Anastas J, Floersch J, et al. The realist frame: scientific realism and critical realism. In Brekke J, Anastas J, eds. *Shaping a Science of Social Work: Professional Knowledge and Identity*. Online Edition New York: Oxford University Academic; 2019: 22–40.

11. Palermo C, Reidlinger DP, Rees CE. Internal coherence matters: lessons for nutrition and dietetics research. *Nutr Diet*. 2021;78(3):252–267.

12. Lincoln YS, Lynham SA, Guba EG. Paradigmatic controversies, contradictions, and emerging confluences revisited. In Denzin NK, Lincoln YS, eds. *The Sage Handbook of Qualitative Research*. 5th ed. Thousand Oaks, Calif.: SAGE; 2018: 108–150.

13. Tuhiwai Smith L. *Decolonizing Methodologies: Research and Indigenous Peoples*. 2nd ed. London: Zed Books; 2012.

14. Braun KL, Browne CV, Ka'opua LS, et al. Research on Indigenous elders: from positivistic to decolonizing methodologies. *Gerontol*. 2014;54(1):117–126.

15. Freire P. *Pedagogy of the Oppressed*. 20th Anniversary Ed. New York: Continuum, 1993.

16. Bunniss S, Kelly DR. Research paradigms in medical education research. *Med Educ*. 2010;44(4):358–366.

17. O'Connor S, Zhang M, Trout KK, et al. Co-production in nursing and midwifery education: a systematic review of the literature. *Nurs Educ Today*. 2021;102:104900.

18. Stringer E. *Action Research in Education*. Upper Saddle River, NJ: Pearson Prentice Hall; 2008.

19. Jaiswal D, To MJ, Hunter H, et al. Twelve tips for medical students to facilitate a photovoice project. *Med Teach*. 2016;38(10):981–986.

20. Rees C. Drawing on drawings: moving beyond text in health professions education research. *Perspect Med Educ*. 2018;7(3):166–173.

21. Gordon L, Rees C, Ker J, et al. Using video-reflexive ethnography to capture the complexity of leadership enactment in the healthcare workplace. *Adv Health Sci Educ*. 2017;22(5):1101–1121.

22. Smith JL. Critical discourse analysis for nursing research. *Nurs Inquiry*. 2007; 14(1):60–70.

23. McGaghie WC, Issenberg SB, Barsuk JH, et al. A critical review of simulation-based mastery learning with translational outcomes. *Med Educ*. 2014;48(4):375–385.

24. Cook KE. Using critical ethnography to explore issues in health promotion. *Qual Health Res*. 2005;15(1):129–138.

25. Tuhiwai Smith L. *Decolonizing Methodologies: Research and Indigenous Peoples*, 3rd ed. London: Bloomsbury; 2021.

26. Jackson CL, Greenhalgh T. Co-creation: a new approach to optimising research impact. *Med J Aust*. 2015;203(7):283–284.

27. Towle A, Farrell C, Gaines ME, et al. The patient's voice in health and social care professional education: the Vancouver Statement. *Int J of Hth Gov*. 2016;21(1):18–25.

28. Nhemachena A, Mlambo N, Kaundjua M. The notion of the "field" and the practices of researching and writing Africa: towards decolonial praxis. *Africology: The J Pan Afr Studies*. 2016;9(7):15–36.

29. Khupe C, Keane M. Towards an African education research methodology: decolonising new knowledge. *Educ Res Soc Change*. 2017;6(1):25–37.

30. Redvers N, Wilkinson M, Fischer C. Colorectal cancer community engagement: a qualitative exploration of American Indian voices from North Dakota. *BMC Cancer*. 2022;9(1):158.

31. Geia LK, Hayes B, Usher K. Yarning/Aboriginal storytelling: towards an understanding of an Indigenous perspective and its implications for research practice. *Contemp Nurse*. 2013;46(1):13–17.

32. Ungunmerr-Baumann MR, Brennan F. Reverencing the earth in the Australia dreaming. *The Way*. 1989;29:38–45.

33. Ferrazzi P, Tagalik S, Christie P, et al. Aajiiqatigiingniq: an Inuit consensus methodology in qualitative health research. *Int J Qual Meth*. 2019;18: 1–9

34. Wexler L, White J, Trainor B. Why an alternative to suicide prevention gatekeeper training is needed for rural Indigenous communities: presenting an empowering community storytelling approach. *Critical Public Health*. 2015;25(2):205–217.

35. Redvers N, Yellow Bird M, Quinn D, et al. Molecular decolonization: an Indigenous microcosm perspective of planetary health. *Int J Environ Res Pub Hlth*. 2020;17(12):4586.

36. Walker M, Fredericks B, Mills K, et al. "Yarning" as a method for community-based health research with Indigenous women: the Indigenous Women's Wellness Research Program. *Health Care Women Int*. 2014;35(10):1216–1226.

37. Brearley L. Deep listening and leadership: an Indigenous model of leadership and community development in Australia. In Voyageur C, Brearley L, Calliou B, eds. *Restorying Indigenous Leadership: Wise Practices in Community Development*, 2nd ed. Banff: Banff Centre Press; 2015: 91–127.

38. Rees CE. Identities as performances: encouraging visual methodologies in medical education research. *Med Educ*. 2010;44(1):5–7.

39. Iedema R, Mesman J, Carroll K. *Visualising Health Care Practice Improvement: Innovation from Within*. London: Radcliffe Publishing; 2013.

40. Mesman J, Walsh K, Kinsman L, et al. Blending video-reflexive ethnography with solution-focused approach: a strengths-based approach to practice improvement in health care. *Int J Qual Meth*. 2019;18:1–10.

41. Ajjawi R, Hilder J, Noble C, et al. Using video-reflexive ethnography to understand complexity and change practice. *Med Educ*. 2020;54(10):908–914.

42. Iedema R. Research paradigm that tackles the complexity of in situ care: video reflexivity. *BMJ Qual Safe*. 2019;28(2):89–90.

43. Carroll K. Outsider, insider, alongsider: examining reflexivity in hospital-based video research. *Int J Mult Res Approaches*. 2009;3(3):246–263.

44. Carroll K, Mesman J. Multiple researcher roles in video-reflexive ethnography. *Qual Health Res*. 2018;28(7):1145–1156.

45. Ellis C, Adams T, Bochner AP. Autoethnography: an overview. *Histor Soc Res*. 2011;12(4):273–290.

46. Adams T, Ellis C, Jones S. Autoethnography. In Matthes J, Davis CS, Potter RF, eds. *The International Encyclopedia of Communication Research Methods*. Hoboken: John Wiley & Sons, Inc; 2017: 1–11.

47. Tachine AR, Yellow Bird E, Cabrera NL. Sharing circles: an Indigenous methodological approach for researching with groups of Indigenous peoples. *Int Rev Qual Res*. 2016;9(3):277–295.

48. Foot KA. Cultural-historical activity theory: exploring a theory to inform practice and research. *J Hum Behav Soc Environ*. 2013;24(3):329–347.

49. Liamputtong P. *Qualitative Research Methods*, 5th ed. Melbourne: Oxford University Press; 2019.

50. Strydom P. *Contemporary Critical Theory and Methodology*. London and New York: Routledge; 2011.

51. Kitto SC, Chesters J, Grbich C. Quality in qualitative research. *Med J Aust*. 2008;188(4):243–246.

52. Cassell C, Radcliffe LS, Malik F. Participant reflexivity in organizational research design. *Org Res Meth*. 2020;23(4):750–773.

53. Barry CA, Britten N, Barber N, et al. Using reflexivity to optimize teamwork in qualitative research. *Qual Health Res*. 1999;9(1):26–44.

54. Carroll KF, Mesman J. Ethnographic context meets ethnographic biography: a challenge for the mores of doing fieldwork. *Int J Mult Res Approaches*. 2011;5(2):155–168.

55. Horsfall D, Higgs J. Boundary riding and shaping research spaces. In Higgs J, Titchen A, Horsfall D, et al., eds. *Creative Spaces for Qualitative Researching*. Rotterdam: Sense Publishers; 2011: 45–54.

56. McCartan J, Brimblecombe J, Adams K. Methodological tensions for non-Indigenous people in Indigenous research: a critique of critical discourse analysis in the Australian context. *Soc Sci Hum Open*. 2022;6(1): 100282.

57. Enosh G, Ben-Ari A. Reflexivity: the creation of liminal spaces – researchers, participants, and research encounters. *Qual Health Res*. 2016;26(4):578–584.

58. Gordon L. Making space for relational reflexivity in longitudinal qualitative research. *Med Educ*. 2021;55(11):1223–1224.

59. Buus N, Agdal R. Can the use of reporting guidelines in peer-review damage the quality and contribution of qualitative health care research? *Int J Nurs Stand*. 2013;50(10):1289–1291.

60. Goodman D, Ogrinc G, Davies L, et al. Explanation and elaboration of the SQUIRE (Standards for QUality Improvement Reporting Excellence) Guidelines V.2.0: examples of SQUIRE elements in the healthcare improvement literature. *BMJ Qual Safe*. 2016;25(12):e7.

61. Ogrinc G, Armstrong GE, Dolansky MA, et al. SQUIRE-EDU (Standards for QUality Improvement Reporting Excellence in Education): publication guidelines for educational improvement. *Acad Med*. 2019;94(10):1461–1470.

62. Abelson J, Li K, Wilson G, et al. Supporting quality public and patient engagement in health system organizations: development and usability testing of the Public and Patient Engagement Evaluation Tool. *Health Exp*. 2016;19(4):817–827.

63. Staniszewska S, Brett J, Simera I, et al. GRIPP2 reporting checklists: tools to improve reporting of patient and public involvement in research. *BMJ*. 2017;358:j3453.

64. National Health and Medical Research Council (NHMRC). Statement on consumer and community involvement in health and medical research. 2016. https://www.nhmrc.gov.au/about-us/publications/statement-consumer-and-community-involvement-health-and-medical-research (accessed 3 September 2022).

65. Australian Commission of Safety and Quality in Health Care. *National Safety and Quality Health Service (NSQHS) Standards: Partnering with Consumers Standard*. Sydney, NSW: 2022.

66. Halman M, Baker L, Ng S. Using critical consciousness to inform health professions education. *Perspect Med Educ*. 2017;6(1):12–20.

67. Baum F, MacDougall C, Smith D. Participatory action research. *J Epidemiol Community Health*. 2006;60(10):854–857.

68. Crampton PES, McLachlan JC, Illing JC. A systematic literature review of undergraduate clinical placements in underserved areas. *Med Educ*. 2013;47(10):969–978.

69. Hudon C, Loignon C, Grabovschi C, et al. Medical education for equity in health: a participatory action research involving persons living in poverty and healthcare professionals. *BMC Med Educ*. 2016;16:106.

70. Mitchell P, Nightingale J. Sonography culture: power and protectionism. *Radiography*. 2019;25(3):227–234.

71. Finn GM, Brown MEL. Ova-looking feminist theory: a call for consideration within health professions education and research. *Adv Health Sci Educ*. 2022;27(3):893–913.

72. Grumbach K, Mendoza R. Disparities in human resources: addressing the lack of diversity in the health professions. *Health Aff (Millwood)*. 2008;27(2):413–422.

73. Matias CE. *The Handbook of Critical Theoretical Research Methods in Education*. London and New York: Routledge; 2021.

74. Paradis EL, Nimmon L, Wondimagegn D, et al. Critical theory: broadening our thinking to explore the structural factors at play in health professions education. *Acad Med*. 2020;95(6):842–845.

75. Cleland J, Razack S. When I say ... privilege. *Med Educ*. 2021;55(12):1347–1349.

Introducing Pragmatic Approaches in Health Professions Education Research

Bridget C. O'Brien[1], Louise Allen[2], Ahsan Sethi[3], Marieke van der Schaaf[4], and Claire Palermo[2]

[1] University of California San Francisco, San Francisco, California, USA
[2] Monash University, Clayton, Victoria, Australia
[3] Qatar University, Doha, Qatar
[4] University Medical Centre Utrecht, Utrecht, Netherlands

Box 9.1 Chapter 9 learning objectives: After reading this chapter you should be able to ...

- Describe the philosophical underpinnings (axiology, ontology, and epistemology) of pragmatic approaches
- Summarise common pragmatic methodologies and methods in health professions education research (HPER)
- Explain the main indicators of quality employed in pragmatic approaches
- Evaluate the strengths and challenges of pragmatic approaches for HPER
- Reflect on the applicability of pragmatic approaches to your own HPER

9.1 INTRODUCING CHAPTER 9

Pragmatism is not a recipe for educational research and educational researchers; it does not offer prescriptions. It is ... a way of un-thinking certain false dichotomies, certain assumptions, certain traditional practices and ways of doing things, and in this it can open up new possibilities for thought. [1 p. 114]

You have likely heard people describe themselves or their approach as pragmatic. The term connotes a practical or sensible orientation that draws on experience to

---

guide action and solve problems. While this usage captures the general orientation of pragmatism, our discussion of pragmatic approaches in this chapter considers the philosophical roots of pragmatism and its development as an approach to educational research. As reflected in the initial quote, pragmatic approaches are best characterised by their shared commitment to 'open up new possibilities' [1 p. 114], through enquiry grounded in practical experiences, actions, and consequences [2, 3]. Pragmatic approaches are not wedded to certain theories and methodologies; instead, they welcome conversations across approaches and value pluralism – the position that multiple theories can be true and that multiple methodologies can contribute to these truths [4]. In this chapter, we discuss pragmatic approaches as a form of research that prioritises the purpose and actionable consequences of research over adherence to conventions. The sections of this chapter aim to help you think through the hows and whys of taking a pragmatic approach to health professions education research (HPER) (see Box 9.1). In section 9.2, we describe the philosophical underpinnings of pragmatic approaches, and in section 9.3, we summarise common characteristics of methodologies and methods used in pragmatic approaches to HPER. We discuss the key markers of quality in pragmatic research in section 9.4, and in section 9.5, we evaluate the challenges and strengths of pragmatic approaches for HPER before summarising the chapter in section 9.6. Throughout this chapter we use four case studies (see Box 9.2) to illustrate important issues and considerations when using a pragmatic approach and to highlight when a pragmatic approach may be useful to consider in HPER. We hope this chapter helps you understand that using a pragmatic approach is not just about asking what works or finding practical solutions, and that the chapter helps you appreciate the fundamental values associated with pragmatic approaches and how to use them to guide rigorous research.

Box 9.2   Case studies: An overview

Explanatory Mixed Methods [5–7]: We investigated the impact of postgraduate qualifications in medical education on health professionals' educational identities, practices, and career progression by employing mixed methods. The professional identity of healthcare educators is a new and complex concept, so we chose a pragmatic approach given our desire to ensure the relevance and applicability of our findings. Mixed methods allowed us to explore the relationship between postgraduate qualifications and identities in depth. Understanding these identities have implications for improving health professionals' experiences as educators and furthering the professionalisation of medical education. Our findings also informed policy and practice, thereby justifying the time and resources requested. Our study comprised an online survey of graduates working in diverse contexts worldwide [5], combined sequentially with semi-structured interviews [6, 7].

Adapted Exploratory Mixed Methods [8–10]: We explored the broad range of impacts of continuing professional development (CPD) on individuals, organisations, and systems. Our approach was pragmatic in that we sought to better understand what these broad impacts were, and to determine how to measure them. We conducted a systematic scoping review and a qualitative study that utilised semi-structured interviews and thematic analysis. The results from these two studies then informed the development of a survey to measure the broad impacts of CPD. This was deemed important to practice as the systematic scoping review showed

(continued)

(continued)

that unvalidated surveys were the most common means of measuring CPD impacts, and that while some validated surveys existed, they focused on one category of impact. We determined that developing and validating a survey measuring broad CPD impacts would be a useful next step.

Action Research [11]: We selected a pragmatic approach to examine how professional and educational development activities (lesson study) contributed to changes in teachers' pedagogical content knowledge (PCK) about research supervision. Lesson study is a type of action research with a pragmatic orientation in which teachers seek to improve students' learning by engaging in collaborative professional development [12]. Multiple types of data are collected (e.g., artefacts, observation, interviews) from multiple sources (e.g., teachers, learners), and contexts (e.g., different classes or clinics). Teachers used data from their own teaching experiences as evidence to guide their discussion and professional development [13]. Lesson study can help teachers to develop the (practical) knowledge and (collaborative) action they need to improve education in practice (e.g., teaching students) [14]. Our lesson study approach engaged a team of teachers in regular meetings to (re)design research education and supervision through collaborative inquiry and evaluation. We gained insight into how teachers developed their PCK in research supervision by collecting and analysing data from: nine videotaped observations of lesson study group meetings, four reports from students of each teacher supervising their research, and one interview with each teacher.

Constructivist Grounded Theory [15]: Our medical school aims to prepare physicians for lifelong learning through curricula on enquiry and mastery learning. Most of the learning sessions focus on skills applied in structured activities and discussions rather than in actual clinical practice. We conducted a constructivist grounded theory study to explore co-learning as a potential way in which lifelong learning might be taught and reinforced during clinical practice. The study aimed to develop a conceptual model for co-learning that could inform faculty development for clinical teachers.

9.2   PHILOSOPHICAL UNDERPINNINGS OF PRAGMATIC APPROACHES

Pragmatism can be challenging to navigate given the variety of scholars and perspectives clustered under its umbrella. Figure 9.1 provides a brief history of pragmatism highlighting multiple theorists' contributions to the philosophy. Some scholars consider pragmatism a theoretical perspective or paradigm along with positivism/postpositivism, constructivism/interpretivism, and critical/transformative [16–18]. Others prefer not to associate pragmatism with specific ontological, epistemological, and methodological positions typically associated with other research approaches [19]. Given the multitude of philosophers and schools of thought that constitute pragmatism, pragmatism cannot easily be described as a singular or homogeneous approach [20]. Nonetheless, there are some common philosophical features that distinguish pragmatic approaches from others. These include: (1) viewing enquiry as an experiential process; (2) recognising experience, knowing, and acting as interconnected; and (3) valuing knowledge that is actionable [21]. Based on these features, pragmatic approaches can be described as those using an: 'experience-based, action-orientated framework' where enquiry takes a practical focus, centred on how we experience and

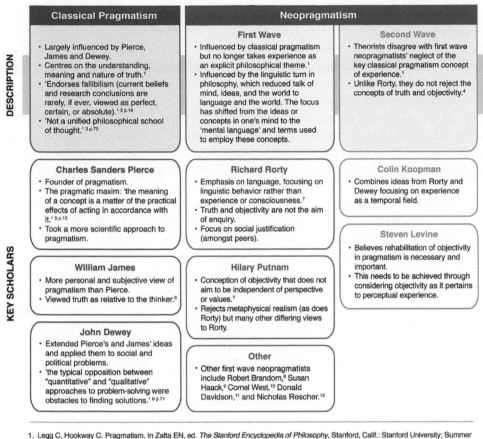

FIGURE 9.1   A brief overview of pragmatism.

come to understand the world [22 p. 864]. This grounding in experience and action means that philosophically, pragmatism tends to view reality as dynamic rather than fixed; truth as provisional, contextual, and temporal rather than absolute; and knowledge as situated [23]. Philosophically, pragmatic approaches align well with health professions education as a practice-orientated field that values actionable knowledge based on thoughtful analysis of problems that matter in practice [24]. In other words, the goal of HPER is not (solely) to advance knowledge or generate theoretical or conceptual understanding; it generally also offers practical implications.

As we describe these philosophical underpinnings of pragmatism, we encourage you to consider whether and how each element – axiology (what we value), ontology (nature of reality), epistemology (nature of knowing), and methodology (how we come to know) – aligns with your personal philosophies. To read more about these elements, you may wish to revisit Chapter 2. You may also find it helpful to review the book glossary for terms commonly used in pragmatic philosophy.

9.2.1 Axiology – Values or Value Judgements Guide Beliefs and Actions

We begin our discussion of pragmatic philosophies with axiology because we view this as the core element of pragmatism. While pragmatists differ in their perspectives on the nature and relevance of ontology and epistemology, most philosophers of pragmatism fundamentally value action, application, and improvement of human experience. Biesta and Burbles characterise the pragmatist's approach to educational research as more than a: 'technical enterprise where educators simply "apply" the findings of educational research. In education, questions about "how" are inseparable from questions about "why" and "what for"' [1 p. 22]. In a pragmatic approach, considerable attention is given to the consequences of enquiry upfront, rather than at the end of the study as a discussion of implications derived from findings. Some scholars view pragmatism as an approach that embraces agency, or an individual's ability to direct their action, and collective responsibility for action [1]. In this way, pragmatism is sometimes considered to be value-orientated rather than value-neutral [17, 23]. Similar to the critical approaches considered in Chapter 8, pragmatic approaches value inclusion and engagement of multiple constituencies or members of a community to foster understanding of multiple perspectives and joint action [17, 18].

9.2.2 Ontology – Single and Multiple Realities

Unlike most of the other research approaches covered in Part II of this book, pragmatism does not take a singular, predetermined position on the nature of reality and thereby avoids the dichotomised view of reality as either objective or subjective [25]. This perspective opens up epistemological and methodological possibilities precluded by the ontological positions of scientific and interpretivist approaches, allowing thoughtful combinations of methodologies premised on different assumptions about reality. Morgan [18] describes the pragmatic approach as intersubjective, viewing reality as neither completely objective nor completely subjective, with emphasis on the need for mutual understanding of different ways of viewing reality. Some pragmatists endorse both singular and multiple realities, meaning they accept a view of reality as external to individuals and existing independent of human experience, and they acknowledge that reality is dynamic and negotiated, and always filtered through human experience [18]. This view has implications for the type of data collected and how data are analysed and interpreted, which we discuss further in section 9.2.4 [14]. Other pragmatists have argued for abandoning questions about reality entirely, viewing these questions as unnecessary or even unhelpful to achieving the goals of pragmatic approaches [26, 27].

9.2.3 Epistemology – Knowledge Is Dynamic, Incomplete, and Temporary

Consistent with a view of reality as dynamic, pragmatists generally identify knowledge as situated, contextualised, and constructed for a practical purpose based on the reality of the world we live in and interact with [23]. As such, knowledge can also be seen as dynamic. That is, the process of generating knowledge (e.g., through experimentation) changes the world. Biesta described a pragmatic approach as one in which people pursue knowledge as participants in 'an ever-evolving universe', rather than as 'spectators of a finished universe' [28 p. 495]. Similar to critical realist approaches discussed in Chapter 6, truth is grounded in social, political, economic, and historical contexts – it is what works at a given time and place, with a particular group of people, and truth is derived from perception and experience in context [26, 29]. The implication of this perspective for researchers who choose a pragmatic approach is that knowledge is viewed as incomplete and temporary, so enquiry should be viewed as an ongoing cycle of investigation and action: 'forcing us to change our knowledge of the world and our ways of acting within it (which, in turn, can yield new experiences to learn from)' [1 p. 13]. You may find it helpful to think of knowledge produced through pragmatic research as warranted assertions (beliefs that guide behaviours and actions) rather than absolute truths [18]. These assertions are based on taking lines of action (behaviours or actions taken as part of the enquiry process) [18], and experiencing the consequences or outcomes of these actions (workability) [3]. In Box 9.3 you can read about the philosophical underpinnings of the four case studies.

Box 9.3   Case studies: A summary of their philosophical underpinnings

Explanatory Mixed Methods [5–7]: We rejected rigid views of reality as either objective and singular or subjective and multiple. Instead, we believed reality could exist apart from experience (objective ontology) and could be encountered through human experience (subjective ontology). We believed knowledge consisted of both unique and socially shared experiences (epistemology) and we supported the use of pluralistic methods to achieve actionable research purposes (axiology). Thus, the survey in our first paper [5] and interviews with participants in the second paper [6] took an agnostic view towards reality (ontology). We combined these methods based on socially shared research experiences to assess and understand the phenomenon in the best possible way (methodology).

Adapted Exploratory Mixed Methods [8–10]: We used a pragmatic approach that valued the generation of knowledge reflecting the views of researchers and participants, as well as producing outputs that were useful in practice (axiology). This pragmatic approach acknowledged both singular and multiple realities (ontology), and that knowledge was seen to be both constructed, as well as based on the reality of the world we live in and interact with (epistemology). How we came to know reality was through research tools generating objective and subjective evidence (methodology) [30]. In addition to this truth, knowledge and meaning were not fixed; they changed over time. The truth, knowledge, and meaning gained through our research was seen as temporary, flexible, contextual, and subject to change (epistemology) [23].

Action Research [11]: We valued research and lesson study as a formative intervention in teachers' collaborative work context to support teachers' development, improve educational practice, and enrich students' learning (axiology). We took the stance that reality exists in the dynamics of teachers' collaborative action, experience, and transformation in their educational practice (ontology). The consequences of this process included changes in personal professional knowledge and beliefs (e.g., PCK), and transformed practice. This socially constructed knowledge was personalised, not fixed (epistemology), and was based on collective enquiry, including teachers' reflections on observations of lesson-related activities of self and colleagues, and identification and understanding of actions that are needed to improve practice (methodology). Research and activity to develop insight into reality were interrelated.

(continued)

(continued)

<u>Constructivist Grounded Theory</u> [15]: Our study reflected the core value that research should provide insights that can both improve practice in the local context and offer concepts for use in health professions education more broadly (axiology). We studied a phenomenon (co-learning) that was inherently intersubjective, meaning it involved a dynamic relationship where multiple realities (ontology) may exist (e.g., teachers and learners may share an experience and understand it in different ways). While we recognised that the knowledge generated through our study was situated in a specific time and context (epistemology), we also anticipated finding patterns using constant comparative techniques that would allow us to describe a general model of co-learning that would account for most of our data on co-learning (methodology).

9.2.4 Methodology – Pluralism

Pragmatism focuses on the importance of the phenomenon of interest, the questions asked about the phenomenon, and the likelihood that progress can be made towards a goal or purpose associated with the phenomenon by studying it via the questions posed. While pragmatic approaches may employ scientific methods such as experimentation to generate technical knowledge about processes, or how things work, pragmatic approaches do not privilege this form of knowledge as superior to knowledge about human beliefs and experiences such as values, emotions, and purpose [1]. Instead, pragmatic approaches create opportunities for different philosophical perspectives, theoretical assumptions, and methodological approaches to occupy: 'the same inquiry space for the purposes of respectful conversation, dialogue, and learning from one another' [31 p. 13]. Pluralism describes the position that multiple methodologies can contribute to knowledge and truths [4]. In pragmatic approaches, researchers often consider multiple ways of collecting and analysing data rather than relying on one best way [23]. This methodological stance welcomes thoughtful combinations of different types of data (e.g., quantitative and qualitative) and analytic techniques. Methodologically, pragmatism offers a flexible and reflexive approach to research design that is typically based on the purpose and action-orientated goals motivating research [18, 32].

Pragmatism is often associated with abductive reasoning – a form of reasoning that moves back and forth between induction (making inferences or generating hypotheses based on observations) and deduction (making inferences or generating hypotheses based on facts or premises) [18]. Abductive reasoning enables researchers to combine the potential of both approaches in a single study [18]. John Dewey and scholars of his work provide much of the methodological foundation for pragmatic approaches in education. Core tenets of the methodology include:

1. Enquiry begins and ends with educational practice – the purpose is to transform educators in ways that make their practice or performance: 'more enlightened, more humane, and more truly educational than it was before' [33 p. 39].
2. Enquiry is a sequential and iterative process that involves studying the relationship between actions and consequences in a systematic and reflective way, which distinguishes it from trial and error.
3. The knowledge, or warranted assertion, generated through enquiry is temporal and contextual – yielding changes and solutions for a given situation that cannot be assumed to work in future situations (similar to realist approaches described in Chapter 6). This tenet captures the continuous, iterative nature of enquiry in dynamic environments [22].

9.3 COMMON PRAGMATIC METHODOLOGIES AND METHODS IN HPER

The methodologies and methods found in studies taking a pragmatic approach are diverse, reflecting methodological pluralism and theoretical inclusivity [22]. They often combine multiple types of data and analytic techniques. Pragmatic approaches begin by considering the desired type of knowledge to be produced (what outcome for what purpose), then by comparing which methodologies can best produce such knowledge by asking why this way and not that way [34]. While other approaches might ask similar questions, they rarely consider the full range of methodologies and the possibility of mixing them like you would in a pragmatic approach. Researchers using a pragmatic approach base their methodological choices on the plausibility of achieving desired outcomes, meeting identified needs, and guiding future action rather than on assumptions about the philosophical underpinnings of a methodology or method (e.g., experiments assume a single reality, phenomenological interviews assume multiple, individual realities) [34].

In this chapter, we have selected three methodologies compatible with pragmatic approaches: mixed methods, action research, and constructivist grounded theory. Note that while these methodologies align well with pragmatic approaches, they can also be used in other types of approaches discussed in Part II of this book. The methodologies and methods are fundamentally similar when used in pragmatic approaches and other approaches; the differences appear in the purposes and outcomes (e.g., action versus theory), and composition of the research team (e.g., pragmatic approaches often engage practitioners or stakeholders in study design, data collection, and/or data analysis).

9.3.1 Mixed Methods

Based on a review and synthesis of many descriptions of mixed methods research, Johnson et al [35]. defined mixed methods research as: 'the type of research in which a researcher or team of researchers combines elements of qualitative and quantitative research approaches (e.g., use of qualitative and quantitative viewpoints, data collection, analysis, inference techniques) for the broad purposes of breadth and depth of understanding and corroboration' [35 p. 123]. Creswell and Plano Clark [36] identify core characteristics of mixed methods research that include collecting, analysing, and integrating or combining qualitative and quantitative data in a rigorous way to address research questions, organising study procedures according to designs that explain the logic behind the conduct of studies, and using theory and philosophy (pragmatism, for this chapter) to frame study methodologies. The mixing of methods can occur within a single study or across multiple studies within a research programme, as in our case studies (see Box 9.4). The decision to use mixed methods can occur upfront as part of the planned study design (fixed mixed methods design) or during the research process based on insights or questions arising during the research, suggesting the need to add a quantitative or qualitative approach (emergent mixed methods design) [36].

There are multiple typologies that describe mixed methods research designs [31, 36–40]. When you choose a design, several elements must be considered, including the timing of the quantitative and qualitative strands (parallel/concurrent or sequential), the weight placed on the quantitative and qualitative strands (equivalent or qualitatively/quantitatively driven), the degree of interaction between the quantitative and qualitative strands (independent or dependent, component or integrated), and the intent of the design (validation/confirmatory, exploratory, explanatory, developmental) [36].

We recommend starting with the three core mixed methods designs described by Creswell and Plano Clark [36]: (1) convergent, (2) explanatory sequential; and (3) exploratory sequential. These designs focus on the intent of the research, which aligns well with pragmatic approaches. You would likely select a convergent design if your study aims to compare or combine quantitative and qualitative data to gain more complete understandings of a problem or phenomenon. In convergent designs, the findings from one strand are used to validate or confirm those of another, or to identify similarities and differences in findings when participants respond to questions through different methods (e.g., survey and interview). If your goal is to better understand the reasons or causes of findings, you might choose an explanatory sequential design in which you begin with quantitative data analysis and use the findings to guide the collection and analysis of qualitative data. This design is often used to explain surprising findings or add depth to findings. If you are working on a problem that requires further description and understanding to guide development of interventions or actions, you would likely choose an exploratory sequential design. This design typically begins with and often prioritises qualitative data analysis. It then uses the findings to develop quantitative strands involving testing interventions experimentally or conducting surveys to further explore the frequency or prevalence of identified variables or the probability of hypothetical relationships. Beginning with the qualitative strand allows the design of an intervention or a quantitative study to be customised to context [36]. Researchers using pragmatic approaches can select from these three designs based on study goals. All three value the combination of quantitative and qualitative methodologies; the difference is in how they configure the collection, analysis, and application or integration of the quantitative and qualitative data. Pragmatic approaches that seek to integrate qualitative and quantitative data or findings through compare/contrast or merging techniques generally have a convergent design with either parallel/concurrent data collection and analysis in each strand followed by comparison as the means of integration, or interactive data collection and analysis using iterative cycles in which initial quantitative and qualitative data collection and analysis informs subsequent phases [41]. Pragmatic approaches that seek to use one phase of research to guide another (as in the examples used throughout the chapter) typically use explanatory or exploratory sequential designs. These designs offer much flexibility to accommodate research goals, which is a key reason mixed methods suit pragmatic philosophies.

9.3.2 Action Research

Action research can take many forms and be described in various ways (e.g., participatory action research, community-engaged research, collaborative enquiry). For this chapter, we selected a definition that aligns well with pragmatic philosophy – a methodology that brings together: 'action and reflection, as well as theory and practice, in participation with others, in the pursuit of practical solutions to issues of pressing concern' [42 p. 1]. In a widely cited article on action research, Meyer [43] describes three primary features of action research as participatory, democratic, and contributing to both social science and social change. Participatory reflects the relational nature of action research and the engagement of participants and community stakeholders in the design, conduct, dissemination, and implementation of the research findings and products [43, 44]. In action research, the boundaries between researchers and participants blur such that co-generative learning occurs [45]. Democratic conveys the importance of partnership, dialogue, and collaboration between the researchers and participants. The researchers play an active role in facilitating change. They are conducting research with, rather than on, participants [44]. The contributions of action research typically offer insights beyond the local context and community in which the research occurs, offering general insights that can be useful and informative to practitioners and researchers alike. Sometimes this is described as bridging the theory–practice gap [43].

Action research is often described as a cyclical or iterative process that involves planning, observing, reflecting, and acting [46]. These phases can be interpreted in a variety of ways depending on the context and issues or problems to be addressed. In general, they involve building relationships, identifying challenges, exploring possible actions to move towards a shared goal and desired future state, working together to take action and observe the consequences, evaluating the consequences through collective assessment and reflection, and deciding how to proceed based on this evaluation of consequences [44].

9.3.3 Constructivist Grounded Theory

As mentioned in Chapter 2 (see section 2.3.3), the original version of grounded theory, introduced by sociologists Glaser and Strauss [47], offered a specific set of strategies to make the methods of qualitative analysis more systematic, and to establish the development of theory as a viable goal of research. Glaser and Strauss' grounded theory retained some of the philosophical assumptions of scientific approaches (e.g., objectivity, empiricism, post-positivism). Over time, researchers retained many of the core analytic strategies associated with grounded theory such as coding, memowriting, and constant comparative techniques while shifting towards a pragmatic orientation drawing on philosophical assumptions associated with interpretivist approaches (e.g., subjectivity, relativism, constructivism). Charmaz articulated the core elements of constructivist grounded theory and identified the methodology as pragmatic in nature based on: 'the dual emphases on action and meaning' [48 p. 13], and on 'process and change' [48 p. 265]. She further describes the pragmatic underpinnings of constructivist grounded theory as evident in its emphasis on problemsolving, on capturing multiple perspectives, on the actions people take in response to emergent problems, on the combination of facts and values, and on views of truth as provisional. These philosophical underpinnings help explain the core strategies that comprise constructivist grounded theory methodology.

The fundamentals of constructivist grounded theory include: (1) a simultaneous and iterative process of data collection and data analysis; (2) analysis (coding, memoing) of actions and processes rather than themes or structures; (3) use of systematic comparative techniques to develop inductive abstract analytic categories and search for variation within these categories; (4) engagement in theoretical sampling – a form of sampling used to elaborate tentative theoretical categories derived from data by defining: 'the properties, boundaries, and relevance of this category or set of categories' [48 p. 345]; and (5) production of a theoretical account of a phenomenon rather than a descriptive account or application of existing theories to the phenomenon [48 p. 15].

9.3.4 Methods

In a pragmatic approach, the methodologies described in sections 9.3.1 to 9.3.3 can use almost any method or combination of methods for data collection (e.g., focus groups, interviews, observations, surveys, document analysis) and analysis (e.g., descriptive, narrative, statistical, thematic), so long as you provide justification based on alignment with study goals, questions, and values. Before moving on to the next section, pause and reflect on how you might apply pragmatic approaches to your HPER (see Box 9.5). See Box 9.4 for a summary of the case studies' methodology and methods.

Box 9.4   Case studies: A summary of their methodologies and methods

Explanatory Mixed Methods [5–7]: We used an explanatory mixed methods design to explore the long-term effects of a degree-awarding programme in medical education on the transformational changes and development of educational identities among health professionals worldwide. Different methods were mixed to increase the range and scope of enquiry, and explore areas of overlap and uniqueness. Using a questionnaire survey, we found that qualifications in medical education enhance theoretical foundations in educational practices resulting in increased self-efficacy and engagement in scholarly activities. These insights into impacts of qualifications on educational identities and careers of health professionals were comprehensively explored in the subsequent qualitative study. We then used a constructivist grounded theory approach and conducted semi-structured interviews to collect data in an iterative manner. This methodology helped reveal that health professionals experience transformational changes and epistemological development as educators with various performance attainments after undertaking medical education qualifications.

Adapted Exploratory Mixed Methods [8–10]: We used an exploratory sequential design to explore the broad impacts of CPD, where the qualitative study was conducted first to inform the subsequent quantitative study. We added a systematic scoping review to the exploratory sequential design that ran alongside the qualitative study. This allowed the collection of multiple types of data: a summary of the literature and qualitative interview data, ultimately providing additional insights into the impacts of CPD in the health professions. Due to the iterative nature of the exploratory sequential design and the pragmatic approach to the research, the type of quantitative study to be conducted was not determined at the outset of the research. Rather, the results of the systematic scoping review and qualitative study were used to inform the type of quantitative study to be conducted, with the decision based on choosing a study that would produce outputs useful to practice. The systematic scoping review showed that unvalidated surveys were the most common means of measuring the impacts of CPD, and that while some validated surveys existed, they focused on one category of impact. As both the scoping review and qualitative study showed that there were a large range of impacts of CPD, we determined that developing and validating a survey measuring a broad range of impacts of CPD would be a useful next step.

Action Research [11]: Our study occurred over a four-month period. Our goal in the research was to learn how teachers' participation in the lesson study approach contributed to their development of PCK related to research supervision. Over the study, teachers collaboratively designed research supervision protocols and experimented with techniques outlined in the protocols (e.g., open questioning and giving positive feedback to their students). To study the effects of this lesson study approach, we collected multiple types of data including video-recordings of lesson study meetings, learner reports of sessions with their research supervisor (teachers in the study), and interviews with the teachers. Our analysis involved coding video and interview transcripts for types of learning activities and indicators of change in PCK components based on constructs identified in previous work by Bakkenes et al. [49], Magnusson et al. [50], and Wongsopawiro et al. [51], and coding student reports for evidence of change in students' experiences of and learning through research supervision. Results showed that the lesson study project contributed to the development of supervisors' PCK on instructional strategies.

Constructivist Grounded Theory [15]: Our study was conducted in a single institution, which allowed us to have in-depth understandings of the contexts and cultures. The research team consisted of clinician-educators interested in the phenomenon of co-learning and non-clinicians committed to improving faculty development to support lifelong learning. Given that our goal was to develop a conceptual model for co-learning, we chose to interview faculty as clinical teachers from multiple specialties and with varying years of experience who worked in a variety of clinical settings (e.g., inpatient, ambulatory, operating room, emergency). We began our initial data analysis after the first interviews were conducted and continued this analysis throughout data collection. This enabled us to focus on sampling in ways that would allow comparison of our early conceptualisations of co-learning processes with subsequent data collected from participants who might offer different perspectives. Members of the research team met regularly to discuss their interpretations and compare them based on their different perspectives as clinician-educators and non-clinical faculty developers. As we moved into the focused coding and finalisation of the conceptual model, we discussed the implications of the model for clinical teaching and faculty development. We began translating our findings into plans for a faculty development workshop.

Box 9.5   Pause and reflect: Selecting a pragmatic approach and appropriate methodologies/methods for your research

- Think about a topic of enquiry in health professions education that you are especially interested in researching. This may relate to a challenge regarding your own teaching or learning, or it may link to previous research you have done, or could relate to key gaps in the literature.

- What research question could you develop relating to this topic that would lend itself well to pragmatic approaches and why? (Hint: see if you can identify the research question in the case studies and model a pragmatic question from these examples).

- What methodologies/methods would be appropriate for this question and why?

- Now think of a research question pertaining to your chosen topic that does not lend itself well to pragmatic approaches. What other methodologies/methods are more appropriate for this question and why? What other chapters should you therefore read next?

- Revisit this pause and reflect box once you have read the other chapters in Part II, and further developed your research ideas.

9.4   KEY QUALITY INDICATORS IN PRAGMATIC APPROACHES

Pragmatic approaches have been criticised as lacking rigour, at least when compared to the well-defined criteria used to evaluate the quality and rigour of scientific approaches [52]. Mumford described pragmatism as an: 'attitude of compromise and accommodation' [53 p. 39], implying that quality is whatever works in a given situation. Others have argued that an approach that views truth as transient defies efforts to evaluate quality and rigour because the knowledge generated cannot be objectively verified or falsified [52]. Such critiques seem to fundamentally misunderstand pragmatic approaches, holding them to the same standards as scientific approaches, rather than appreciating the distinctive philosophical orientation of pragmatic approaches. Instead, the quality of pragmatic approaches should be judged on the actionability of insights they produce and the processes used to produce them. That is: (a) are the insights useful and impactful for the intended audience? (b) do they offer description or explanation in ways that support creation or achievement of desired outcomes? [54] and (c) are the processes used to gain these insights inclusive, iterative, and/or transformative? [55].

We are not aware of any guidelines or universal indicators used to gauge the quality of pragmatic approaches. We can, however, identify important features of studies conducted from a pragmatic approach, which can be helpful for you to use when designing and reviewing pragmatic research. First, pragmatic approaches both aim to, and actually do, produce actionable knowledge, or knowledge that is useful and has practical relevance and consequences [21, 55]. We can evaluate this feature based on the study purposes and aims articulated by the researchers (e.g., do they: seek transformation and change; address a problem or need that stakeholders view as relevant and important; strive for practical solutions to real-life problems?) and on the discussion of consequences and implications of their findings (e.g., specific actions taken and plans for subsequent action and inquiry?). Second, pragmatic approaches employ participatory and inclusive enquiry practices [55]. We can evaluate these features by looking for evidence of relationships and dialogue between researchers and stakeholders to achieve shared understanding (particularly among those holding disparate views) and ensure mutual relevance of aims, actions, and consequences. Third, pragmatic approaches use iterative processes that tend to use abductive, rather than purely inductive or deductive, reasoning [18]. When evaluating studies that use pragmatic approaches we can look for a clear description of the research process, including evidence of reflexivity and collaborative discussion throughout the process, and rationale for theoretical and methodological choices (e.g., how and why key decisions were made regarding conceptual or theoretical frameworks, sampling, types of data, timing of data collection, analytic and integrative techniques, what values and ethical principles guided decisions). The type of evidence selected as the basis for interpretation and the quality requirements used to ensure evidence is of sufficient quality to warrant the findings or assertions must be clear. As the meaning or impact of the research findings are essential to pragmatic approaches, the findings must address the goals of the study in a useful or actionable and impactful way.

From a methodological standpoint, you may find it helpful to draw on guidelines for specific methodologies. These exist for mixed methods, action research, and constructivist grounded theory. When considering these guidelines, keep in mind that most are not specific to a pragmatic philosophy. Thus, they should be considered in conjunction with the features of pragmatic approaches mentioned above.

9.4.1   Quality in Mixed Methods

Few mixed methods researchers contest the need for criteria to evaluate the quality of mixed methods research, though they may suggest different terms and perspectives on appropriate criteria [56]. Some recommend using the methodological criteria for quality that apply to each methodology used in the study [57]. Others argue that while this may work to evaluate the quality of design, data collection, and some aspects of data analysis, it omits the most important and distinguishing feature of mixed methods research – the integrative component that yields the meta-inferences and insights that prompted the selection of mixed methods [58]. We recommend the framework proposed in the Mixed Methods Appraisal Tool (MMAT) [59] as a comprehensive synthesis of various proposed quality criteria for mixed methods research. This framework includes both unique features of mixed methods studies (e.g., rationale for the mixed methods design, integration of qualitative and quantitative components in interpretation, and addressing differences between qualitative and quantitative results) and provides criteria for appraising the quality of the study's qualitative and quantitative components. As use of mixed methods research has grown in health services and clinical research, you may also find it helpful to review O'Cathain and colleagues' [60] guidelines for Good Reporting of A Mixed Methods Study (GRAMMS) in health services research and Gaglio and colleagues' [61] methodological standards for qualitative and mixed methods patient-centered outcomes research.

9.4.2 Quality in Action Research

Action research seeks transformation and change through: 'co-creation of scientific and practical knowledge with, not on, those people with a stake in the issues at hand' [62 p. 12]. This orientation is critical to understanding the concept of quality in action research. Quality criteria pay particular attention to the processes used to define the purpose or objectives of the research, the engagement of stakeholders throughout the research process, and the production of outcomes that change practice. Conventional markers of rigour for research methods (e.g., validity evidence of the data collection instruments, compliance with prescribed techniques for data analysis) are important considerations, but perhaps less so than demonstrating the values associated with action research. Bradbury et al. [62] describe seven requirements for quality in action research, emphasising the integration of objective, intersubjective, and subjective perspectives in each of these requirements. The requirements emphasise: (1) clear articulation of the objectives of the research so stakeholders, as well as other reviewers, can evaluate whether the research achieved the objectives; (2) evidence of the partnership and participation of stakeholders in alignment with the participatory values and relational aspects of action research; (3) researcher reflexivity throughout the research process; and (4) the contributions of the research in ways that both guide action in the local context and add practical knowledge or theory useful beyond the local context. Audit procedures offer one way to demonstrate how the research team meets these quality requirements. In an audit procedure, the research team documents the entire research process in an audit trail, which they then share with a designated auditor (external to the research team) who reviews the audit trail and produces a report on key markers of research quality such as transparency, comprehensibility, and acceptability [63, 64].

9.4.3 Quality in Constructivist Grounded Theory

Quality in constructivist grounded theory considers both the process and the product of the methodology. Charmaz acknowledges that disciplines vary in the standards they set for rigorous research conduct and acceptable forms of evidence [48]. Nonetheless, she offers four general criteria that researchers can use to reflect on their work and that reviewers can consider when evaluating the research: (1) credibility; (2) originality; (3) resonance; and (4) usefulness. Credibility considers whether the research demonstrates intimate familiarity with the topic of study and the context in which it was studied. Such familiarity depends on sufficient data (based on range, number, and depth of content) to support the argument or theory put forth and evidence of systematic comparisons within and across categories and data sources. Originality refers to the novelty of the categories and the conceptual or theoretical insights produced by the research. The grounded theory constructed from the study should 'challenge, extend, or refine current ideas, concepts, and practices' [48 p. 337]. Resonance considers the connection between the study findings and the experiences and circumstances of participants or people similar to the participants. Research with resonance should make sense to participants and intended audiences, and give them insights about their lives, experiences, and situations. Usefulness indicates that the analysis and resulting theory contributes both knowledge and practical implications that can lead to change and improvement for individuals, institutions, and/or society [48].

Now that you have read about different ways of evaluating the quality of studies using pragmatic approaches and methodologies, take a moment to read our reflections on quality in our own studies (see Box 9.6) and to appraise quality in a published study (see Box 9.7).

Box 9.6   Case studies: A summary of their quality

Explanatory Mixed Methods [5–7]: To enhance the transparency and credibility of research, we explained the philosophical approach (i.e., pragmatism) as well as provided justifications for employing mixed methods. We explained and used specific terms such as development, complementarity, and expansion [65]. The sequential nature of studies and their individual contribution towards primary and secondary research questions was also explained. We presented study findings individually, then discussed them collectively. Experts reviewed our questionnaire and we pilot-tested it with colleagues. Due to the Data Protection Act in the UK, it was difficult to ensure the representativeness of the sample. Based on available data, we selected a diverse range of participants in each study to explore similarities and differences, and to capture unique and deviant experiences. For coherence, the philosophical assumptions, methods, and methodology aligned, which made the outcomes robust, defensible, and credible. The data interpretation was thoroughly discussed and agreed upon. Our influence (reflexivity), our context, and any other factors affecting the interpretations were also thoroughly discussed to enhance the transferability of the findings.

Adapted Exploratory Mixed Methods [8–10]: We used a different method for each study, therefore, the key indicators of quality varied across the studies. As a whole, our key goal regarding quality was to ensure the methods used in each component of the research programme were reported clearly. Our research team also continued to return to what the product of the research would be – something useful to practice. In our scoping review, we found no surveys with validity evidence to measure a broad range of impacts, so our research aimed to produce such a survey measure. When considering quality, categories 1 (qualitative), 4 (quantitative descriptive), and 5 (mixed methods) of the MMAT were employed. This allowed the quality of the individual studies to be considered, and the research to be reviewed holistically. In the qualitative study the method was clearly described, as well as a rationale for why the qualitative approach was appropriate. We used quotes to support the findings and describe our results. We linked results to literature and theory. In the quantitative study, the sampling strategy was clearly described, and the sample deemed similar to the target population based on age, profession, and gender. In addition, while not explicitly stated in the paper, the risk of non-response bias was deemed low. We described the measurement used (survey) and how it was developed, including use of Principal Component Analysis for initial validity evidence. We described the rationale for our specific mixed methods approach and made connections between each of the three studies forming our research programme. We integrated the results of the studies in a final thesis chapter by using the categories from the systematic scoping review, the themes from the qualitative study, and the components from the quantitative study to develop a framework that could be used to help conceptualise the different levels of impacts of CPD programmes.

Action Research [11]: We checked the quality of the study by conducting an audit [63, 64]. The audit was carried out by an independent researcher and considered all steps of the methods, including data gathering and analysis. The auditor verified the research design, data gathering, and analysis according to the following criteria: transparency; comprehensibility; and acceptability. The main researcher acted as auditee and presented all findings to the auditor, accompanied with justifications of all decisions made during the research process. After the audit, the auditor presented her findings to the auditee. There were some discrepancies in the auditor's claims. The audit was used formatively to improve the study. Transparency in the methods section was improved and some steps in data analysis reporting were adapted. The auditor finished the assessment and provided a final written report on the trustworthiness of the study.

Constructivist Grounded Theory [15]: We established credibility by using an analytic process consistent with Charmaz [48], and by conducting interviews with 34 faculty members offering a range of perspectives to enrich our model. Throughout analyses we reviewed participants' examples and descriptions of co-learning multiple times to compare them with our model and ensure that we captured a range of experiences. We established the originality of our work by identifying gaps in related literature on workplace learning and clinical teaching, and by noting that the few instances where the term 'co-learning' was used lacked a description of processes and supporting conditions. For resonance, we shared our findings with clinical educators and education researchers locally and at national conferences. The comments and feedback we received suggested that the model made sense and offered new insights on clinical teaching. For usefulness, we designed our study with the goal of producing findings that educators could use to enhance the teaching of lifelong learning in clinical practice and we remained committed to this goal throughout the research process.

Box 9.7   Stop and do: Appraising the quality of a paper using a pragmatic approach

Read the abstract of the following open-access paper: Bowen et al. Exploring current physicians' failure to communicate clinical feedback back to transferring physicians after transitions of patient care responsibility: A mixed methods study. *Perspect Med Educ.* 2020;9(4):236–244. https://www.ncbi.nlm.nih.gov/pmc/articles/PMC7459044.

(continued)

(continued)

- Based on the quality indicators and resources described in section 9.4, select the quality indicators you think best suit this paper (e.g., MMAT – available from: http://mixedmethodsappraisaltoolpublic.pbworks.com/w/file/fetch/127916259/MMAT_2018_criteria-manual_2018-08-01_ENG.pdf)
- Read the paper and note where quality indicators are addressed. Revisit these alongside the indicators you selected. How strong would you rate each indicator? Are there any quality indicators that are not addressed?
- How would you rate the overall quality of the study based on your evaluation of these indicators?

9.5 CHALLENGES AND STRENGTHS OF EMPLOYING PRAGMATIC APPROACHES IN HPER

If you are considering a pragmatic approach for your research, you must be aware of both the challenges and strengths of this approach. One of the primary challenges in HPER is that few studies identify their approach as pragmatic. This absence makes it difficult to find good examples and models to guide the write up of your work. It also means that journal peer reviewers may be less familiar with the approach and unsure what criteria to use to evaluate the quality of your research. You may need to provide more detailed explanations of your research process, including justification for key decisions and clarification of important criteria such as usefulness, workability, or actionability in the context of your study. Providing this level of detail may require more words, which can be challenging in reporting pragmatic approaches. Many journals allow more words with reasonable justification and others have no word limits. Supplemental materials and appendices can also be used to provide additional information without adding length to a manuscript. A related challenge is deciding how to present the findings generated through pragmatic approaches. This challenge relates both to considerations of audience and research standards (e.g., wanting to present findings in ways that are useful and actionable for educators and that meet the expectations of various research communities that may hold different standards of quality) [66]. The research may generate findings that are highly important, meaningful, and valuable to local stakeholders, but may be of less interest beyond this audience. Having few published high-quality examples of pragmatic approaches in HPER poses a challenge for novice researchers in deciding how to present methods and findings in a coherent manner. Finally, as described in section 9.3, pragmatic approaches often involve combinations of methodologies, methods, and types of data that come from different philosophical perspectives. As such, pragmatic research often engages a team of researchers and stakeholders who hold diverse views on the nature of research, the types of evidence that hold most value, and the ways of demonstrating rigour. Managing these diverse perspectives to achieve mutual understanding and acceptance of findings can yield formidable challenges and requires a research plan that allows ample time for the team to share perspectives, engage in reflexivity, and agree on findings, implications, and actions to take as a result of the research.

While these challenges are not trivial, they must be considered alongside several strengths of pragmatic approaches. Pragmatic approaches suit HPER due to the practice-orientated field valuing actionable knowledge [24]. One of the greatest strengths of pragmatic approaches is the ability to generate transformative and mutually relevant knowledge (warranted assertions), and consequences (outcomes) that are meaningful and valued by educators and stakeholders – often because they are engaged throughout the research process. This aspect of the research often makes it motivating and rewarding for the researchers. A related strength of pragmatic approaches is their ability to bridge the gap between research and practice. HPER is often described as an applied field that aims to improve the education of health professionals [67, 68], yet studies describe various challenges of translating knowledge and evidence produced through research into evidence-informed actions of educators [69–71]. These include limited time for educators to search and access the large body of literature, difficulty penetrating the language of HPER without training in the field, and resistance to changing practice [69–71]. Pragmatic approaches address some of these challenges by encouraging interaction and relationships between researchers and educators that involve sharing different types of expertise, identifying mutually relevant problems and desired outcomes, and working together throughout the research process to co-construct knowledge and meaning through iterative processes of enquiry and action.

As we sum up the balance of these challenges and strengths, we see promising opportunities for pragmatic approaches to expand and advance HPER. The challenges are not insurmountable, as we show by discussing how we overcame various challenges encountered in our case studies (see Box 9.8). After reviewing these case studies, review Box 9.9 to practise evaluating the strengths and challenges of a published study.

Box 9.8   Case studies: A summary of their strengths and challenges

Explanatory Mixed Methods [5–7]: Using a mixed methods approach, we explored overlapping as well as different facets of the phenomenon. Our use of both quantitative and qualitative methods helped strengthen our study by offsetting the weaknesses of each method and also brought completeness to our account. The qualitative findings helped to complement, clarify, and extend the quantitative results. We needed to be familiar with both quantitative and qualitative methodologies and methods. Our mixed methods approach required extensive data collection, management, and analysis in multiple stages. We reported different parts of the study in separate publications considering the extensive detail of these parts and journal word count limitations. In each journal, these studies were briefly mentioned as part of a bigger mixed methods research project underpinned by pragmatism. As the publications were separate, justifications for using mixed methods were not explicitly discussed. However, each paper cited the other. Blending our methods required expertise and resilience among clashing expectations and cultures within our team. Discussions and reflexivity on perspectives and other factors affecting the interpretations helped enhance the transferability of findings.

Adapted Exploratory Mixed Methods [8–10]: The exploratory nature of our work was its key strength. Conducting the research in this way meant that each part of the research flowed onto and linked with the next. This meant each stage of the research was able to inform subsequent stages, as well as link back to previous stages. This led to choosing the quantitative study – the development of a validated survey – to measure the broad impacts of CPD, something which was identified as a gap in the literature and which was useful in

(continued)

(continued)

practice. The number of words needed to explain each of these studies in sufficient detail was a key challenge given journal limitations. It meant that the three studies were published separately. In each case, the manuscript word count was over the journal word limit. To overcome this, an explanation was included in the manuscript cover letter to explain why the additional word count was necessary. Also, the previous works were referred to and referenced in latter works.

Action Research [11]: Our study's combination of professional development activities, design of new instructional approaches, and collection of evidence about impact on students' learning was a strength in that our research directly benefited multiple stakeholders. Our findings also contributed new insights into how teachers can use learning activities such as lesson study to advance their PCK. Researchers and participants completed multiple rounds of co-design, data gathering, inquiry, and analysis. Our study also required substantial planning for a systematic approach to manage boundaries between professional development and research, which easily blur in action research. The findings of our study are not generalisable given that lesson studies are local and small-scale, so disseminating the work was challenging.

Constructivist Grounded Theory [15]: Our study explored a phenomenon (co-learning) that educators found important and useful to understand, with practical implications for clinical teaching. At the same time, our study expanded the literature on workplace learning and lifelong learning by articulating intentional processes by which teachers and learners acknowledge learning needs and contribute to learning outcomes. Our research team brought multiple perspectives to the analysis and our sampling strategy ensured our model was inclusive of multiple educator perspectives and contexts. We recognised the need to collect trainees' perspectives to inform our model of co-learning, but given the original scope of our project and the limited capacity of our research team, we decided to conduct interviews with trainees after completing faculty interviews and initial analyses. We also decided to publish faculty and trainee perspectives on co-learning as separate studies because combining the two would have made for a very long paper and would likely require sacrificing details we felt were important to include from each perspective. We intended to deliver a workshop to help translate our findings into concrete tools and strategies educators could use, but our workshop was cancelled due to unforeseen circumstances.

Box 9.9   Stop and do: Evaluating the strengths/challenges of a paper using a pragmatic approach

- Read the following open-access paper: Miyachi et al. A collaborative clinical case conference model for teaching social and behavioral science in medicine: an action research study. *BMC Med Educ.* 2021;21(1):574. https://bmcmededuc.biomedcentral.com/articles/10.1186/s12909-021-03009-8.

- Note the strengths of the pragmatic approach employed in this study in terms of addressing the purpose and research aims.

- Note the challenges of the pragmatic approach for addressing the research aims.
- What alternative approaches may have addressed these research questions? You may need to revisit this query after reading other chapters in Part II.

9.6 CHAPTER SUMMARY

Pragmatism unstiffens all of our theories, limbers them up and sets each one to work. William James, quoted in Dickstein [72 p. 7]

We began this chapter with a brief description of the history and various philosophical views of pragmatism. We then discussed how these philosophical perspectives inform pragmatic approaches to research, namely the value placed on processes that are grounded in experience, inclusive of multiple perspectives and experiences (intersubjective, mutually relevant), action-orientated (actionable), and that understand knowledge as fallible and reality, as both internal and external – knowable but filtered through human experience – and dynamic. The pluralistic nature of pragmatic approaches is a strength that may provide a way to address some of the challenges associated with the multilayered and dynamic nature of educational concepts and phenomena that often demand a multimethod or mixed methods approach. We described mixed methods and action research as two methodologies commonly associated with pragmatic approaches, with the caveat that pragmatic approaches emphasise the goals and purposes of the research and therefore are less prescriptive about methodological choices and associated methods. Correspondingly, the indicators for quality focus less on technical aspects of the research process and more on the contextual, intersubjective or relational, and purposeful aspects. We identified commonly used frameworks to guide and assess quality in mixed methods [56, 60], action research [62], and constructivist grounded theory[48]. To guide your decisions about which approach best suits your research, we discussed several challenges and strengths of pragmatic approaches and provided examples of how we addressed these challenges and benefited from the strengths of pragmatic approaches in our own research. We see a pragmatic approach as well-aligned with the goals of HPER and rich in potential for further development within HPER. We invite you to consider the merits of this approach and to learn more about pragmatic approaches by pursuing the recommended readings in Box 9.10.

Box 9.10   Recommended reading for pragmatic approaches in HPER

Biesta GJJ, Burbles NC. *Pragmatism and Educational Research*. Lanham, Md: Rowman & Littlefield Publishers Inc.; 2003 [1].

Bradbury H, Lewis R, Embury DC. Education action research: with and for the next generation. In Mertler CA, ed. *The Wiley Handbook of Action Research in Education*. Hoboken, NJ: John Wiley & Sons Inc; 2019: 7–28 [62].

Charmaz K. *Constructing Grounded Theory*, 2nd ed. Thousand Oaks, Calif.: SAGE; 2014 [48].

(continued)

(continued)

Creswell JW, Plano Clark VL. *Designing and Conducting Mixed Methods Research*, 3rd ed. Thousand Oaks, Calif.: SAGE; 2017 [36].

Hothersall SJ. Epistemology and social work: enhancing the integration of theory, practice and research through philosophical pragmatism, *Eur J Soc Work*. 2019;22(5):860–870 [22].

Mertler CA. *The Wiley Handbook of Action Research in Education*. Hoboken, NJ: John Wiley & Sons Inc.; 2019 [44].

Morgan DL. Paradigms lost and pragmatism regained: methodological implications of combining qualitative and quantitative methods. *J Mix Meth Res*. 2007; 1(1):48–76 [18].

Morgan DL. Pragmatism as a paradigm for social research. *Qual Inq*. 2014; 20(8):1045–1053 [3].

O'Cathain A. Assessing the quality of mixed methods research: toward a comprehensive framework. In Tashakkori A, Teddlie C, eds. *SAGE Handbook of Mixed Methods in Social & Behavioral Research*, 2nd ed. Thousand Oaks, Calif.: SAGE; 2010: 531–556 [56].

Watling CJ, Lingard L. Grounded theory in medical education research: AMEE Guide no. 70. *Med Teach*. 2012;34(10):850–861 [73].

REFERENCES

1. Biesta GJJ, Burbles NC. *Pragmatism and Educational Research*. Lanham, Md: Rowman & Littlefield Publishers Inc.; 2003.

2. Kaushik V, Walsh CA. Pragmatism as a research paradigm and its implications for social work research. *Soc Sci*. 2019;8(9):255.

3. Morgan DL. Pragmatism as a paradigm for social research. *Qual Inq*. 2014;20 (8):1045–1053.

4. Johnson RB, Gray R. A history of philosophical and theoretical issues for mixed methods research. In Tashakkori A, Teddlie C, eds. *SAGE Handbook of Mixed Methods in Social & Behavioral Research*, 2nd ed. Thousand Oaks, Calif.: SAGE; 2010: 69–94.

5. Sethi A, Schofield S, Ajjawi R, et al. How do postgraduate qualifications in medical education impact on health professionals? *Med Teach*. 2016;38(2):162–167.

6. Sethi A, Ajjawi R, McAleer S, et al. Exploring the tensions of being and becoming a medical educator. *BMC Med Educ*. 2017;17(1):62.

7. Sethi A, Schofield S, McAleer S, et al. The influence of postgraduate qualifications on educational identity formation of healthcare professionals. *Adv Health Sci Educ*. 2018;23(3):567–585.

8. Allen LM, Palermo C, Armstrong E, et al. Categorising the broad impacts of continuing professional development: a scoping review. *Med Educ*. 2019;53(11):1087–1099.

9. Allen LM, Hay M, Armstrong E, et al. Applying a social theory of learning to explain the possible impacts of continuing professional development (CPD) programs. *Med Teach*. 2020;42(10):1140–1147.

10. Allen LM, Palermo C, Armstrong E, et al. Measuring impacts of continuing professional development (CPD): the development of the CPD impacts survey (CPDIS). *Med Teach*. 2021;43(6):677–685.

11. Agricola BT, van der Schaaf MF, Prins FJ, et al. The development of research supervisors' pedagogical content knowledge in a lesson study project. *Educ Action Res*. 2022;30(2):261–280.

12. Dudley P. Teacher learning in lesson study: what interaction-level discourse analysis revealed about how teachers utilised imagination, tacit knowledge of teaching and fresh evidence of pupils learning, to develop practice knowledge and so enhance their pupils' learning. *Teach Educ.* 2013;34:107–121.

13. Cajkler W, Wood P, Norton J, et al. Lesson study as a vehicle for collaborative teacher learning in a secondary school. *Prof Dev Edu.* 2014;40(4):511–529.

14. Lewis CC, Hurd J. *Lesson Study Step by Step: How Teacher Learning Communities Improve Instruction.* Portsmouth: Heinemann; 2011.

15. Haddock LM, Rivera J, O'Brien BC. Learning together: co-learning among faculty and trainees in the clinical workplace. *Acad Med.* 2023;98(2):228–236.

16. Denzin NK, Lincoln YS. *The Sage Handbook of Qualitative Research*, 3rd ed. Thousand Oaks, Calif.: SAGE; 2005.

17. Mertens DM. *Research and Evaluation in Education and Psychology: Integrating Diversity with Quantitative, Qualitative, and Mixed Methods*, 5th ed. Thousand Oaks, Calif.: SAGE; 2019.

18. Morgan DL. Paradigms lost and pragmatism regained: methodological implications of combining qualitative and quantitative methods. *J Mix Methods Res.* 2007;1(1):48–76.

19. Biesta GJJ. Pragmatism and the philosophical foundations of mixed methods research. In Tashakkori A, Teddlie C, eds. *SAGE Handbook of Mixed Methods in Social & Behavioral Research*, 2nd ed. Thousand Oaks, Calif.: SAGE; 2010: 95–118.

20. Legg C, Hookway C. Pragmatism. In Zalta EN, ed. *The Stanford Encyclopedia of Philosophy.* Stanford, Calif.: Stanford University; Summer 2021 ed. https://plato.stanford.edu/archives/sum2021/entries/pragmatism (accessed 25 January 2022).

21. Kelly LM, Cordeiro M. Three principles of pragmatism for research on organizational processes. *Method Innov.* 2020;13(2):1–10.

22. Hothersall SJ. Epistemology and social work: enhancing the integration of theory, practice and research through philosophical pragmatism. *Eur J Soc Work.* 2019;22(5):860–870.

23. Johnson RB, Onwuegbuzie AJ. Mixed methods research: a research paradigm whose time has come. *Educ Res.* 2004;33(7):14–26.

24. Regehr G. It's NOT rocket science: rethinking our metaphors for research in health professions education. *Med Educ.* 2010;44(1):31–39.

25. Biddle C, Schafft KA. Axiology and anomaly in the practice of mixed methods work: pragmatism, valuation, and the transformative paradigm. *J Mix Methods Res.* 2015;9(4):320–334.

26. Cherryholmes CH. Notes on pragmatism and scientific realism. *Educ Res.* 1992; 21(6):13–17.

27. Rorty R. Pragmatism as anti-representationalism. In Murphy JP, Murphy AR, eds. *Pragmatism: From Peirce to Davidson.* Boulder, Col.: Westview Press; 1990; 1–6.

28. Biesta GJJ. Why 'what works' still won't work: from evidence-based education to value-based education. *Stud Philos Educ.* 2010;29:491–503.

29. Rossman GB, Wilson BL. Numbers and words: combining quantitative and qualitative methods in a single large-scale evaluation study. *Eval Rev.* 1985;9(5):627–643.

30. Creswell J, Poth C. *Qualitative Inquiry and Research Design: Choosing among Five Approaches*, 4th ed. Thousand Oaks, Calif.: SAGE; 2018.

31. Greene JC. *Mixed Methods in Social Inquiry.* San Francisco: Jossey-Bass; 2007.

32. Feilzer MY. Doing mixed methods research pragmatically: implications for the rediscovery of pragmatism as a research paradigm. *J Mix Methods Res.* 2010;4(1):6–16.

33. Dewey J. The sources of a science of education. In Boydston JA, ed. *John Dewey: The Later Works (1925-1953) Volume 5: 1929–1930.* Carbondale, Ill.: Southern Illinois University Press; 2011: 1–40.

34. Morgan DL. *Integrating Qualitative and Quantitative Methods: A Pragmatic Approach.* Thousand Oaks, Calif.: SAGE; 2013.

35. Johnson RB, Onwuegbuzie AJ, Turner LA. Towards a definition of mixed methods research. *J Mix Methods Res.* 2007;1(2):112–133.

36. Creswell JW, Plano Clark VL. *Designing and Conducting Mixed Methods Research*, 3rd ed. Thousand Oaks, Calif.: SAGE; 2017.

37. Leech NL, Onwuegbuzie AJ. A typology of mixed methods research designs. *Qual Quant.* 2009;43(2):265–275.

38. Morse JM, Niehaus L. *Mixed Method Design: Principles and Procedures.* Walnut Creek, Calif.: Left Coast Press; 2009.

39. Schifferdecker KE, Reed VA. Using mixed methods research in medical education: basic guidelines for researchers. *Med Educ.* 2009;43(7):637–644.

40. Teddlie CB, Tashakkori A. *Foundations of Mixed Methods Research: Integrating Quantitative and Qualitative Approaches in the Social and Behavioral Sciences.* Thousand Oaks, Calif.: SAGE; 2009.

41. Fetters MD, Curry LA, Creswell JW. Achieving integration in mixed methods designs – principles and practices. *Health Serv Res.* 2013;48(6Part II):2134–2156.

42. Bradbury H. ed. *The Handbook of Action Research*, 3rd ed. Thousand Oaks, Calif.: SAGE; 2015.

43. Meyer J. Qualitative research in health care: using qualitative methods in health action research. *BMJ.* 2000;320(7228):178–181.

44. Mertler CA. *The Wiley Handbook of Action Research in Education.* Hoboken, NJ: John Wiley & Sons Inc.; 2019.

45. Greenwood DJ. Pragmatic action research. In Coghlan D, Brydon-Miller M, eds. *The SAGE Encyclopedia of Action Research.* Thousand Oaks, Calif.: SAGE; 2014: 645–647.

46. Cohen L, Manion L, Morrison K. *Research Methods in Education*, 6th ed. London and New York: Routledge; 2007.

47. Glaser BG, Strauss AL. *The Discovery of Grounded Theory: Strategies for Qualitative Research.* Chicago: Aldine; 1967.

48. Charmaz K. *Constructing Grounded Theory*, 2nd ed. Thousand Oaks, Calif.: SAGE; 2014.

49. Bakkenes I, Vermunt JD, Wubbels T. Teacher learning in the context of educational innovation: learning activities and learning outcomes of experienced teachers. *Learn Instr.* 2010;20(6):533–548.

50. Magnusson S, Krajcik J, Borko H. Nature, sources, and development of pedagogical content knowledge for science teaching. In Gess-Newsome J, Lederman NG, eds. *Examining Pedagogical Content Knowledge: The Construct and its Implications for Science Education.* Dordrecht: Kluwer Academic Publishers; 1999: 95–132.

51. Wongsopawiro DS, Zwart RC, van Driel JH. Identifying pathways of teachers' PCK development. *Teachers and Teaching.* 2017;23(2):191–210.

52. Biesenthal C. Pragmatism. In Coghlan D, Brydon-Miller M, eds. *The SAGE Encyclopedia of Action Research.* Thousand Oaks, Calif.: SAGE; 2014: 648–650.

53. Mumford L. The pragmatic acquiescence. In Kennedy G, ed. *Pragmatism and American Culture.* Boston: DC Heath and Company; 1950: 36–49.

54. Argyris C. Actionable knowledge: design causality in the service of consequential theory. *J Appl Behav Sci.* 1996;32(4):390–406.

55. Bradbury H. Quality and "Actionability": what action researchers offer from the tradition of pragmatism. In Shani AB, Mohrman SA, Pasmore W, et al., eds. *Handbook of Collaborative Management Research.* Thousand Oaks, Calif.: SAGE; 2008: 583–600.

56. O'Cathain A. Assessing the quality of mixed methods research: toward a comprehensive framework. In Tashakkori A, Teddlie C, eds. *SAGE Handbook of Mixed Methods in Social & Behavioral Research*, 2nd ed. Thousand Oaks, Calif.: SAGE; 2010: 531–556.

57. Bryman A. Paradigm peace and the implications for quality. *Int J Soc Res Methodol.* 2006;9(2):111–126.

58. Tashakkori A, Teddlie C. Quality of inferences in mixed methods research: calling for an integrative framework. In Bergman MM, ed. *Advances in Mixed Methods Research: Theories and Applications.* London: SAGE; 2008: 101–119.

59. Hong QN, Pluye P, Fàbregues S, et al. Mixed Methods Appraisal Tool (MMAT), version 2018. Registration of Copyright (#1148552);Industry Canada: Canadian Intellectual Property Office2018.

60. O'Cathain A, Murphy E, Nicholl J. The quality of mixed methods studies in health services research. *J Health Serv Res Policy.* 2008;13(2):92–98.

61. Gaglio B, Henton M, Barbeau A, et al. Methodological standards for qualitative and mixed methods patient centered outcomes research. *BMJ.* 2020;371:m4435.

62. Bradbury H, Lewis R, Embury DC. Education action research: with and for the next generation. In Mertler CA, ed. *The Wiley Handbook of Action Research in Education.* Hoboken: John Wiley & Sons Inc; 2019: 7–28.

63. Akkerman S, Admiraal W, Brekelmans M, et al. Auditing quality of research in social sciences. *Qual Quant.* 2008;42(2):257–274.

64. de Kleijn R, van Leeuwen A. Reflections and review on the audit procedure: guidelines for more transparency. *Int J Qual Methods.* 2018;17(1):1–7.

65. Greene JC, Caracelli VJ, Graham WF. Toward a conceptual framework for mixed-method evaluation designs. *Educ Eval Policy Anal.* 1989;11(3):255–274.

66. Greene JC. Is mixed methods social inquiry a distinctive methodology? *J Mix Method Res.* 2008;2(1):7–22.

67. Albert M, Hodges B, Regehr G. Research in medical education: balancing service and science. *Adv Health Sci Educ.* 2007;12(1):103–115.

68. van Enk A, Regehr G. HPE as a field: implications for the production of compelling knowledge. *Teach Learn Med.* 2018;30(3):337–344.

69. Doja A, Lavin Venegas C, Cowley L, et al. Barriers and facilitators to program directors' use of the medical education literature: a qualitative study. *BMC Med Educ.* 2022;22(1):45.

70. Onyura B, Légaré F, Baker L, et al. Affordances of knowledge translation in medical education: a qualitative exploration of empirical knowledge use among medical educators. *Acad Med.* 2015;90(4):518–524.

71. Thomas A, D Gruppen L, van der Vleuten C, et al. Use of evidence in health professions education: attitudes, practices, barriers and supports. *Med Teach.* 2019;41(9):1012–1022.

72. Dickstein M. *The Revival of Pragmatism: New Essays on Social Thought, Law, and Culture.* Durham, NC: Duke University Press; 1998.

73. Watling CJ, Lingard L. Grounded theory in medical education research: AMEE Guide no. 70. *Med Teach.* 2012;34(10):850–861.

Bringing together principles and perspectives, this image represents
strong, unique and impactful practices. Being both intended and emergent
in its design. Reflecting our creative research practices, this pebble
pathway leads to (imagined) possibilities

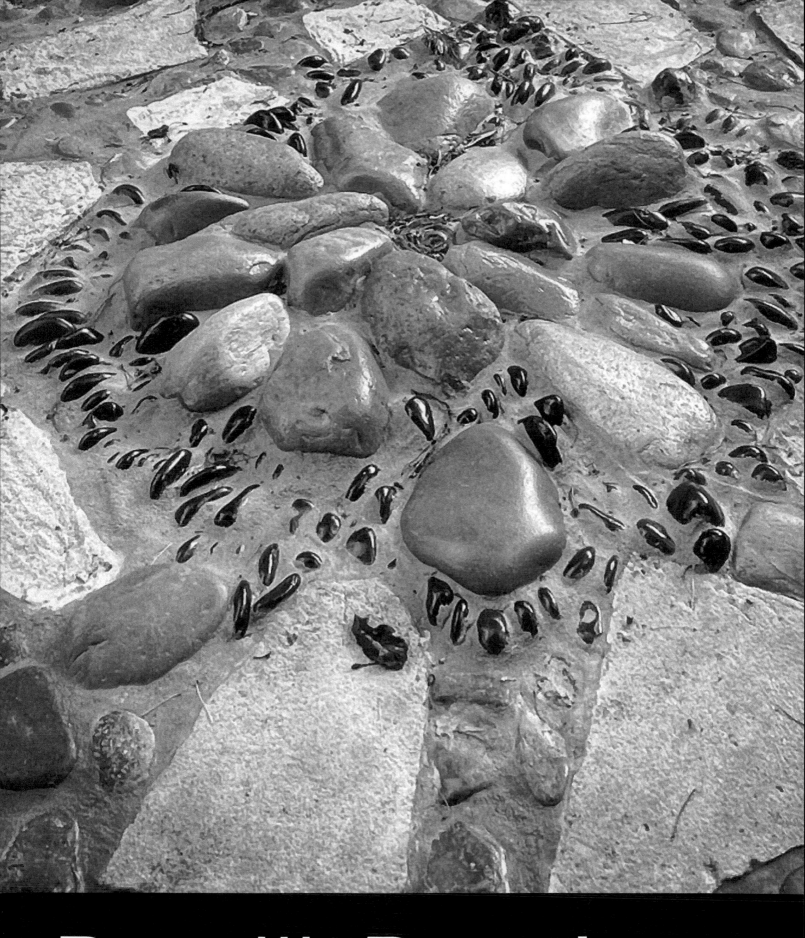

Part III: Practices

Proposals in Health Professions Education Research

Maria A. Blanco[1], Mahbub Sarkar[2], and Claire Palermo[2]

[1] *Tufts University, Boston, Massachusetts, USA*
[2] *Monash University, Clayton, Victoria, Australia*

Box 10.1 Chapter 10 learning objectives: After reading this chapter you should be able to ...

- Describe the different purposes of health professions education research (HPER) proposals
- Explore the key phases for drafting a high-quality HPER proposal including the key components of high-quality educational research proposals
- Discuss the style of writing required for HPER proposals
- Explore common errors made in HPER proposals
- Critically appraise research proposals for their strengths and areas for improvement

---

10.1 INTRODUCING CHAPTER 10

Preparing a research proposal is arguably the central creative act underpinning the development of new research. [1 p. 62]

A research proposal is a detailed written plan for a research project [1]. It describes why the research is important and how it will be carried out, including the project timeline and resources needed [1]. A research proposal identifies an issue or problem, intellectual or practical, for which more information is needed. At the same time it explains and justifies study designs, and theoretical and conceptual

---

Foundations of Health Professions Education Research: Principles, Perspectives and Practices,
First Edition. Edited by Charlotte E. Rees, Lynn V. Monrouxe, Bridget C. O'Brien, Lisi J. Gordon, and Claire Palermo.
© 2023 John Wiley & Sons Ltd. Published 2023 by John Wiley & Sons Ltd.

frameworks, therefore portraying an argument or the need for research [2]. Research proposals should clearly articulate the problem to be addressed, why the study needs to be conducted, what it will achieve, who will benefit, what will happen (how, where, and when), and why this is significant from a practical and societal perspective [3]. Research proposals are a key first step in commencing any research and can be challenging for health professions education research (HPER) as they require researchers to conceptualise the research in its entirety and write in a way that convinces the reader that the work should be undertaken [4, 5]. A good research proposal places the research team in good stead for the successful conduct of research [4].

Research proposals are an essential part of the research process. There are many reasons for writing a research proposal. First, writing a research proposal allows researchers to focus their thinking on the project, while putting their ideas down on paper and checking for the soundness and feasibility of the project. Second, it gives an opportunity to seek and get constructive feedback for improvement from colleagues and other relevant stakeholders by sharing written drafts. Research proposals are also needed to obtain formal approval for the project by supervisors and/or ethical committees (see Chapter 3, section 3.3.1), and to apply for funding. Finally, a detailed research proposal serves as a guide throughout the research planning and implementation, and as an audit document upon completion of projects [1].

In this chapter, we walk you through the steps for writing research proposals while describing their essential components, highlighting high-quality features, and illustrating common mistakes made by authors (see Box 10.1). Along the way, we provide you with writing tips and concrete examples. As stated above, there are many reasons for writing a research proposal and while there is no single approach, there are common features. In this chapter, we focus on generic aspects of writing any type of research proposal and offer some recommendations for seeking funding and ethical approval. In the following sections, we present three key phases for writing a research proposal. In section 10.2, we present preparing to write a proposal (phase one), then move on to drafting a proposal in section 10.3 (phase two). In section 10.4, we discuss reviewing your research proposal (phase three), before moving on to a more detailed breakdown of the typical components of a research proposal in section 10.5. Finally, we discuss the challenges and benefits of proposal writing in section 10.6, before summarising the chapter in section 10.7. Throughout this chapter, we draw on two case study examples from our own work to illustrate key points – an unpublished successful grant application and a published research protocol – providing our critical reflection on these examples (see Box 10.2). We recommend further review of existing HPER literature on writing grant proposals for more information on grant writing (see Box 10.19) [4, 6]. We also refer you to our book glossary for definitions of complex terms used in this chapter.

Box 10.2   Case studies: An overview

Underlined grant application*: Sarkar and colleagues submitted this grant proposal to a small, external health professions education grant scheme (AU$5000). The project aimed to explore how health professions educators perceive the use of pedagogical content knowledge (PCK) as a framework for capturing and developing the professional knowledge required for high-quality teaching.

Published research protocol [7]: This protocol describes a convergent mixed methods study that aims to evaluate the impact of shifting to online education during the COVID-19 pandemic on learners and faculty across a range of health professions education courses.

*While references/citations have been removed from this example, for ease of reading, proposals should always be referenced and thus evidence-based.

10.2 PHASE ONE: PREPARING TO WRITE A RESEARCH PROPOSAL

In HPER, a phenomenon of interest is typically identified through practice, from discussions with others in the field, or in the broader HPER community as discussed earlier in Chapter 1. The first step to writing a research proposal is immersion in existing literature that might speak to the phenomenon of interest. Consultation with experts or other reliable sources of information about these ideas is common. This will not only support the refinement of ideas, but also ensures that the proposal will address a need in the field [4]. If possible, consult with a librarian for assistance with literature searching to ensure that previous literature published on the topic is captured [8]. Searching the Internet for literature reviews published on the topic is a useful starting point (e.g., systematic reviews published in open-access journals). The purpose of this phase is to identify relevant theories and theoretical frameworks that inform the research project (see Chapter 2, section 2.5.2.1 for suggestions about searching the literature for theory). Talking to others about the idea, especially seeking input from scholars who have done work in your area of interest, attending conferences, and engaging with credible discussions on relevant social media (e.g., Twitter, LinkedIn) will also help you to refine your idea. This process helps you to build the research conceptual framework right from the inception of the project. This is also a good time for you to identify and invite collaborators, if applicable. There are no rules for collaboration. However, it can be useful to ensure a breadth of experience and expertise across your team. Before starting the writing process, meet with your collaborators to go over a writing strategy and timeline, while discussing important deadlines (e.g., ethics committee deadlines), and assigning roles and responsibilities among members of the team [4].

Research ethics protect the integrity of three distinct areas of the research endeavour: science, research participants, and authorship [9]. When it comes to planning a submission to the ethics committee, become familiar with the submission processes at your local institution that correspond to the type of study proposed. Contact the local ethics committee directly to check submission plans and seek their guidance with multi-site research projects if needed. Similarly, if applying for funding, ensure your familiarity with any funder instructions by working with your institutional research division and contact the funding programme manager directly with any questions related to the grant call and application. Contacting previous awardees to get their insights from their grant proposal experiences with the funder may also be useful [9].

10.3 PHASE TWO: DRAFTING A RESEARCH PROPOSAL

In this phase, start by drafting an outline of the proposal with the main headings and subheadings (see Box 10.3). Then proceed by adding bulleted ideas for each section, which can subsequently be elaborated upon. Be aware that there are multiple templates for writing research proposals that suggest different ways of labelling or organising the proposal components (e.g., grant or ethics applications that lump the background and conceptual framework together into one introductory section). Different study designs and research approaches may also require different headings and subheadings. Regardless of the proposal template outline, the components described below need to be addressed.

Proposals targeting HPER are typically written using the future tense, active voice, and first person singular or plural. While some disciplines may prefer the use of the passive voice and third person, as in scientific approaches, the HPER field has been a proponent of the active voice and first person pronouns [4]. In a research proposal, the use of the third person in scientific language may downplay the research team's involvement and communicate a neutral observation, while the use of the first person singular or plural underscores the subjective nature of the research approach (see Chapters 5 and 7). Ensure sentences are clear and concise, avoiding or explaining technical jargon. Pretend to write to non-experts in the area. For example, the following sentence: 'We used a qualitative lens, informed by sociocultural perspectives of learning activity, to focus on how academic literacy was infused into the lecture', can be rephrased for clarity as follows: 'Sociocultural perspectives of learning maintain that social interaction plays a fundamental role in the development of understanding. Using participant observations, we will explore qualitatively interactions between the teacher and the students that facilitate students' acquisition of literacy skills.'

Your writing style should be consistent throughout your proposal [3]. This requires special attention when there is more than one person involved in the writing process. When the drafting of the proposal is complete, we suggest that you ask senior mentors not involved in the research project to read the proposal for clarity and consistency. An existing network of peer/grant reviewers may be available or you may choose to set up a group at your institution. Consultation with end-users of your research may also be important at this stage, especially in certain types of research approaches valuing co-design. Box 10.3 provides an overview of the typical components of a research proposal that we further elaborate on later in section 10.5.

Box 10.3   Typical components of a research proposal

- Title page
- Abstract/Summary
- Introduction
- Conceptual and/or theoretical framework
- Methodology and methods (including study aims and research questions)
- Educational implications/significance/impact
- Dissemination plan
- Timeline
- Budget
- Research team and roles and responsibilities
- References

10.4   PHASE THREE: REVIEWING YOUR RESEARCH PROPOSAL

As mentioned in section 10.3, once your proposal is drafted, it can be useful to have it reviewed by experienced researchers who can provide feedback on its appropriateness and soundness [4]. Recruit a non-experienced reviewer (e.g., an end-user of the research findings), who can provide feedback on clarity and overall writing style. It can also be useful to serve as a reviewer of paper proposals that are submitted for presentation at professional meetings. This scholarly activity provides insights into research proposals across a spectrum of quality, while providing useful insights on how to approach writing your own research proposals. We propose using a checklist to assess proposals (see Box 10.4), as this is aligned with the typical components of research proposals [1].

Box 10.4 Checklist for assessing proposals*

Section	Description and guidance
General points	☐ Includes all necessary sections and subsections in a logical manner
	☐ Presents an easy-to-follow sequence
	☐ Shows appropriate formatting and layout, including grammar and spelling
	☐ Includes a reference list that is consistent in style, accurate, and complete
Abstract	☐ Describes the purpose/goal, study design, and methods
Introduction	☐ Defines feasible aims, purpose, and objectives of the study
	☐ Gives convincing information to justify the need for and importance of the study
	☐ Includes a literature review that is relevant to the topic and presents information
Conceptual framework	☐ Describes the state of existing knowledge
	☐ Identifies gaps in understanding of a phenomenon or problem
	☐ Outlines the methodological underpinnings of the research project
	☐ Describes relevant theoretical frameworks if applicable
Methodology and methods	☐ Outlines the study approach and methodology
	☐ Describes the study context with enough detail
	☐ Shows good understanding of research terminology and techniques
	☐ Presents a detailed, well-organised description of the sampling approach, data collection methods, and analysis plans
	☐ Conveys research procedures that are appropriate to the project objectives, and are feasible and achievable
	☐ Indicates ethical requirements
	☐ Clearly stated aims and research questions
Educational implications	☐ Clearly outlines the impacts of the research and beneficiaries
Dissemination plan	☐ A feasible plan for dissemination is stated

(continued)

(continued)

Section	Description and guidance
Timelines and budget	☐ Provides clear details on project management, specific roles of the research team, and resources required
	☐ Includes a timeline that is logical and consistent
	☐ Provides an estimation of financial resources needed that is well-considered, realistic, and sufficiently detailed
Formatting	☐ Cover includes all important contact information
	☐ All pages after the cover are numbered
	☐ Complies with required guidance, if prescribed
	☐ References are consistent and accurate

*Adapted from Thomas and Hodges [1].

10.5   TYPICAL COMPONENTS OF A RESEARCH PROPOSAL

In this section, we discuss in more detail the typical components of a research proposal (already outlined in Box 10.3). Associated with this, we present in boxes examples of how these components have been written in successful grants.

10.5.1   Title Page

The first page of a proposal typically includes the title, the name of the author(s) with their contact information and institutional affiliations, and the version number and date of the completed proposal. It can also include the name and contact information of the addressee, if applicable. Pay considerable attention to the title. Start with a general title and come back to refine it as you develop your study design. The title is the first component of the proposal that readers will notice to determine whether they would be willing to invest time in reading the rest of the work. Therefore, the title should not only provide a clear and concise snapshot of the research proposal, but also grab the attention of the reader [10]. This is especially important when applying for funding. Adding a catchy phrase to the title can be effective, but make sure that the title includes all key features of the study design, (i.e., the phenomenon of study, study design, participants, and setting). Before moving on to the next section, pause and reflect on how to write a high-quality proposal title (see Box 10.5).

Box 10.5   Pause and reflect: Writing a high-quality proposal title

Consider the titles: 'Exploring the value of pedagogical content knowledge in health professions educators and its impact on improving teaching practice,' and 'Impact of the COVID-19 pandemic on teaching and learning in health professional education: a mixed methods study protocol.'

- What are the strengths of these titles?
- What could be improved?
- Consider a research project you are working on. What is your current title? How could you improve this?

10.5.2   Abstract/Summary

The abstract or summary provides a succinct description of the main features of the research proposal, including the purpose/goal, the study design, and the methods (see Box 10.6) [4]. It should start with a problem statement, explain the need for the research in light of existing literature and current understandings, and convince readers that this needs to be addressed [11]. Conveying the educational implications of your research project may also be important here. The length of the abstract may vary, and may be structured with defined subheadings or unstructured. We suggest that you follow the application guidelines wherever possible. Write the abstract or summary once you finish writing the proposal. Avoid using acronyms in the abstract. These may frustrate the reader who is unfamiliar with the term or acronym [4].

Box 10.6   Case studies: Example abstract/summary

Unpublished grant application*:

Problem: Pedagogical content knowledge is defined as the particular knowledge possessed by educators that combines knowledge of discipline-specific content and knowledge of pedagogical approaches used to teach that content to enhance student learning. The concept of pedagogical content knowledge has been applied over the past several decades mostly in teacher education settings, to understand and improve teaching and learning. There is a paucity of research investigating the use of pedagogical content knowledge in the context of health professions education.

Purpose: The proposed project aims to explore how health professions educators perceive the use of pedagogical content knowledge as a framework for capturing and developing the professional knowledge required for high-quality teaching in the context of health professions education.

Design: Using a qualitative design, underpinned by social constructionism, the study will engage educators in the process of collaborative content representation design and refinement through a series of meetings facilitated by experts in pedagogical content knowledge and content representation design. Analysing focus group interviews and content representation design artefacts, the study will then explore how this process contributes to stimulating explicit reflection on practice and enhancing professional teaching knowledge in the form of enhanced pedagogical content knowledge.

Implications: The value of this project lies in making explicit what is usually tacit – that is, the planning for, reasoning behind, and enactment of health professions educators' pedagogical decision-making in teaching specific health-related content. This explicit decision-making process can support both their professional development and practice, and be communicated among other health professions educators for collective improvement.

*While references/citations have been removed from this example, for ease of reading, proposals should always be referenced and thus evidence-based.

10.5.3   Introduction

A clear and compelling introduction sets the stage for the research proposal and justifies its importance (see Box 10.7) [12]. The introduction should briefly consider the problems that need to be addressed in light of existing literature, or issues with the existing literature related to this problem, the purpose of the proposed research, and the significance of the research [3, 4, 11]. You will then further elaborate on these aspects in the conceptual framework, and educational implications sections of your proposal. The statement of the problems should describe the key features and causes of the problems followed by what has been done to address them, while citing the relevant literature to date and what further research is needed as a result. While citing this literature, make sure that you do not provide a summary of it, but rather a critical analysis of it based on your literature review, clearly highlighting existing understandings from the literature and how your proposal will address these and advance understanding [4]. In the justification for the research, also consider the social and educational importance of the work and its potential impacts (see Chapter 12 for further details on research impact).

The purpose of your study will then flow as a logical and necessary next step to advance the area. To describe the purpose of your research, paraphrase your research questions. This section will also summarise the goal and provide a list of the objectives or hypothesis depending on the study design. End this section briefly stating the contributions that the research will make and who will benefit from it. You will have an opportunity to further elaborate on the educational implications of your research at the end of your proposal. After reading an introduction, the proposal reviewers should be convinced that your team members have complementary expertise on the topic and that the problem highlighted needs addressing.

Box 10.7   Case studies: Example introduction

Unpublished grant application*:
Typically, in university educational settings, subject matter expertise of teachers is highly valued, regardless of their expertise in *teaching* [original emphasis] that subject matter. Just knowing content and general pedagogy is *not* sufficient to be an effective teacher. Rather, effective teaching requires: 'the blending of content and pedagogy into an understanding of how particular topics, problems, or issues are organised, represented, and adapted to the diverse interests and abilities of learners, and presented for instruction' [i p. 9]. This: 'special amalgam of content and pedagogy' [i p. 9], which Shulman termed pedagogical content knowledge (PCK) over three decades ago, has attracted a great deal of research attention in the field of education, through its attempts to explain the complex, nuanced, and sophisticated work of teaching. The majority of research in the area originated from primary and secondary school contexts, with few studies focused on tertiary educators, particularly in STEM-related disciplines. There is a paucity of research investigating the use of PCK in the context of health professions education.

There are different forms of knowledge for clinical teaching in medicine that need to be mastered. Targeted professional development to facilitate this knowledge transformation process, suggestive of a PCK-infused health professions' educational philosophy, is recommended. A dialogue between science educators and medical educators in order to move medical education away from teacher-dominated and cognitive-centric approaches is needed. This dialogue might support medical educators to develop their professional knowledge for high-quality teaching using the PCK framework. High-quality teaching is defined as: 'the purposeful and deliberate planning of instruction that results in a coherent learning experience for students' [ii p. 945]. Drawing on these views, the proposed study aims to explore how health professions educators perceive the use of PCK as a framework for capturing and developing the professional knowledge required for high-quality teaching in the context of health professions education.

   (i) Shulman LS. Knowledge and teaching: foundations of the new reform. *Harvard Educ Rev.* 1987;57:1–22.
   (ii) Gess-Newsome J, Taylor JA, Carlson J, et al. Teacher pedagogical content knowledge, practice, and student achievement. *Int J Sci Educ.* 2019;41(7):944–963.

*While the majority of references/citations have been removed from this example, for ease of reading, proposals should always be referenced and thus evidence-based.

10.5.4 Conceptual and Theoretical Frameworks

A research proposal must include a clear conceptual framework and its associated theoretical framework (see Chapter 2 for more details on theory) [4]. Even though some researchers use the terms conceptual framework and theoretical framework interchangeably, they do have different meanings [12, 13]. While a theoretical framework is a logically developed and connected set of concepts established from one or more theories, a conceptual framework is the justification for why a given study should be conducted [12]. A conceptual framework is then a tentative theory that informs the rest of the design [2]. A thoughtful conceptual framework helps to assess and refine the goals of your research, develop realistic and relevant research questions, select appropriate methods, and identify potential alternate explanations to your conclusions [2].

Construct the conceptual framework by: (1) employing existing theories that speak to the phenomenon of study wherever possible; (2) conducting a critical synthesis of empirical literature and other relevant sources; and (3) reflecting on experiences with the phenomenon of study [13, 14]. Thus, the conceptual framework describes the state of known knowledge, identifies your current understanding of a phenomenon or problem and areas for development, and outlines the methodological underpinnings of your research project [12].

In this section, you will further elaborate on the synthesis of the empirical literature that you reviewed to craft your introduction, while further explaining how this literature helped you to define the phenomenon of study. You should also explain how the research team's professional experiences and personal beliefs will shape the research (for example, when using interpretive approaches). Thus, in writing your conceptual framework, the purpose is not only descriptive, but also critical. It demonstrates your understanding of the problems with previous research and theory, what contradictions or holes there are in existing views, and how your study can make an original contribution or offer new perspectives [2]. Furthermore, it may be useful to bring ideas from outside traditionally defined study fields, integrate different approaches, lines of investigation, or theories that nobody has previously connected within the conceptual framework [2].

If you identified a relevant theory or theories to ground your research, then also reflect on how that theory will be used in your study by describing the theoretical framework. Thus, a theoretical framework articulates the logic of why a particular theory is being used (see Box 10.8) [12]. The articulation of your conceptual and theoretical frameworks may differ based on your research approach (as indicated in Part II of this book). For example, scientific and realist approaches may finalise the conceptual framework prior to the study and rarely modify it once data collection has started, while with some interpretivist approaches, the conceptual framework may evolve during data collection or analysis [12].

Box 10.8   Case studies: Example conceptual framework

<u>Unpublished grant application*</u>:

PCK refers to the particular knowledge possessed by teachers that combines: (i) knowledge of specific content, and (ii) knowledge of teaching that content in ways which enhance student learning. PCK also comprises the collective knowledge that is widely agreed upon and formed through research and/or collective expert wisdom of practice related to the teaching of specific topics. PCK can be used to understand how teachers transform their subject matter knowledge into forms and representations (e.g., analogies, illustrations) that are meaningful and comprehensible to students at a level that matches their development. The construct of PCK also considers the personal and contextual features of teaching and student learning, including: teachers' beliefs, teaching orientation and learning context, along with students' beliefs, prior knowledge, and behaviours that can greatly influence the teaching and learning that takes place.

PCK appears to be a stronger predictor for the success of teachers' practice to support student learning as compared to content knowledge. The value of a PCK-informed approach lies in teachers being able to articulate both their approach to, and the reasoning behind, their pedagogical choices in teaching specific content. Making explicit that which is normally a tacit component of teachers' practice (i.e., how and why teachers do what they do to support student learning of content) can be valuable for both promoting the specialised knowledge development of individual teachers (personal PCK) and supporting the collective knowledge of the profession (collective PCK). Capturing and developing PCK may therefore be considered as a central component of teachers' professional development.

Based on the theoretical underpinnings described above, our study will utilise the Content Representation (CoRe) tool, in order to capture and develop health professions educators' PCK. Previous research in the STEM education context suggests that the CoRe tool offers a meaningful way to conceptualise and capture PCK as professional practice knowledge. The CoRe tool engages teachers in reflecting on a specific content topic, asking them to identify the central concepts (i.e., big ideas) associated with that topic. Once identified, teachers provide written responses to a series of prompts including: what students should learn about each big idea; why that idea is important to know; what students typically struggle to conceptualise related to the idea; specific teaching strategies designed to promote students' learning about the idea; and ways of assessing student understanding of the idea. Used in this way, the CoRe tool offers a method for eliciting PCK as teachers document and reflect on their teaching goals and practices. When used with a group of teachers, the CoRe tool provides a sharing platform for practice wisdom about how to teach particular content and a process for building collective professional knowledge. Thus, the CoRe tool can simultaneously collect sophisticated PCK from expert teachers, accelerate PCK development among novice teachers, and promote collective professional practice knowledge within a community of teachers.

Drawing upon the conceptual framework, discussed above, the project will explore these research questions (RQs):

1. How can the construct of PCK be used by health professions educators to capture their wisdom of practice?
2. How can health professions educators develop their teaching expertise individually and collectively through the use of the CoRe tool?

3. What value do health professions educators see in the construct of PCK/content representation for their ongoing professional learning and development?

It is worth noting that as part of our conceptual framework, we used PCK as a theoretical framework to explore educators' professional knowledge required for high-quality teaching in health professions education (HPE). We used PCK as a theoretical framework due to its success in explaining the complex, nuanced, and sophisticated work of teaching in school education contexts.

*While references/citations have been removed from this example, for ease of reading, proposals should always be referenced and thus evidence-based.

10.5.5 Methodology and Methods

The methods section of the proposal includes a description of the study design, the context of the study, and the study participants, together with the ethical review plan, and the methods of sampling, data collection, and analysis (see Box 10.9 for study design). Start this section by clearly articulating your study design, while making the research approach explicit for readers [4]. The research approach will frame the rationale for the choice of your methods. High-quality research proposals attend to the internal coherence among epistemology, methodology, and methods [15].

Box 10.9   Case studies: Example study design

Unpublished grant application*:
Study design: Underpinned by social constructionism, acknowledging that individuals make sense of their experiences through social interactions and the surrounding environment, this research will adopt a qualitative methodology and take an interpretivist approach.

*While references/citations have been removed from this example, for ease of reading, proposals should always be referenced and thus evidence-based.

Clearly articulating your research questions guiding your study is key. If your research is being approached from a scientific perspective, associated research hypotheses may be included in this section. Approaching research from an interpretivist standpoint may instead explain the assumptions being brought to the research, while revealing researcher reflexivity. Subsequently, regardless of approach, the context of the study will be described. A thorough description of the study context will allow reflection on contextual factors (e.g., health professions discipline, country, setting) at play. For example, conducting an interprofessional education study involving health professions schools that belong to the same university, versus conducting an interprofessional education study involving health professions schools from different academic institutions. The description of the study context will also allow readers to better judge the usefulness of the study to their local contexts.

The portrayal of study participants should include the sampling strategy, together with any inclusion and exclusion criteria [4]. You should also clarify how your participants will be recruited and protected from any risks that could be associated with their study participation (see Box 10.10) [4]. Please be aware that although educational research might qualify for exemption from full ethics committee review status (for example, in some settings where research may be considered as standard audit or quality assurance processes), such a status must be determined by the corresponding ethics committee after their review of the study application. Drafting a thorough research protocol first will support completion of any ethics applications. A copy of the data collection instruments and data management plan will also need to be submitted with ethics applications. If applying for funding, you need to understand the rules of your institution and/or funder – you may either need to have ethics approval before applying to the funder, or you may need to wait for the funder's decision before submitting your ethics application.

Box 10.10   Case studies: Example participant recruitment

Unpublished grant application*:
Participant recruitment: Given the project team's disciplinary expertise, the study will include four health disciplines: medicine, biomedical sciences, medical imaging and radiation sciences, and public health. Co-investigators representing each of these disciplines will purposively recruit 4–5 educators, including both expert and novice educators. With the total sample of 16–20 educators, the study aims to achieve depth and rigour of collected data using our proposed qualitative methodology. For the purpose of this study, we consider expert educators as those known for their teaching excellence within their discipline (e.g., evidenced by receipt of teaching excellence awards, as listed on the university database) with a premise that they may have more articulated PCK to share within the education community. We consider novice educators the ones with less than five years of teaching experience in the university context.

*While references/citations have been removed from this example, for ease of reading, proposals should always be referenced and thus evidence-based.

Finally, the methods of sampling, data collection, and analysis must be described in as much detail as word counts permit (see Box 10.11). The description of the methods section should clearly illustrate to readers the feasibility and transferability of the study. When describing the methods of data analysis, remember to clarify not only the analytic procedures and approaches being conducted, but also any research software you are planning to use. Remark on how the research will address quality indicators relevant to the approach (see Chapter 4, Box 4.3 for a summary of eight dimensions of quality). Once the methods are clear, assess whether the team has the skills necessary to execute the project. Attesting to the researchers' qualifications is particularly important when applying for funding.

Box 10.11   Case studies: Example sampling, data collection, and analysis

Unpublished grant application*:
A five-phase method for data collection will be used:

Phase I: Meeting 1 will include the sample of all selected educators (4–5 educators purposively recruited by collaborators) across participating disciplines. Workshops will be designed and delivered to introduce PCK and the CoRe tool coinciding with an explanation of the study aims and expectations. Following this, each participant (individually or as a group) will select a topic that is typically difficult for students to understand and that will be taught during 2021–2022. Based on the chosen topic for that health profession group, each participant will individually complete the CoRe tool.

Phase II: Participants will come back to their discipline speciality area (e.g., biomedical science) and discuss the results of the CoRe tool with their disciplinary colleagues and make some agreements on what is in their content representation and what is not. A collective content representation will be developed from this process and shared with members of the group (Meeting 2).

Phase III: Participants will teach the chosen topic, annotating the collective content representation as they teach the topic to capture teaching-related or student learning insights of the chosen topic, prior to Meeting 3.

Phase IV: Meeting 3 will focus on the process of making and annotating the content representation, and discussing views on the process, focusing on how it influenced thinking about teaching and learning and classroom practice, and how it influenced their understanding of PCK more generally. Prompts will be provided to stimulate the group discussion (group interview 1), for example, how useful (or not) the content representation development process is for meaningful teaching in a manner supportive of student understanding; benefits and challenges related to the content representation development process; and what relationships are identified between content representation and PCK.

Phase V: Group interview 2, to be conducted about 2–3 months after Meeting 3, will explore the participants' final views on the entire process, including content representation and PCK and how they believe this may (or has) impacted, or influenced, their professional practice.

Data collection: Data will be collected in the form of audio-recorded focus group interviews and participant artefacts (CoRe tool). Focus group interviews are chosen as the main data source to enable dialogue and a joint exploration of participants' experiences and their emerging understandings. The nature of the interviews will be semi-structured, allowing the interviewer to explore participants' answers to gain deeper insights and seek clarification to ensure the research questions are addressed.

Data analysis: Focus group interview data will be analysed using Ritchie and Spencer's team-based, five-stage framework analysis, which includes: familiarisation; identifying the coding framework; indexing; charting; and mapping and interpretation. Both group interview 1 and 2 data will be analysed to answer RQ1, while RQ2 and RQ3 will be answered from group interview 1 and 2 respectively. Content representation (both initial and annotated) will be used as an additional data source for RQ2 and analysed thematically.

Our five-member research team is diverse in terms of disciplinary background (e.g., medicine, health sciences, science education), experiences with (and orientations to) qualitative methodologies, and demographics (e.g., age, gender). We completed a team reflexivity exercise at the beginning of developing this proposal, which supports researchers to share their backgrounds and experiences, and fears about the project. This provided us with a valuable opportunity to understand each other's perspectives and served to surface our backgrounds and experiences, and thus potential influences over data collection, analysis, and interpretation based on our social constructionism worldview. Diversity within our team will

(continued)

(continued)

support more rigorous data interpretation with team members contributing different perspectives and insights into the data analysis and reporting.

*While references/citations have been removed from this example, for ease of reading, proposals should always be referenced and thus evidence-based.

10.5.6 Educational Implications, Significance, and Impact

In this section, the goals of your project should be restated, together with expected contributions to the field from conducting your study (see Box 10.12). The practical and/or theoretical significance of the research project should also be stated. The potential impacts of your research on beneficiaries (e.g., students, educators, patients), together with any translation into education practice or policy should also be stated (see Chapter 12 for further details about research impact). For example, the work might discover new knowledge related to an educational phenomenon and/or cast light on new ways of approaching education. The next steps, as well as areas for further research, should also be stated. Before you move on, undertake the stop and do activity in Box 10.13.

Box 10.12   Case studies: Example educational implications

Unpublished grant application*:
This project will provide novel evidence on the use of PCK in the field of health professions education. Expected outcomes of this project include educators' increased ability to articulate both their approach to, and the reasoning behind, their pedagogical choices in teaching specific health-related content that may support their professional development and enhance their practice. The findings will help develop a framework for teaching specific content that will be communicated among other health professions educators for collective improvement. The project will facilitate the exploration of PCK across other health disciplines, with future research collaborations with other institutions. This novel insight will provide the basis for the development of a PCK framework that can be generalised to the broader field of health professions education.

*While references/citations have been removed from this example, for ease of reading, proposals should always be referenced and thus evidence-based.

Box 10.13   Stop and do: Critique a study protocol

- Read the following open-access paper: Kumar A, et al. Impact of the COVID-19 pandemic on teaching and learning in health professional education: a mixed methods study protocol. *BMC Med Educ.* 2021;21(1):439. https://doi.org/10.1186/s12909-021-02871-w. [7]
- Consider the following questions:
  - What was the proposal's conceptual framework?
  - In what ways do the authors describe clearly the research approach, methodology, and methods?
  - In what ways could the proposal have been clearer? After reading the proposal, do you think it is an important piece of research to conduct?

10.5.7   Dissemination Plan

Applications for funding typically require a dissemination plan (see Box 10.14). This involves submitting manuscripts for publication, as well as presentations at professional meetings or engaging key users of your research as part of a reference group [4]. Even if you are not applying for funding, outlining your dissemination plan helps to strengthen the plan for developing endurable scholarly products from your project (see Chapter 11 for more details on publishing). Dissemination of your work not only communicates it, but more importantly, begins its translation into practice, policy, and future research. For further details on how you might plan for research impact, see Chapter 12.

Box 10.14   Case studies: Example dissemination plan

Unpublished grant application*:
The proposed research will be disseminated through professional presentations and academic publications.

- Presentations: (a) relevant discipline-specific (e.g., seminar, faculty education workshop series); (b) university-wide learning and teaching conference; and (c) stakeholder and participant meetings/sharing events.
- National and international conference presentations.
- Academic publications in relevant journals.
- Social media (e.g., Twitter, LinkedIn).

*While references/citations have been removed from this example, for ease of reading, proposals should always be referenced and thus evidence-based.

10.5.8   Timeline

Drafting comprehensive and realistic timelines are essential for projects to be judged as feasible [4]. Gantt charts are a useful tool that assist in summarising timelines and tasks [16]. Including a specific timeline with a grant application is almost always required and we strongly encourage you to draft such a study project timeline regardless (see Box 10.15). This will also help your research team stay on track and remain accountable throughout the process. While allocating time frames, we suggest that you allocate a generous amount of time to each phase of the project to account for unexpected events, like ethical approval delays, global events, or participant changes in availability. Some funders require the completion of a risk analysis, including an estimation of the chance of the risk of events occurring (high, medium, low) together with a mitigation strategy per risk. This demonstrates to the reader that your team is well prepared to deal with challenges that may arise, and understands the complexity of the research process and how challenges may impact study timelines.

10.5.9   Budget

The budget is a key component of grant proposals [3, 4]. Having a detailed budget section will help you to identify the potential resources needed. Proposal readers might also benefit from learning about the resources used to repeat the study. If you are applying for funding, pay special attention to what items are fundable and non-fundable by the grant programme, working with your institutional research division.

Box 10.15   Case studies: Example timeline

<u>Unpublished grant application*:</u>

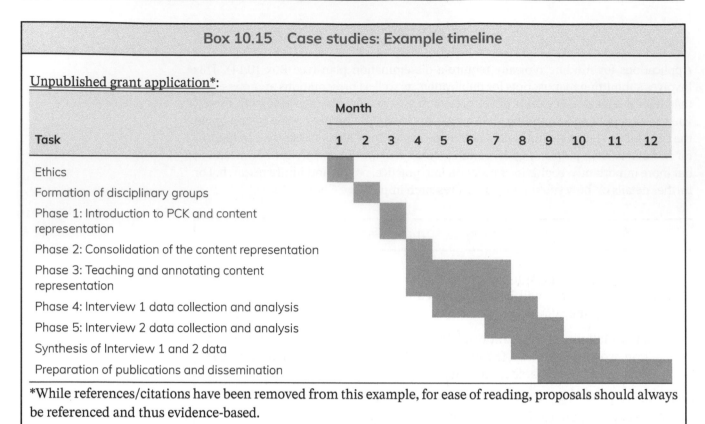

	Month
Task	1 2 3 4 5 6 7 8 9 10 11 12
Ethics	
Formation of disciplinary groups	
Phase 1: Introduction to PCK and content representation	
Phase 2: Consolidation of the content representation	
Phase 3: Teaching and annotating content representation	
Phase 4: Interview 1 data collection and analysis	
Phase 5: Interview 2 data collection and analysis	
Synthesis of Interview 1 and 2 data	
Preparation of publications and dissemination	

*While references/citations have been removed from this example, for ease of reading, proposals should always be referenced and thus evidence-based.

Budget guidelines vary greatly across educational grant programmes. If this information is not clearly available from the grant call, we strongly suggest you contact the funder to double-check fundable items. The requested budget should be realistic and reflect what is required to complete the proposed work. This is particularly important in highly competitive calls (see Box 10.16).

Box 10.16   Case studies: Example budget

<u>Unpublished grant application*:</u>

Cost purpose	Amount (AU$)
Personnel:	
(1) Casual research assistant (RA) non-PhD salary (as of 21/12/2020): (AU$45.21 per hour + 16%) = AU$52.44 for 90 hours	4719.60
RA will assist in collecting and analysing data, and writing report.	
(2) Principal and co-investigators – Level B, D and E academics	In kind
Transcription:	
Interview transcriptions approx. 16 hours @AU$2.00 per minute	1920
The research team has existing transcription service access	– 1920
Catering for workshop: approx. 20 participants @AU$10 per head	200
Total requested funding	4919.60

*While references/citations have been removed from this example, for ease of reading, proposals should always be referenced and thus evidence-based.

10.5.10   Research Team and Roles and Responsibilities

This section lists the members of the research team with a brief description of their research background and experiences, specifically those related to the research project to justify why these particular people are on the team and how they complement each other [4]. This section can also include each team member's specific tasks and responsibilities, as well as how the work of the team will be structured and managed (see Box 10.17) [4].

Box 10.17   Case studies: Example research team and roles and responsibilities

Unpublished grant application*:
The five-person research team involves researchers from two faculties (Medicine, Nursing and Health Sciences, and Education), and four health disciplines (medicine, biomedical sciences, medical imaging and radiation sciences, and public health) demonstrating interfaculty and interdisciplinary collaboration. The principal investigator, Sarkar, will oversee and manage the project, including ethics, supervise the research assistant and support co-investigators, and assist with data collection, analysis, and dissemination of findings. The co-investigator, Berry, brings to this project expertise in science education, teacher learning, and PCK. In addition, she brings experience in leading large-scale research grants, working with multidisciplinary teams, and successfully delivering research outcomes. Other co-investigators (Ilic, Lazarus, and Wright) bring discipline expertise and will lead the discipline-specific community of practices. They will contribute to recruiting potential research participants from their respective disciplines and organising meetings with them, supporting the research assistant in data collection, assisting with data analysis and research dissemination, and developing outputs.

*While references/citations have been removed from this example, for ease of reading, proposals should always be referenced and thus evidence-based.

10.5.11   References

The references used throughout the written proposal must adhere to a standard referencing format or that prescribed by the funder, and you should ensure that this format is followed consistently. Ideally use reference manager software to keep track of the citations, like EndNote, Reference Manager, or Mendeley. Ensure adherence to the requirement of the funder or audience of the proposal.

10.6   CHALLENGES AND BENEFITS OF PREPARING AN HPER PROPOSAL

HPER proposals are a key part of the research process, yet there are several challenges associated with preparing proposals. Health professions education researchers have often transitioned into HPER from other non-education/social sciences backgrounds such as basic or clinical sciences. Therefore, making shifts to writing proposals in HPER may be challenging, particularly because of HPER's greater emphasis on theory [5, 9]. In addition, writing a proposal is different from a research paper in terms of the purpose, audience, and format. Research proposals aim to convince the reader that the work should be done, and research papers present the process and outcomes of the research that has been done. The writing in proposals may be more provocative and convincing than that usually found in a research paper [5]. Another key challenge is time. Writing grant proposals is one of the core activities of research work and probably the most time-consuming [5, 9]. Many researchers feel a low return on investment with only a few proposals obtaining funding. Further, grant writing demands logistics, management, and leadership. Despite these challenges, when written well, proposals provide research teams with a clear plan and pathways to research success (see Box 10.18).

Box 10.18   Case studies: Reflections on lessons learnt from proposals

Unpublished grant application*: We submitted our PCK proposal for an external research grant scheme. It was only for AU$5000, but required significant time and effort to develop. Since there are few external grant schemes available for HPER, it was competitive: there were 23 submissions, five of which were funded, ours being one of these. Given the small budget, the investigators needed to commit to spending in-kind time (cost) to deliver the project, increasing our workloads. Participation in this project required prolonged engagement, so we had difficulty in recruiting and engaging study participants. However, there are high stakes for the investigators of this grant as they are representing disciplines that supported the recruitment and retention of study participants.

Published study protocol [7]: We had a large team of researchers across various health disciplines collaborating on the COVID-19 project, which made the project management challenging (e.g., working through busy diaries). Given our multidisciplinary backgrounds, we had considerable variations in our orientations to research and underpinning methodological preferences (e.g., scientific, interpretivist, pragmatist). We did not have a robust discussion among the team on our philosophical positioning and assumptions when we conceived and designed the project. While we were excited about working in a multidisciplinary team and not in silos, various sites and professions have used different teaching approaches online, which created considerable variations in the data and made our analysis challenging. Also, there is a plethora of research exploring the impacts of the COVID-19 pandemic on learning and teaching since the pandemic started that challenged the publication potential of our study. However, with our longitudinal mixed-methods design and voluminous quantitative and qualitative data from key stakeholders across various health professional courses, we could provide a unique contribution of the long-term impact of the pandemic on health professional education.

*While references/citations have been removed from this example, for ease of reading, proposals should always be referenced and thus evidence-based.

10.7   CHAPTER SUMMARY

In this chapter, we have provided a brief overview of the reasons you would prepare a research proposal and outlined the key steps for preparing a HPER proposal, providing some guidance on typical proposal sections. We have outlined a checklist for proposal content, and provided an example HPER grant proposal to illustrate key points, as well as a research protocol to further expand your learning. We have outlined the challenges in preparing proposals in educational research. After reading this chapter, we hope that you have reflected on the many reasons for writing a research proposal, and we hope this chapter has clearly articulated the key tips for writing high-quality research proposals. To extend your reading, work through the key references in Box 10.19.

Box 10.19   Recommended reading for writing HPER proposals

Blanco MA, Gruppen LD, Artino Jr AR, et.al. How to write an educational research grant: AMEE Guiden. 101. *Med Teach.* 2016;38(2):113–122 [4].

Blanco MA, Lee MY. Twelve tips for writing educational research grant proposals. *Med Teach.* 2012;34(6):450–453 [10].

Hofmann AH. *Scientific Writing and Communication Papers, Proposals, and Presentations*, 4th ed. New York: Oxford University Press; 2019 [3].

Lingard L. Bonfire red titles. *Perspect Med Educ.* 2016;5(3):179–181 [10].

Lingard L, Watling C. *Story, Not Study: 30 Brief Lessons to Inspire Health Researchers as Writers*. Cham: Springer; 2021 [17].

Palermo C, Reidlinger DP, Rees CE. Internal coherence matters: lessons for nutrition and dietetics research. *Nutr Diet.* 2021;78(3):252–267 [15].

Porter R. Why academics have a hard time writing good grant proposals. *J Res Adm.* 2007;38(2):37–43 [5].

Wong G. Literature reviews: who is the audience? In Cleland J, Durning SJ, eds. *Researching Medical Education*. Chichester: Wiley Blackwell; 2015: 25–34 [8].

REFERENCES

1. Thomas DR, Hodges ID. *Designing and Managing Your Research Project: Core Knowledge for Social and Health Researchers*. Thousand Oaks, Calif.: SAGE; 2010.

2. Maxwell JA. *Qualitative Research Design: An Interactive Approach*, 2nd ed. Thousand Oaks, Calif.: SAGE; 2005.

3. Hofmann A. *Scientific Writing and Communication Papers, Proposals, and Presentations*, 4th ed. New York: Oxford University Press; 2019.

4. Blanco MA, Gruppen LD, Artino Jr AR, et al. How to write an educational research grant: AMEE Guide no. 101. *Med Teach.* 2016;38(2):113–122.

5. Porter R. Why academics have a hard time writing good grant proposals. *J Res Admin.* 2007;38(2):37–43.

6. Wisdom J, Riley H, Myers N. Recommendations for writing successful grant proposals: an information synthesis. *Acad Med.* 2015;90(12):1720–1725.

7. Kumar A, Sarkar M, Davis E, et al. Impact of the COVID-19 pandemic on teaching and learning in health professional education: a mixed methods study protocol. *BMC Med Educ.* 2021;21(1):439.

8. Wong G. Literature reviews: who is the audience? In Cleland J, Durning S, eds. *Researching Medical Education*. Chichester: Wiley Blackwell; 2015: 25–34.

9. Blanco MA, Lee MY. Twelve tips for writing educational research grant proposals. *Med Teach.* 2012;34(6):450–453.

10. Lingard L. Bonfire red titles. *PerspectMed Educ.* 2016;5(3):179–181.

11. Lingard L. Joining a conversation: the problem/gap/hook heuristic. *Perspect Med Educ*. 2015;4(5):252–253.

12. Varpio L, Paradis E, Uijtdehaage S, et al. The distinctions between theory, theoretical framework, and conceptual framework. *Acad Med*. 2020;95(7):989–994.

13. Bordage G, Lineberry M, Yudkowsky R. Conceptual frameworks to guide research and development (R&D) in health professions education. *Acad Med*. 2016;91(12):e2.

14. Ringsted C, Hodges B, Scherpbier A. 'The research compass': an introduction to research in medical education: AMEE Guide no. 56. *Med Teach*. 2011;33(9):695–709.

15. Palermo C, Reidlinger DP, Rees CE. Internal coherence matters: lessons for nutrition and dietetics research. *Nutr Diet*. 2021;78(3):252–267.

16. Geraldi J, Lechter T. Gantt charts revisited: a critical analysis of its roots and implications to the management of projects today. *Int J Manag Proj Bus*. 2012;5(4):578–594.

17. Lingard L, Watling C. *Story, Not Study: 30 Brief Lessons to Inspire Health Researchers as Writers*. Cham: Springer; 2021.

CHAPTER 11

Publishing in Health Professions Education Research

Lisi J. Gordon[1], Anique Atherley[2], Anna T. Cianciolo[3], and Bridget C. O'Brien[4]

[1] University of Dundee, Dundee, Scotland, UK
[2] Ross University School of Medicine, Bridgetown, Barbados
[3] Southern Illinois University School of Medicine, Springfield, Illinois, USA
[4] University of California San Francisco, San Francisco, CA, California, USA

> **Box 11.1 Chapter 11 learning objectives: After reading this chapter you should be able to ...**
>
> - Conceptualise publishing as a multifaceted research dissemination process in health professions education research (HPER)
> - Recognise different forms of research dissemination in HPER
> - Summarise common approaches in preparing your HPER for dissemination
> - Describe HPER dissemination processes via conferences, peer-reviewed journals, and alternative formats, from submission to final decision

11.1 INTRODUCING CHAPTER 11

We tend to think that journals exist to publish scholarly manuscripts. But they don't. They do publish scholarly manuscripts, yes, but that's done in service of a higher purpose: they exist to promote scholarly conversations. [1 p. 252]

So far, the chapters of this book have provided the foundations on how to conceptualise, conduct, and evaluate health professions education research (HPER). In this chapter, we turn to the critically important step of sharing your research findings (see Box 11.1). This can feel both invigorating and terrifying – invigorating as you

---

consider end-users' learning from the products of your hard work; terrifying as you imagine how peers may evaluate it. Identifying reasons and goals for publishing, knowing the options, developing a plan, and familiarising yourself with publication processes can help you feel more comfortable and confident. In this chapter, we first discuss publishing as a broad concept including multiple forms of research dissemination (section 11.2). We describe key considerations when sharing your work at conferences (section 11.3), in peer-reviewed journals (section 11.4), and, in section 11.5, through creative (e.g., visual), conversational (e.g., dialogues on Twitter), and alternative formats (e.g., academic blogs). We then recommend ways to plan a publishing approach incorporating multiple forms of dissemination (section 11.6). We discuss characterising publishing as a career-long pursuit and aspirational competency, and offer suggestions for continuous engagement (section 11.7), before summarising the chapter in section 11.8.

Our chapter reflects the literature on publishing, as well as our own experiences as HPER authors, reviewers, and editors. Our backgrounds include education, medicine, organisational behaviour, engineering psychology, and physiotherapy before our migration to HPER. We range from early career to 18 years of HPER experience, and have published our research in multiple forms. We have each celebrated successes, weathered disappointments, and learned reflexively from our perseverance in publishing our research. We introduce four case studies in Box 11.2 and discuss them in detail in specific sections to illustrate research publication journeys. Please see our book glossary for definitions of publishing-related terms employed across this chapter.

Box 11.2   Case studies: An overview

Scenario 1: Choosing the right journal for your manuscript [2]: This example highlights how it took three cycles for the research team to find the right journal.

Scenario 2: Moving beyond desk rejection [3]: This example highlights how support, reflection, and persistence are key to moving beyond desk rejection. The publication was the first, first-author publication of original research by an early career researcher.

Scenario 3: Revising a manuscript [4]: This example highlights the complexities of undertaking an effective manuscript revision using feedback from four reviewers and engaging in dialogue with the editor to successfully publish a journal article by a doctoral student.

Scenario 4: Planning a dissemination approach [5–7]: This example highlights a planned approach to multiple forms of dissemination from the same research project (The Scottish Doctors' Wellbeing Study) demonstrating the reasoning around a conference workshop [5], a journal paper [6], and an infographic [7].

11.2   PUBLISHING: DIFFERENT WAYS OF UNDERSTANDING PUBLISHING AND ITS PURPOSES

At first, the term publishing may make you think of books or peer-reviewed journal articles. Such publications are, after all, the building blocks used by researchers to construct reputations and networks [8]. While these forms of publishing remain important, there are many ways to share your research [9]. As some journals transition to open-access and online-only formats, new opportunities arise for creative, interactive presentations of findings [8, 9].

In this chapter, the term publishing includes many forms of dissemination: journal articles, conference abstracts, posters, and presentations; visual abstracts; preprints; white papers or reports; infographics; blog posts; podcasts; videos; and social media [10]. We emphasise the scholarly nature of these research outputs, meaning they must have clear goals or purposes; involve adequate preparation including review of relevant literature, evidence, and resources; use appropriate methods (e.g., ethical, rigorous, aligned with purpose); share meaningful and valuable findings; be accessible for others to use, evaluate, and provide feedback on; and show evidence of reflective critique and improvement [10, 11]. This last item, reflective critique and improvement, aligns with our view of publishing as a dynamic, iterative process in which publications are launching points for conversations rather than end points [1]. In other words, publishing is generative – it sparks conversation, new insights (theoretical, conceptual, practical, methodological), new research directions, and practice change (see Chapter 12 for an in-depth discussion of research impact) [1]. While you might initially think of publishing as a necessary activity that helps you achieve career milestones and improves your chances of securing grant funding, we hope this chapter also encourages you to view publishing as a means of putting new knowledge to good use and sharing it in ways that appropriate audiences will access and interact with [12]. The sections that follow encompass a diverse range of credible ways to disseminate research findings [13]. Each of these engages the peer-review process in different ways – some begin with peer review to select submissions for presentation or publication, while others involve an ongoing peer-review process whereby others interact with the publication (e.g., comments on blogs or social media posts).

11.3 CONFERENCE PRESENTATIONS

Conference presentations offer opportunities to introduce your recent HPER to peers. They can raise a project's profile, prompting your audience to search for related publications. Presentations can also help you anticipate feedback from peer reviewers as the audience will likely ask questions and/or make suggestions to help you refine your conceptual framing, identify the compelling aspects of your study, and enhance understanding of your target audience [14, 15]. Conferences also expose you to others' current ideas and thinking [16].

11.3.1 Choosing the Right Conference

Because conference presentations and journal articles can overlap, being strategic with these dissemination opportunities is important. There are multiple types of local, national, and international conferences [15]. Each serves a particular audience. For example, the Developing Excellence in Medical Education Conference (DEMEC: see https://www.demec.org.uk) targets those involved in medical education across the UK, the Asia Pacific Medical Education Conference (APMEC: https://medicine.nus.edu.sg/cenmed/apmec2023) targets medical and health professions educators from the Asia-Pacific region, and the American Educational Research Association meeting (AERA: see https://www.aera.net/Events-Meetings/Annual-Meeting) draws international, interdisciplinary education researchers. Each differs in size and competitiveness in terms of getting your abstract accepted (typically, the larger the conference, the greater the competition) [16]. See Box 11.3 to explore possible HPER conferences.

Box 11.3   Stop and do: Exploring conferences

Explore and choose a conference that you think your HPER work is best suited to. Use the following tips to help with your choice:

- Ask colleagues about conferences they have attended – who was there and what was the research quality like? If you belong to a professional society associated with your HPER (e.g., the Association for the Study of Medical Education: ASME; the Australian & New Zealand Association for Health Professional Educators: ANZAHPE) check out their website for upcoming conferences.
- What do you want to achieve by presenting at this conference?
- Who should your audience be? For example, is it clinical educators, HPE researchers, or education researchers more generally?
- Is the conference in-person, online, or hybrid? What are the benefits of attending in-person or online?
- What is your budget? Consider conference fees, travel, accommodation, meals, and other expenses.
- Who is attending the conference? Is there a conference theme? Look at the conference website for information about keynotes. Consider how your HPER can be articulated in relation to the conference theme.

11.3.2   Choosing the Right Type of Presentation

There are multiple ways to present at health professions education (HPE) conferences (e.g., short communications, research presentations, posters or ePosters, workshops, seminars, lightning talks). When choosing a presentation type, be clear about your goals for the session. For example, if the aim is to test a new idea or share work in progress, then a roundtable or poster session giving you opportunities for longer discussions and peer feedback might work best. Closely read the description of each type of conference session to ensure that your submission is fit for purpose.

11.3.3   Preparing Your Submission

A conference submission (often in the form of an abstract) needs to concisely convey fundamental information about your HPER project [15]. Reviewers will evaluate the content of your submission according to selection criteria and others' submissions, and make a decision as to its suitability for inclusion in the conference [15]. Varpio and colleagues describe three core aspects of abstract writing: (1) the purpose – to effectively present the fundamentals of your study; (2) the audience; and (3) selection committee expectations for abstract structure. Box 11.4 offers a task to help you consider how to prepare a good abstract [15].

Box 11.4   Stop and do: Preparing an abstract

The aim of this task is to get you to practise preparing a conference abstract:

- Based on a current HPER project, write a 300-word abstract using the following headings: introduction, methods, results, and discussion.

- Now read: Varpio L, Amiel J, Richards BF. Writing competitive research conference abstracts: AMEE Guide no. 108. *Med Teach.* 2016;38(9):863–871.

- Go back to your abstract and consider how it might be improved (you may even want to try rewriting it).

11.3.4 Preparing Your Presentation

Preparing a presentation narrative that engages your audience takes time, so be sure to plan sufficient time to prepare and practise [14]. Additionally, the visual aspects of your presentation (e.g., a poster or slides) require thought to ensure connection to your narrative [14, 17]. Typically, a conference presentation is more limited in scope than a full journal paper, maybe addressing a single element of a complex analysis or highlighting a subset of findings. Deciding the scope of your presentation (regardless of format) should be purpose driven, based on the following: study status (e.g., complete or incomplete); what findings you wish to present (all or an interesting subset); who is your audience (e.g., practitioners, theorists; national or international colleagues); and what you covered in your abstract. Do not worry if your study is incomplete; feedback on your partially completed study can reveal timely ways to refine your approach and reflect on your study narrative.

11.3.5 Attending the Conference

An enjoyable aspect of conferences is networking with scholars with mutual interests and engaging in constructive, knowledge-building conversations [16]. Conferences are places where you can truly feel like part of the living, breathing HPER community. However, networking can feel daunting. Planning which sessions or events to attend, arranging meetings with people whose work piques your curiosity or relates to your own, and knowing what you will say when people ask you about your work can help you make the most of your conference time [16]. Authentically and enthusiastically discussing your ideas can stimulate new collaborations and associated dissemination efforts. See Box 11.5 for an activity that asks you to prepare a brief description of your work, and Box 11.6 for tips on getting started with conferences.

Box 11.5 Stop and do: Craft your elevator pitch

Imagine you are walking through the conference venue and you bump into an admired colleague. They ask you what you are working on. What would you say?

- Prepare a 30-second version and a 2-minute version of your response.

- Consider what would make your work interesting and compelling to others.

- Make sure to include what is important about this work and why it matters.

- Share your elevator pitch with other researchers (e.g. peers, supervisors) and/or end-users and ask them to summarise what they heard you say, what they found interesting, and what strikes them as important about your work.

> **Box 11.6   Pause and reflect: Tips for getting started with attending conferences**
>
> - Start with local and regional conferences, which can cost less and have more manageable agendas.
> - Initially, go to conferences with a mentor (e.g., supervisor) or more experienced peer who can help you acclimatise and provide introductions.
> - Participate in scholarly service at the conference, such as moderating a session and judging posters.
> - Participate in small-group activities designed to stimulate networking, such as special interest groups and newcomer welcome sessions.

11.4   JOURNAL ARTICLES

Journal articles give you the opportunity to situate your work more fully in the scholarly landscape, by elaborating on how your work contributes to current problems and conversations, explaining your methodology, and presenting more detailed and nuanced findings. In addition to conferences, journal articles are the most common way for HPE researchers to disseminate findings.

11.4.1   Choosing a Journal

An important aspect of publication is choosing the right journal [18]. This task can be harder than it seems as there are many factors to consider when choosing a journal (see Box 11.7). A recent large, international survey of published HPE scholars identified six factors that influence journal choice: fit (between manuscript and journal mission, target audience, and submission categories); advice from others (e.g., respected colleagues, mentors); decision-making by editors about acceptance, acceptance rate, and publishing speed; journal impact; and breadth of readership (e.g., national, international) [18]. Selecting a journal is about how best to achieve impact by joining knowledge-building conversations most likely to amplify your message [19]. Selecting well will increase the likelihood of receiving feedback on your manuscript and decrease the number of rejection letters (and the time and effort of reformatting for submissions elsewhere).

> **Box 11.7   Factors to consider when choosing a journal**
>
> - Mission/scope: The journal's statement of purpose and description of its publication priorities.
> - Target audience: The journal's intended readership (e.g., clinician-educators, researchers, educational leaders).
> - Submission categories: The types of articles the journal publishes (e.g., research reports, conceptual analyses, commentaries, reviews, personal reflections, poetry).
> - Open solicitations: Active requests for submissions on specific topics or from particular author types (e.g., students, trainees, scholars underrepresented in medicine). However, beware of predatory journals.

- Publication access: The journal's approach to dissemination, which may be subscription only or include a range of open-access options.

- Publication fees: The journal's fees, charged to authors, for publishing an article; some journals may also charge fees upon submission to cover processing costs.

- Author guidelines: Each journal will have these on their website which gives insight into the types of submissions accepted, limits for words and exhibits (e.g., tables), and restrictions on prior publications (e.g., pre-prints, conferences).

- Time to decision: The average amount of time it takes journals to make initial decisions on submissions (e.g., reject a manuscript without peer review or return a manuscript with an editorial decision based on peer reviews).

- Time to publication: The average amount of time it takes a journal to publish a manuscript following acceptance including whether they publish online early.

- Editorial approach: The approach the journal's editorship takes to cultivating manuscripts collaboratively with authors, which may range from essentially hands-off to writing mentorship.

- Journal impact factor/quality rankings: Reflected by several different metrics, this is the extent to which the journal's publications are cited in other publications. Quality rankings are based on factors like the journal's acceptance rate, journal impact factor, altmetrics from social media, and expert opinion, among others. Different countries have different ways to articulate quality rankings (e.g., in Australia, indicators of journal quality are linked to what journal quartile they belong). Websites such as Scimago (https://www.scimagojr.com/index.php) and Clarivate (https://jcr.clarivate.com/jcr/home) rank journals by quartile.

- Altmetrics: Reflected by several different metrics, this is the amount of attention the journal's publications receive online (e.g., number of Twitter mentions) [11].

- Legitimacy: The journal's dedication of editorial services to rigorous peer review and publication quality assurance (contrasted with predatory journals, whose purpose is to seek profit via publication fees without editorial attention to scientific integrity or merit).

To choose a journal, we recommend engaging in the 3Rs: (1) Research – familiarise yourself with the array of legitimate HPER journals, read articles written by editors to provide guidance to authors [20–23]; (2) Reflect – consider how your work fits with a journal based on the information you have gathered; and (3) Respond – choose a journal based on the alignment of your motivations, constraints, and goals with journal characteristics. The 3Rs can empower you to make informed decisions about your manuscript and help you avoid setbacks (e.g., accidentally selecting a predatory journal or discovering your target journal has a publication fee you are unable to pay). Box 11.8 provides a brief exercise in applying the 3Rs, and Box 11.9 presents a case study of how an international team of authors applied the 3Rs to get their work published.

Box 11.8   Stop and do: Applying the 3Rs

Think of a study you are working on and a potential paper you might write. Use the 3Rs described above (Research, Reflect, Respond) and the factors presented in Box 11.7 to help you select your top journal choices for publishing the manuscript.

Compile a list of possible journals by:

- listing journals that publish articles you cite frequently or that inform your work;
- asking co-authors and colleagues who publish HPER and serve on editorial teams for suggestions;
- exploring the Annotated Bibliography of Journals for Educational Scholarship: https://www.aamc.org/professional-development/affinity-groups/group-educational-affairs/mesre-section;
- ascertaining the quality of the journal using the indicators provided by Scimago (https://www.scimagojr.com/index.php).

Box 11.9   Case study: Choosing the right journal for our manuscript

Scenario 1: It took three cycles of applying the 3Rs to find the right journal for our manuscript [2]. Our paper reports findings from a multinational interview study used an integrated theoretical framework (Social Cognitive Career Theory and Professional Identity Formation) and appreciative enquiry to explore the interplay of professional identification and research context in shaping post-training research success narratives.

Cycle 1: Research: With decades of collective HPER experience, our research team leadership was already familiar with the diverse array of legitimate HPER journals.

Reflect: The task was to explore what we knew of these journals (see Box 11.7). We considered only legitimate journals, and aimed to publish in a high-quality journal whose mission/scope, target audience, and author guidelines were aligned with the work we had performed.

Respond: Initially, we selected a top-tier HPER journal [Journal A], thinking that our study's topic was highly relevant to Journal A's readers. We knew that most of the articles we cited in our introduction were published in Journal A. Our study was multi-institutional, and we believed our results had sufficiently broad implications to assist medical school deans of research (part of Journal A's readership). Our submission was rejected without review or editorial feedback.

Cycle 2: Reflect: After this desk rejection, we had to reflect on what made our work ill-suited to Journal A's mission/scope, target audience, or author guidelines. Our manuscript presented a multinational, qualitative interview study, which required a somewhat longer than usual word count and involved a participant subgroup (Pakistani researchers) that was perhaps outside the concern of Journal A's typical readers.

Respond: With this in mind, we shortened the manuscript and submitted it to another top HPER journal with a highly international readership [Journal B], although we were less sure that physician scientists would be a topic of interest to the editors. Journal B sent our manuscript out to peer review, but the editor rejected it based on reviewer feedback.

Cycle 3: Reflect: The reviewers' comments were very helpful for improving two key aspects of our work that related to reaching a target audience of fellow HPE researchers: (1) clarifying the conceptual framing; and (2) streamlining the results to better convey the patterns we identified in our data.

Research: We chose *Advances in Health Sciences Education* [Journal C] because the journal has an international readership, no word limit, and we thought the editors would appreciate our theoretical development. Finally, because time to publication was becoming a priority, we appreciated that the journal had a fast-track submission category, to which authors can submit a revised manuscript (with tracked changes) along with the original peer reviews from Journal B and a detailed response letter. Authors generally received an accept or reject decision in less time than they would for a regular submission.

Respond: Based on Journal B reviewers' positive tone, we carefully and thoroughly revised the manuscript, submitting it to Journal C where it was ultimately published.

Lessons learned: In hindsight, perhaps we should have selected this journal first, factoring it into our planning process. However, we learned that finding a suitable journal involved more than prioritising the right journal selection criteria; it also required being thoughtful and adaptive in how we connected with readers.

11.4.2 Submitting Your Manuscript

Submitting a manuscript takes time. Journals' style, standards, and author guidelines vary, and following each journal's specific guidelines is key to submitting successfully. Editors expect authors to comply with their guidelines to facilitate manuscript processing and peer review. When submitting, it is important to budget enough time – often several hours – to navigate the journal's online submission portal and re-review the author guidelines to ensure that your submission meets the journal's requirements.

11.4.3 The Decision Letter

Your initial submission will be reviewed by the journal editor and at this point a judgement will be made relating to your paper's relevance to the journal, its quality, and its originality [24]. Your paper might be desk-rejected if the editor deems that any of these aspects are not met, or it might be sent for peer review [24]. You will receive a decision letter from the journal editor by email, which may take between a few days to a few months. The decision letter can have varying levels of detail depending on the decision and the journal's style [25]. The decision letter generally states one of three decisions: (1) reject (most common), with or without feedback; (2) revise, often further specified as minor or major revisions; or (3) accept (extremely rare for initial decisions; more common following revisions, although not guaranteed: see Figure 11.1). You may be tempted to think any decision other than accept indicates your paper is unworthy of publication. This is untrue. Receiving a revise decision should be celebrated as it gives you the opportunity to improve the quality of your paper. As seen in Figure 11.1, a revise decision can lead to acceptance if you revise your paper effectively.

If the decision is reject, do not be disheartened. Everyone, regardless of career stage, receives rejections. Research shows a paper is often rejected for the following reasons: having an ineffective study question and/or design (92%); suboptimal data

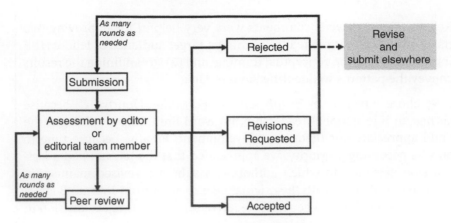

FIGURE 11.1   Pathway from submission to journal decision.

collection (49%); or a topic unimportant or irrelevant to the journal's mission (37%) [26]. Desk rejections can come with minimal feedback about why the manuscript was rejected. If your paper is rejected after peer review, feedback will provide some insight into the reasons for rejection; this feedback can be leveraged to improve the manuscript for submission to another journal [27]. As demonstrated in Box 11.9, a decision letter requesting major revisions is a good sign [28]. The editor has decided your paper fits the journal's scope and that your work has the potential to reach sufficient quality to be published. Reviewer feedback generally identifies serious but not fatal concerns and editors may indicate certain items that must be addressed for a successful revision. A first decision letter rarely suggests minor revisions. This decision tends to follow major revisions [28]. Minor revisions can include requests to clarify content, streamline arguments, and/or restructure sections [29]. If you stick close to the feedback requested in a minor revision, your manuscript is likely to be accepted. With persistence and hard work, most papers presenting rigorous studies can eventually reach acceptance by a journal, even if it's not your first or second choice. After acceptance, you will often receive instructions from the journal about timelines and next steps for final publication, including copy-editing and review of the typeset manuscript.

11.4.4   Moving on from a Challenging Decision Letter

Receiving a reject or major revision decision letter can be psychologically difficult [30]. Researchers can expend a lot of mental energy anticipating poor outcomes [31]. Studies show that this anxiety declines over careers, and it is important that everyone in the research team takes responsibility to plan the next steps for a rejected paper. The ability to see rejection and revisions as an opportunity to bring a paper to its maximum potential comes with time. After informing your research team of the decision, you may find it helpful to take a week or two before regrouping and engaging with the revise and resubmit process. On very rare occasions, research teams may decide to submit an appeal of an editor's decision. Allow emotions to dissolve before taking this route; if you still wish to appeal, be respectful (devoid of emotion and focused on facts), reflective (offer a specific plan to strengthen the work and address shortcomings), and rational (be explicit about the appeal's basis and remember the author's responsibility to write clearly and succinctly, even if reviewers have missed something that you provided in the original manuscript) [24]. Box 11.10 asks you to pause and reflect on your own decision letter experiences, and Box 11.11 describes one of ours.

Box 11.10 Pause and reflect: Decision letter experiences

Imagine or reflect on (if this has already happened to you) this scenario: You are very proud of, and excited about, a HPER paper you submitted. A week later you receive a desk rejection from the journal editor stating that: 'it is not within the journal's scope' without further clarification or feedback. Write down how you would feel about receiving this decision letter. You might even want to make a drawing or write a poem representing these feelings.

Box 11.11 Case study: Moving beyond desk rejection

Scenario 2: Our story highlights how support, reflection, and persistence were key to moving beyond desk rejection. This was my first, lead-author publication of original research [3]. Our paper reports findings from an interview and question-naire study in which we used organisational socialisation theory to explore medical student transitions within the clinical years. First decision: We submitted our manuscript: 'The psychological impact of the "micro-transition" into a final-year medicine clerkship' to a top-tier HPER journal [Journal A]. We received a decision letter within 14 days that began with the words: 'I'm sorry to inform you...' This manuscript was desk rejected, with no tangible feedback.

Moving on: For me, as first author, moving on from this desk rejection required support, reflection, and persistence. Support first came from my mentor (a senior author on the paper). My mentor took the time to turn this into an academic lesson, highlighting the normalcy of rejection in academia. After this, I reflected on the team's decision to submit to Journal A and could recognise that the paper was not a good fit.

Second decision: We resubmitted the manuscript to another HPE journal [Journal B]. This time the manuscript was rejected after peer review.

Moving on again to success: The need for further support and persistence came into play. One research team member noted: 'the critique though blunt and direct, I find very useful for guiding future research and publication, I think we can take many learning points ... the effort at least was not wasted'. Encouraging team discussions led to engaging an external researcher with international HPER experience to provide some feedback. This was used alongside the peer reviews from Journal B to prepare a submission that was ultimately accepted in Journal C.

Lessons learned: Recognise that everyone's support needs look different and if you feel you need more assistance, consider reaching out to peers or even an online community like Twitter for some help as you navigate a rejection. Try to get to a place where you see rejection or a revision request as a redirection and not an impasse.

11.4.5 Revising Your Manuscript: Responding to Reviewers and Editors

While the list of revisions in a decision letter may initially feel overwhelming, having a system to review, organise, and address the comments and a supportive team to encourage, guide, and contribute to the revision makes the process more manageable

[24]. Start by checking the journal website for the required format of resubmissions (e.g., request for clean and tracked-changes versions of the manuscript; format for response to reviewers) and develop a plan with your team. You may find it helpful to read editorials that provide guidance on how to respond to reviewers [32–36]. If any part of the process is unclear, you can contact the journal editor or staff. Clarification upfront saves time and most editorial teams welcome such communication. Occasionally, an editor will invite you to discuss the revision, which is an excellent learning opportunity you should accept.

We suggest three principles to guide you towards an effective revision:

1. Communicate and engage with your co-authors: Ensure all co-authors are aware of the decision and the due date for revisions. Work with co-authors on initial plans, a timeline, and expected roles, responsibilities, and deadlines. Asking co-authors to review your response to reviewers is an excellent way to ensure that you are clear and that the tone is respectful and appreciative. Throughout the revision process, maintain communication about plans, progress, and timelines. All authors must have time to review and approve the revised manuscript before you resubmit.

2. Ensure a systematic and comprehensive response to the review: Absorbing the content of the review takes time and often multiple reads. We recommend starting with the editor's comments, which often summarise the key items the editor identifies as most critical to a successful revision. Then review the reviewers' comments and highlight or create a list of the items you view as most important to address, as well as any conflicting recommendations. You may be able to identify a theme or two among the reviews or in each of the reviewer's comments, which can give you insights into reviewers' perspectives and rationales. If the reviewers identify themselves, it can be worthwhile to look them up to understand more about their perspective, expertise, and publications (particularly if on related topics). You may also notice that the quality, style, and level of detail in reviews varies. While you need to thoughtfully attend to all comments, noticing differences among the reviews may help you decide how to negotiate discordant recommendations. It is also important to identify any recommendations that you disagree with or that you are unable to address and discuss these with your co-authors to ensure agreement on how to respond.

3. Communicate your response thoroughly: You can and should feel empowered to respond to each comment and suggestion in a way that improves your manuscript. While some argue that 'the reviewer is always right' [32], meaning that all comments are informative because they call attention to places where authors need to provide more clarity or information, this maxim does not mean that you must comply with everything the reviewers suggest. If you disagree with a recommendation, are unable to make a suggested change or addition, or decide to make a different change, make sure that your response letter states this and provides your rationale. When recommendations conflict, we suggest drawing the editor's attention to the discrepancy and explaining why you chose one suggestion and not the other.

A potential challenge of revising papers is balancing the word limit with reviewer requests for more information and explanation. Such decisions are a great place to solicit input from co-authors regarding priorities, consequences of omitting certain text, and clever suggestions for ways to reduce words (e.g., move content to tables, figures, or supplementary materials). To conclude this section, we present a case study from our experiences of revising a manuscript (see Box 11.12).

Box 11.12   Case study: Revising a manuscript

Scenario 3: This example highlights the complexities of undertaking an effective manuscript revision using feedback from four reviewers [4]. Our paper reports findings from an interview study which identifies specific personal, social, and physical environmental elements that influence students' perceived use of biochemistry during patient care activities.

First peer review: A doctoral student I supervise submitted the first manuscript from her doctoral research to our top choice HPER journal. This submission was a big milestone and we felt pleased with the manuscript. Several months later, I eagerly opened the email from the journal and was delighted to see a 'major revision' decision. Then I kept reading. And reading. And reading. We received comments from four reviewers, a deputy editor, and the editor-in-chief. The comments spanned 14 pages when pasted into a single document. We had two months to complete our revision and much work to do!

Revising the manuscript: We met as a team to construct a plan, talk through the key points, and decide how to address the comments that: a) conflicted; and b) seemed most challenging (e.g., unclear, required major changes). As first author, the doctoral student took the lead in preparing the revision. She organised the comments by section of the manuscript and clustered them by common points. She then placed these organised comments into a revision table with two columns – one for comments and the other to explain relevant changes or justification for no changes. To make the revision process manageable, she worked through the manuscript section by section, sending the co-authors sections to review as she completed them along with the revision table. As the senior author and primary supervisor, I met with her every week or two to talk through sections and comments that she found particularly challenging. After completing the sections, each co-author read through the whole manuscript, making some further changes for consistency. With this structured approach and weekly goals, we resubmitted the revised manuscript by the deadline.

Second peer review: Given the extent of the revisions, the editor chose to send the paper back out for peer review by one reviewer. A few months later, we received another 'major revision' decision. While we were initially disappointed in this decision because it meant investing substantially more effort to make the manuscript suitable for publication, we decided to persist.

Second revision: The feedback seemed more manageable, and the editor graciously offered to meet with the doctoral student to talk through key points that needed to be addressed in the revision. The doctoral student left the conversation feeling inspired and motivated to persevere. She also felt much clearer about how to simplify the argument, clarify the study's purpose, and restructure the findings to better align with the study's purpose. Since this revision was also quite extensive and came at a busy time for the doctoral student, we needed two months to complete the revision.

Success! Two weeks after submitting the revision, we were thrilled (and relieved) to receive an email from the editorial office stating: 'we are pleased to accept your manuscript for publication' and requesting no further revisions.

(continued)

(continued)

Lessons learned: It can be easy to forget that editors are people dedicated to supporting quality scholarship. This experience taught us the value of having a conversation with the editor. The first author, a doctoral student, felt empowered and motivated to persist after having the opportunity to explain the study as part of a supportive/constructive conversation, including discussing her thought processes for the revision, and her dilemmas. As her PhD supervisor, I deeply appreciated the editor's willingness to offer guidance when our team was stuck and uncertain how to proceed.

11.5   NEW WAYS OF PUBLISHING: CONVERSATIONS AND CREATIVITY

Increasingly, HPE researchers are considering options to publish their work beyond conference presentations and journals. Conversations are emerging about these options as credible ways to disseminate research findings [13]. This evolving area can extend the reach of your work to wide and varied audiences. Some of the types of publishing we have engaged in include: visual abstracts [17], writing blogs [37], podcasts [38–40], designing infographics [41], producing video animations [42], creating comics [43], writing poems [44], developing websites [45], and engaging in social media activities. These forms of publishing can be quick and simple ways to disseminate findings with a focus on concise and practical information [46], often using cognitively appealing visual representations of complex ideas, as in visual abstracts [17, 47]. Using social media to share scholarship with a wide audience has gained popularity. Most journals and scholarly HPER organisations have social media presences [13].

All modes of dissemination require thoughtful actions to ensure credibility and quality. While many of these publications are not considered peer-reviewed in the classic sense because peers are not gatekeepers to publication, peer review occurs as others interact with the content (e.g., comments on a blog or social media post). Perhaps core to these approaches is that more onus is placed on the information user to critically appraise the information that authors share [47]. We suggest that you consider the following criteria when developing your alternative publications to support critical appraisal and enhance the credibility of your outputs: (1) choose professional fora in which to share your work (e.g., webpages within an established website); (2) clearly link to the source of your information (e.g., original papers, datasets); (3) wherever possible, ensure methods for others to provide feedback are transparent (e.g., comments on blogs, workshops using visual materials as a prompt); (4) ensure that authors are named; (5) make sure any images used are not copyrighted, following rules for permissions (see https://creativecommons.org) and are useful (not merely for aesthetics); and (6) consider cost – often developing visual representations such as comics or animated videos will require professionals to ensure that your message is conveyed well. See Box 11.13 for a chance to practise crafting a tweet. See Figure 11.2 for an example of an infographic developed as part of the case study presented in Box 11.2 (scenario 4) and Box 11.15.

Box 11.13   Stop and do: Draft a tweet

Prepare a tweet (statement of 280 characters or less) to inspire others to read about and discuss your work. Use the following top tips by Rzewnicki and Nabavi to prepare your tweet [48]:

- Avoid long threads – stick to short, catchy content.
- Use a hashtag every time (hashtags typically used in HPER include #MedEd and #HPE).
- Ensure relevant Twitter users are tagged.
- Colourful emojis or pictures will draw the eye – use these, but not excessively.

11.6   PLANNING YOUR OVERALL APPROACH TO PUBLISHING

As we have described, there are multiple ways to publish your HPER. Planning is key to success, as a journal article might not always be the best and most appropriate mode of dissemination. A range of different audiences may be interested in your research, and you need to consider the full suite of publishing avenues. You may choose multiple ways to publish the same study. We have devised a set of planning points below to help you consider how to approach publishing your HPER.

11.6.1   Identify Your Audience

A key aspect of planning is identifying your target audience (see Box 11.14). For example, if the target of your message is practicing medical educators, then a journal that focuses on educational theory such as *Advances in Health Sciences Education* might not get to the right audience; *Medical Teacher* or *Clinical Teacher* would be better. Likewise, if you want to target practicing nurse educators with your paper *Nurse Education in Practice* may be a more optimal home than the more theory-centred journal *Nurse Education Today*. Indeed, you may realise that multiple audiences can benefit from your research. For example, if your audience comprises fellow HPE researchers, you might choose to publish in a top-ranking, highly cited HPER journal. If you also wish to share your work with healthcare leaders, presenting a poster at a healthcare leadership conference or using an infographic to share on social media might work better.

Box 11.14   Stop and do: Begin your dissemination plan

Think of a research project that you are currently undertaking or planning. Use these questions to devise your dissemination plan:

- Who is my audience?
- What are the messages from my research that I want to convey?
- What am I contributing to the field?
- Who should be part of the authorship team?
- How should I ensure that I am not salami slicing?

11.6.2   Decide on Your Message

Once you identify your audience, it is important to decide what type of message you want to share. For example, does your work contribute to new theoretical, conceptual, or empirical understandings as part of an academic conversation? If so, you might plan peer-reviewed submissions to conferences and journals. However, if you wish to start a discussion and share information about your research as it unfolds, you might consider developing a social media presence or blog. Alternatively, clear and practical recommendations based on your research might be best conveyed via a briefing paper or seminar.

11.6.3   Position Your Work in the Field

Chapter 4 discusses positioning (see section 4.3.2) and relevance (see section 4.3.3) as key dimensions of quality. Both dimensions emphasise the importance of making novel and relevant contributions with your HPER. Even if they tell the story of a great research study, publications will be rejected or ignored if they do not convey how the study fits into the bigger picture and moves the conversation forward [49]. A contribution can be made in multiple ways (e.g., as theory development or innovative solutions to an HPE problem, or as application of conceptual understanding from one context to another).

11.6.4   Decide Who the Authors Are

This can be the most problematic aspect of research collaboration, often discussed only when there is a dispute about who has contributed what and how much (see section 3.4.5 in Chapter 3 for more discussion about credit breaches) [50]. Many HPE journals use the International Committee of Medical Journal Editors' four criteria to define who qualifies for authorship [51]. We suggest, as a matter of good practice, that teams use these criteria for all forms of publication. We also recommend discussing authorship upfront as a deliberate part of planning [52, 53]. Undertaking a team reflexivity exercise in which team members respond to a series of questions regarding their experience, what they wish to gain from a project, and what their concerns are can be an honest way to clarify what each team member wants from a project and its associated dissemination activities [54].

11.6.5   Consider Impact

When planning a dissemination strategy, it is important to consider impact. As Chapter 12 covers impact, we will not dwell on it here, except to say that you should plan the range and number of publication activities and how you will articulate their interconnection. Each publication should also stand alone as original work. Publication pressure can lead to slicing up research projects to maximise outputs (often termed salami slicing) [55–57]. See Chapter 3 for more details on salami slicing. Some ways to avoid salami slicing include ensuring each publication has a different message and is addressing a different problem, and sharing previous publications with journal editors and explaining what this submission uniquely contributes to the field [58]. However, these guidelines should not prevent you from presenting the same work in different formats (e.g., conference presentation, journal article, blog post, podcast). In Box 11.15, we share a case study drawn from a large, national, multifaceted project to illustrate how planning can be used.

Box 11.15   Case study: Planning dissemination

Scenario 4: Introduction to Scottish Doctor Wellbeing Study [59]: In this Scotland-wide project, we aimed to design and deliver evidence-based interventions to support the well-being of doctors during COVID-related transitions. This six-month project had four concurrent work streams: (1) a scoping review of interventions for healthcare worker well-being during times of crisis; (2) qualitative longitudinal data collection of 120 doctors' experiences during the pandemic; (3) use of data, literature review, and theoretically-based intervention design frameworks to create and implement evidence-based interventions to support doctors' well-being; and (4) intervention evaluation. Due to the short-term but large-scale nature of the project, dissemination planning began early. Publication activities for this project are numerous, wide-ranging, and ongoing, and we regularly discuss further publications and their purpose [55]. This project has elicited more than 20 different outputs (see https://www.scotlanddeanery.nhs.scot/your-development/scottish-medical-education-research-consortium-smerc/research/covid-19-wellbeing-study/). Below we focus on three specific examples: a journal paper [6], a conference workshop [7], and an infographic (see Figure 11.2) [8].

Journal paper: This paper was intended for other health professions scholars (audience). It was the first paper planned from the empirical work stream, and was meant for joining the academic conversation about health professionals' well-being as a core aspect of HPE and to extend the theoretical literature on well-being and transitions (message and contribution to the field). Therefore, we chose the journal *Medical Education* as the most appropriate home for this submission. All project members were authors, as all contributed to the paper (authorship).

Conference workshop: Due to the unusual, fast-paced nature of the study with four concurrent work streams, we wanted to make a methodological contribution of interest to HPE researchers (audience and contribution to the field). We therefore devised a conference workshop abstract, targeting an HPER conference (https://www.asme.org.uk/events/rme2021) focusing on the rapid, rigorous, responsive, and resourced nature of the project, with the aim that HPE researchers might consider similar approaches in their HPER (message to convey). Three project team members who wrote the abstract and ran the workshop were listed as authors (authorship).

Infographic: We developed an infographic to portray a very complex project, showing a summary of its findings and outputs (message) to inform a wide audience (e.g., HPE professionals, healthcare leaders, policymakers, clinicians, the public). We did this to explain the project and raise awareness, and elicit wide conversations about the issues uncovered and the interventions developed (contribution). We worked with a medical illustrator to develop a project infographic (see Figure 11.2). All project team members contributed to this infographic and were therefore authors (authorship). The infographic is easily shared through our website and social media channels (e.g., Twitter). It also makes a great presentation slide!

11.7 PUBLISHING – AN ASPIRATIONAL COMPETENCY

The information and strategies presented in this chapter help make the process of publishing more transparent and can help you approach dissemination in a systematic and thoughtful way. Nonetheless, every research project is different and the environment in which we share our work changes – publication standards, audience needs and

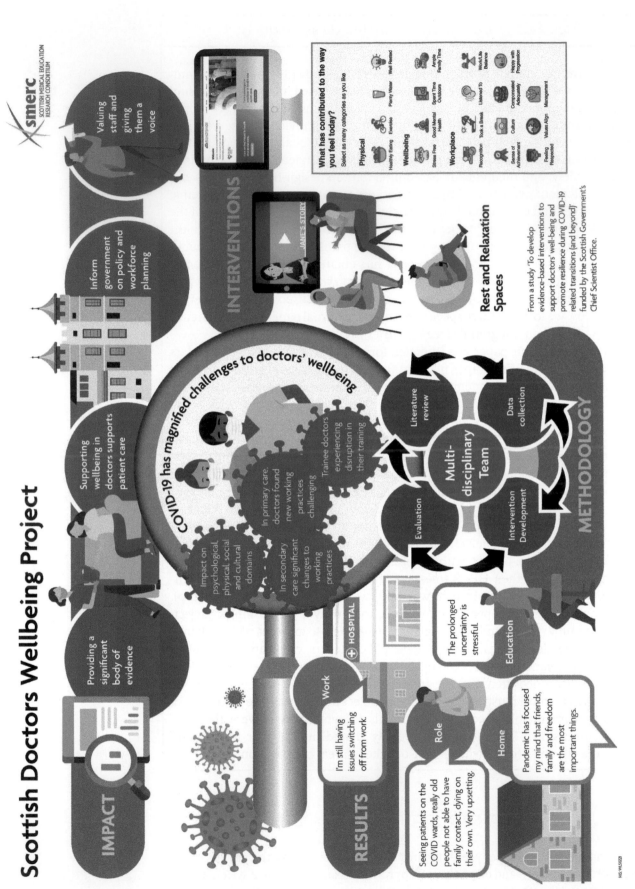

FIGURE 11.2 Infographic for the Scottish Doctor Wellbeing Study [8] (reproduced with author permission).

preferences, opportunities, and formats all change. See Chapter 4, Box 4.7 for reporting guidelines and critical appraisal tools. While many of us dream about the day when publishing our work becomes simple and straightforward, living this dream eludes most of us. For this reason, we suggest viewing publishing as an aspirational competency – one that continues to require effort regardless of experience and prior success. As researchers and authors, we can always improve. Box 11.16 offers some specific strategies for staying engaged in the field and abreast of new ideas and opportunities.

Box 11.16   Stop and do: Activities to support your efforts to publish

There are several activities that can help you keep current with HPER and opportunities for dissemination [60]. Choose and commit to doing at least one of these activities this month:

- Read the latest issues of journals that publish work you value; signing up for table of contents alerts and following the journal on Twitter makes this easier to do.
- Subscribe to or follow a blog, podcast, person, journal, or other forum that will expose you to ideas and formats that are new to you or outside your usual scope.
- Volunteer and accept invitations to peer-review for conferences and journals.
- Pursue multiple ways of sharing your work (e.g., conference presentations, tweets, podcasts, workshops).
- Seek feedback on your work before you submit; choose at least one person who is not familiar with your work so they can give you a fresh perspective.

11.8   CHAPTER SUMMARY

In this chapter, we have discussed publishing as a multifaceted dissemination process and described a variety of ways to engage. While we discussed journals most thoroughly, we emphasise that journals are but one of many components of a comprehensive dissemination plan. We suggested a series of questions to consider when formulating this plan. Conferences, creative (e.g., visual), and conversational (e.g., dialogue via blogs and tweets) formats all reach important audiences and communicate information in ways that can increase the impact of your work (more on impact in Chapter 12). While it may be tempting to think of publishing as a skill that becomes easier with time and experience, the dynamic nature of HPE and of communication media makes it critical to regularly invest effort in learning about and participating in multiple channels for scholarly dissemination. We encourage you to work through the recommended reading in Box 11.17.

Box 11.17   Recommended reading for publishing in HPER

Breu AC, Cooper AZ. Tweetorials: digital scholarship deserving of inclusion in promotion portfolios. *Med Teach.* 2022;44(4):450–452 [13].
Eva KW. The reviewer is always right: peer review of research in Medical Education. *Med Educ.* 2009;43(1):2–4 [33].
Jackson D, Walter G, Daly J, et al. Editorial: Multiple outputs from single studies: acceptable division of findings vs. "salami" slicing. *J Clin Nurs.* 2014;23:1–2 [57].

(continued)

(continued)

Lingard LA. Joining a conversation: problem/gap/hook heuristic. *Perspect Med Educ*. 2015;4(5):252–253 [1].

Regehr G, Varpio L. Conferencing well. *Perspect Med Educ*. 2022;11(2):101–103 [16].

Sullivan GM, Simpson D, Yarris LM, et al. Writing author response letters that get editors to say "yes". *J Grad Med Educ*. 2019;11(2):119–123 [36].

Varpio L, Driessen E, Maggio L, et al. Advice for authors from the editors of Perspectives on Medical Education: getting your research published. *Perspect Med Educ*. 2018;7(6):343–347 [21].

REFERENCES

1. Lingard LA. Joining a conversation: problem/gap/hook heuristic. *Perspect Med Educ*. 2015;4(5):252–253.

2. Cianciolo AT, Mitzelfelt J, Ghareeb A, et al. Physician–scientist or basic scientist? Exploring the nature of clinicians' research engagement. *Adv Health Sci Educ*. 2021;26(2):353–367.

3. Atherley AE, Hambleton IR, Unwin N, et al. Exploring the transition of undergraduate medical students into a clinical clerkship using organizational socialization theory. *Perspect Med Educ*. 2016;5(2):78–87.

4. Fulton TB, Collins S, van der Schaaf M, et al. Connecting biochemistry knowledge to patient care in the clinical workplace: senior medical students' perceptions about facilitators and barriers. *Teach Learn Med*. 2022;1–13. [online ahead of print].

5. Laidlaw A, Gordon L, Walker KA. *Rapid and rigorous: a novel methodological approach to intervention development* (Conference Workshop). ASME Researching Medical Education Conference: London, UK; November 2021.

6. Gordon L, Scanlan G, Tooman T, et al. Heard, valued, supported? Doctors' wellbeing during transitions triggered by COVID-19. *Med Educ*. 2022;56(5):516–526.

7. Walker K, Gibson Smith K, Gordon L, et al. COVID-19 doctor wellbeing study.Scottish doctors wellbeing project [infographic]. Scottish Deanery; 2021. https://www.scotland deanery.nhs.scot/your-development/scottish-medical-education-research-consor tium-smerc/research/covid-19-wellbeing-study (accessed 13 November 2022).

8. ten Cate O. Can you recommend a journal for my paper? *Perspect Med Educ*. 2022;11:146–148.

9. Herman E, Akeroyd J, Bequet G, et al. The changed – and changing – landscape of serials publishing: review of the literature on emerging models. *Learn*. 2020;33(3):213–229.

10. Glassick CE. Boyer's expanded definitions of scholarship, the standards of assessing scholarship, and the elusiveness of the scholarship of teaching. *Acad Med*. 2000;75(9):877–880.

11. Cleland JA, Jamieson S, Kusurkar RA, et al. Redefining scholarship for health professions education: AMEE Guide no. 142. *Med Teach*. 2021;43(7):824–838.

12. Ward V, Smith S, House A, et al. Exploring knowledge exchange: a useful framework for practice and policy. *Soc Sci Med*. 2012;74(3):297–304.

13. Breu AC, Cooper AZ. Tweetorials: digital scholarship deserving of inclusion in promotion portfolios. *Med Teach*. 2022;44(4):450–452.

14. Kulasegaram K, Buller D, Whitehead C. Taking presentations seriously: invoking narrative craft in academic talks. *Perspect Med Educ*. 2017;6:270–272.

15. Varpio L, Amiel J, Richards BF. Writing competitive research conference abstracts: AMEE Guide no. 108. *Med Teach*. 2016;38(9):863–871.

16. Regehr G, Varpio L. Conferencing well. *Perspect Med Educ*. 2022;11(2):101–103.

17. Rees C. Drawing on drawings: moving beyond text in health professions education research. *Perspect Med Educ*. 2018;7(3):166–173.

18. Rees EL, Burton O, Asif A, et al. A method for the madness: an international survey of health professions education authors' journal choice. *Perspect Med Educ.* 2022;11(3):165–172.

19. Ginsburg S, Lynch M, Walsh CM. A fine balance: how authors strategize around journal submission. *Acad Med.* 2018;93(8):1176–1181.

20. Eva KW, Lingard L. What's next? A guiding question for educators engaged in educational research. *Med Educ.* 2008;42(8):752–754.

21. Varpio L, Driessen E, Maggio L, et al. Advice for authors from the editors of Perspectives on Medical Education: getting your research published. *Perspect Med Educ.* 2018;7(6):343–347.

22. Durning SJ, O'Brien BC, West CP, et al. Innovation reports: guidance from the editors. *Acad Med.* 2020;95(11):1623–1625.

23. Thistlethwaite JE, Anderson E. Writing for publication: increasing the likelihood of success. *J Interprof Care.* 2021;35(5):784–790.

24. Lingard L, Watling C. Making every word count: keys to a strong research abstract. In Lingard L, Watling C, *Story, Not Study: 30 Brief Lessons to Inspire Health Researchers as Writers.* Cham: Springer; 2021: 69–74.

25. Lingard L, Watling C. Successfully navigating the peer review process. In Lingard L, Watling C, *Story, Not Study: 30 Brief Lessons to Inspire Health Researchers as Writers.* Cham: Springer; 2021: 209–218.

26. Sullivan GM. What to do when your paper is rejected. *J Grad Med Educ.* 2015;7(1):1–3.

27. Meyer HS, Durning SJ, Sklar DP, et al. Making the first cut: an analysis of academic medicine editors' reasons for not sending manuscripts out for external peer review. *Acad Med.* 2018;93(3):464–470.

28. Ellaway RH. Journal standards. *Adv Health Sci Educ.* 2022;27(1):1–5.

29. Ellaway R, Tolsgaard M, Norman G. Peer review is not a lottery: AHSE's fast track. *Adv Health Sci Educ.* 2020;25(3):519–521.

30. Hayes MM, Fessler HE. How we review a medical education research manuscript. *ATS Sch.* 2022;3(1):38–47.

31. Edwards MS, Ashkanasy NM. Emotions and failure in academic life: normalising the experience and building resilience. *J Manage Organ.* 2018;24(2):167–188.

32. Dooley MD, Sweeny K. The stress of academic publishing. *Chron High Educ.* 2017;12 September.

33. Eva KW. The reviewer is always right: peer review of research in Medical Education. *Med Educ.* 2009;43(1):2–4.

34. Cook DA. Twelve tips for getting your manuscript published. *Med Teach.* 2016;38(1):41–50.

35. Gottlieb M, Lotfipour S, Murphy L, et al. Scholarship in emergency medicine: a primer for junior academics. Part I: writing and publishing. *West J Emerg Med.* 2018;19(6):996–1002.

36. Sullivan GM, Simpson D, Yarris LM, et al. Writing author response letters that get editors to say "yes". *J Grad Med Educ.* 2019;11(2):119–123.

37. Tang KS, Cheng DL, Wu WC, et al. Example-based learning as a guide for revising a peer-reviewed manuscript. *Med Sci Educ.* 2020;30(3):1263–1266.

38. Johnston PW. What is being done to look after doctors during COVID-19 and beyond? *The BMJ Opinion.* BMJ Publishing Group; Mar 11 2021. https://blogs.bmj.com/bmj/2021/03/11/what-is-being-done-to-look-after-doctors-during-covid-19-and-beyond (accessed 13 November 2022).

39. Zaidi Z, O'Brien BC, Eva K. Exploring how physician educators approach politically charged topics with learners. Interview with Zareen Zaidi & Bridget C. O'Brien. Medical Education Podcasts; 2022. https://podcasts.apple.com/us/podcast/exploring-how-physician-educators-approach-politically/id784455563?i=1000542372053 (accessed 13 November 2022).

40. Veen M, Cianciolo A, de la Croix A. Problems no one looked for: philosophical expeditions into medical education. Let me ask you something podcast 2020. https://www.

podbean.com/media/share/pb-3xxm8-e093b5?utm_campaign=w_share_ep&utm_medium=dlink&utm_source=w_share (accessed 13 November 2022).

41. Rietmeijer C, Veen M, Cianciolo A. Discussion of phenomenological research in health professions education: tunneling from both ends. Let me ask you something podcast; 2022. https://www.podbean.com/media/share/pb-34hyw-11cfc64?utm_campaign=w_share_ep&utm_medium=dlink&utm_source=w_share (accessed 13 November 2022).

42. Jindal-Snape D, Gordon L, Innes N, et al. Multiple and multi-dimensional transitions of healthcare graduates due to COVID-19. 2022. https://doi.org/10.15132/10000185 (accessed 13 November 2022).

43. Walker K, Gibson Smith K, Gordon L, et al. COVID-19 doctor wellbeing study. Jane's story [animation]. Scottish Deanery; 2021. https://www.scotlanddeanery.nhs.scot/your-development/scottish-medical-education-research-consortium-smerc/research/covid-19-wellbeing-study (accessed 13 November 2022).

44. Jindal-Snape D, Murray C, Innes N, et al. eds. *THE COVID ROLLERCOASTER: Multiple and Multi-dimensional Transitions of Healthcare Graduates.* Dundee: University of Dundee: UniVerse, 2022.

45. Brown MEL, Kelly M, Finn GM. Thoughts that breathe, and words that burn: poetic inquiry within health professions education. *Perspect Med Educ.* 2021;10(5):257–264.

46. Walker K, Gibson Smith K, Gordon L, et al. COVID-19 doctor wellbeing study. Scottish Deanery; 2021. https://www.scotlanddeanery.nhs.scot/your-development/scottish-medical-education-research-consortium-smerc/research/covid-19-wellbeing-study (accessed 13 November 2022).

47. Chan AKM, Nickson CP, Rudolph JW, et al. Social media for rapid knowledge dissemination: early experience from the COVID-19 pandemic. *Anaesthesia.* 2020;75(12):1579–1582.

48. Rzewnicki D, Nabavi N. Tips and tricks on how to use Twitter. *BMJ.* 2021;375:n2225.

49. Lingard L, Watling C. *Story, Not Study: 30 Brief Lessons to Inspire Health Researchers as Writers.* Cham: Springer; 2021.

50. Dance A. Authorship: who's on first? *Nature.* 2012;489:591–593.

51. International Committee of Medical Journal Editors (ICMJE). Defining the role of authors and contributors. http://www.icmje.org/recommendations/browse/roles-and-responsibilities/defining-the-role-of-authors-and-contributors.html (accessed 13 November 2022).

52. Roberts LW. Addressing authorship issues prospectively: a heuristic approach. *Acad Med.* 2017;92(2):143–146.

53. Regehr G. When names are on the line: negotiating authorship with your team. *Perspect Med Educ.* 2021;10(4):197–199.

54. Barry CA, Britten N, Barber N, et al. Using reflexivity to optimize teamwork in qualitative research. *Qual Health Res.* 1999;9(1):26–44.

55. Eva KW. How would you like your salami? A guide to slicing. *Med Educ.* 2017;51(5):456–457.

56. Norman G. Data dredging, salami-slicing, and other successful strategies to ensure rejection: twelve tips on how to not get your paper published. *Adv Health Sci Educ.* 2014;19(1):1–5.

57. Jackson D, Walter G, Daly J, et al. Editorial: multiple outputs from single studies: acceptable division of findings vs. 'salami' slicing. *J Clin Nurs.* 2014;23(1–2):1–2.

58. Walter G. Salami: kosher and unkosher. *Aust N Z J Psychiatry.* 1999;33(5):766–767.

59. Walker KA, Gibson-Smith K, Gordon L, et al. *To Develop Evidence-based Interventions to Support Doctors' Wellbeing and Promote Resilience during COVID-19 (and Beyond).* Edinburgh: Chief Scientist Office; 2021.

60. Bierer SB, Foshee C, Uijtdehaage S. Strategies to remain current with the medical education field. *Med Sci Educ.* 2015;25(2):163–170.

Impact in Health Professions Education Research

Charlotte E. Rees[1,2], Olivia A. King[2,3], and Lynn V. Monrouxe[4]

[1] The University of Newcastle, Callaghan, New South Wales, Australia
[2] Monash University, Clayton, Victoria, Australia
[3] Western Alliance, Warrnambool, Victoria, Australia
[4] The University of Sydney, Camperdown, New South Wales, Australia

> **Box 12.1 Chapter 12 learning objectives: After reading this chapter, you should be able to ...**
>
> - Summarise different understandings of research impact
> - Explain the philosophical underpinnings of different approaches to research impact
> - Critique research impact pathways within health professions education research (HPER)
> - Evaluate key enablers and barriers of HPER impact
> - Outline the different ways of assessing HPER impact
> - Develop strategies to plan for and enhance impact from your own HPER

12.1 INTRODUCING CHAPTER 12

> In the fields of education and educational psychology ... a primary purpose of research is to generate credible evidence to inform practice, policy, and theory, with the end goal of improving learner outcomes. [1 p. 110]

While research impact has various definitions, in this chapter we describe it as: 'the good that researchers can do in the world' [2 p. 15]. Many of us enjoy research because we are curiosity-driven, but typically we also appreciate research because it can make a positive difference outside of academia. It can have impact. Research impact matters increasingly against a societal backdrop of greater expectations for the accountability of research investment in resource-constrained environments. Indeed, current

Foundations of Health Professions Education Research: Principles, Perspectives and Practices, First Edition. Edited by Charlotte E. Rees, Lynn V. Monrouxe, Bridget C. O'Brien, Lisi J. Gordon, and Claire Palermo.

impact agendas in higher education are driven by desires to simultaneously minimise research waste (i.e., wasted time and money) and maximise research benefits
[3, 4]. Thinking about health professions education research (HPER), this might
mean eschewing poor-quality research that lacks relevance to educational policy or
practice, and instead focusing on high-quality research that should positively impact
on educators' practice, as well as learner and patient outcomes and organisational
success. In this chapter, we aim to help you better understand research impact, as
well as plan for impacts from your own research (see Box 12.1). What we present in
this chapter is based on our reading of the impact literature, in addition to our own
experiences developing and reviewing HPER impacts. In section 12.2, we describe
the diverse ways of understanding research impact, and consider the types of impact
and beneficiaries of HPER. In section 12.3, we unpack the philosophical underpinnings of different approaches to research impact. In section 12.4, we consider research
impact pathways. We evaluate the key barriers and enablers of research impact at the
individual, relational, and organisational levels in section 12.5, and we outline various approaches to assessing HPER impacts in section 12.6. We try to bring these
issues to life throughout this chapter by discussing our own research impact experiences drawing on three illustrative cases: a research programme on healthcare professionalism [5], a research project on dignity during work-integrated learning (WIL)
[6], and a research programme setting priorities for HPER (see Box 12.2) [7, 8]. We
hope this chapter helps you to think critically about research impact, and we invite
you to start developing impact plans for your own HPER.

Box 12.2   Case studies: An overview[*]

Healthcare professionalism: We have undertaken an international programme of
research since 2007 [5], including multiple qualitative (narrative interview) and
quantitative (questionnaire) studies, across more than fifty countries and involving five healthcare student groups: medicine, nursing, pharmacy, physiotherapy,
and dentistry [9, 10]. This work has served to understand the diversity and prevalence of professionalism dilemmas experienced by students during workplace
learning [11, 12]. It has also explored students' reasons for their own professionalism lapses, as well as their compliance with [13], or resistance to seniors' requests
encouraging lapses [14]. We have also examined students' emotional responses
(including moral distress) to participating in professionalism lapses or witnessing
others' lapses [10, 12].

Work-integrated learning (WIL) dignity: We conducted a large qualitative study
including 46 students and 30 supervisors, exploring their understandings and
experiences of dignity during WIL [6, 15, 16]. Employing 58 individual and seven
group interviews with students and WIL supervisors representing multiple disciplines (medicine, nursing, counselling, education, law, and business), we
attempted to better understand dignity practices during WIL to promote positive
dignity experiences and to identify opportunities for improvement.

HPER priorities: We conducted an international programme of studies determining priorities for HPER in the UK [17, 18], Australia [8], and Taiwan [7, 19, 20].
Using mixed methods designs including a scoping review, online qualitative and
quantitative surveys, group or individual interviews, Q-sort methodology, and
Delphi, these studies have ascertained contemporary priorities for HPER as identified by multiple stakeholders, provided stakeholders' rationales for the priorities,
and clustered priorities into higher-order themes, as well as identifying differences
in the priorities identified by different stakeholders.

*While two of these case studies (the first and third) involve research programmes, as impact is more likely from programmatic research [21, 22], it is possible to have impacts from stand-alone studies, as illustrated by the second case.

12.2   DIFFERENT WAYS OF UNDERSTANDING RESEARCH IMPACT

You are likely to come across a multiplicity of different words associated with research impact in the literature. You will quickly find that there is a lack of consistency in the terminology used across the world, and that sometimes different words (e.g., knowledge transfer, knowledge exchange, knowledge translation, implementation science) are employed synonymously but with different meanings [23]. For example, knowledge transfer implies that knowledge is an object that can be moved from one person to the next in a one-way, linear fashion, whereas knowledge exchange implies that knowledge is two-way, interactive, and non-linear [23]. Please see our book glossary for all impact-related (and complex) terms employed in this chapter. However, we employ the term *research impact* throughout this chapter; consistent with that utilised in many national research assessment exercises across the world such as the UK Research Excellence Framework (REF) and the Excellence in Research for Australia (ERA). In terms of the word impact, variation also exists in understandings, with some definitions being broader and more inclusive than others. For example, Friesen et al. [24 p. 955] recently defined research impact in the context of academic medicine as: 'the effect or influence of research, within and beyond academia'. Not only does this definition imply that effects could be in any direction (positive, negative, or neutral), but also that these effects can happen within academia (i.e., influencing other researchers/research), as well as outside academia. Others in education adopt similarly broad/inclusive definitions: 'effect of research on policy, practice, theory, and other research' [1 p. 110]. However, in this chapter we focus on a narrower, more exclusive definition of research impact (from the UK REF), which considers the positive effects of research outside academia: 'an effect on, change or benefit to the economy, society, culture, public policy or services, health, the environment or quality of life, beyond academia... [including] an effect on, change or benefit to: the activity, attitude, awareness, behaviour, capacity, opportunity, performance, policy, practice, process or understanding of an audience, beneficiary, community, constituency, organisation or individuals in any geographic location whether locally, regionally, nationally or internationally... [can also include] the reduction or prevention of harm, risk, cost or other negative effects' [25 p. 90]. In lay terms, Reed has described this as: '... the good that researchers can do in the world' [2 p. 15] (see also Greenhalgh et al. [4]).

Although different scholars and organisations classify impact types in diverse ways, the most recent and arguably most comprehensive classifications involving research from all disciplines include Reed [2 p. 20–21], and UK REF [25 p. 93–109]. While Reed outlines ten different types of impacts, he explicitly excludes pedagogical impacts [2]. So, we instead draw on the REF classification [26], which outlines nine types of impact. This includes two impacts especially relevant to HPER (i.e., impacts on health and well-being, and impacts on practitioners and delivery of professional services), and another four relevant impacts (i.e., impacts on social welfare; commerce and the economy; public policy, law, and services; and understanding, learning, and participation). Speaking of the two more central impacts, often health professions education (HPE) researchers strive for immediate impacts on practitioners, with HPER commonly serving to improve educators' performance, and therefore educational practice. Indeed, HPER can contribute to professional bodies developing training standards or guidelines, continuing professional development (CPD), or educators changing their pedagogical practices [26].

However, HPE researchers' ultimate goal is often to improve the health and well-being of patients through graduating the best possible healthcare professionals who will optimise patient care through improved service delivery based on enhanced training standards or guidelines, educational practices, and CPD [26]. Furthermore, a considerable amount of HPER nowadays also aims to impact positively on the health and well-being of healthcare students, and healthcare professionals [27]. Regarding other impact types, HPER studies on widening participation, or diversity and inclusion issues could have social welfare impacts [28]. Cost-effectiveness or workforce planning studies could also have impacts on commerce and the economy [29]. HPER commissioned by governmental and/or public sector organisations could have impacts on public policy and services [30]. And finally, HPER studies on patient involvement in health education could have impacts on public understanding, learning, and participation [31]. See Box 12.3 for the types of impacts and beneficiaries for the chapter case studies.

Box 12.3   Case studies: Types of impacts and beneficiaries

Healthcare professionalism: This research programme has led to a range of research-related benefits (e.g., conference presentations, workshops, and keynotes; peer-reviewed journal articles and book chapters; grants). It also generated practice-related impacts through the publication of our evidence-based textbook for healthcare students and educators [5], with the book making its way onto reading lists for various courses worldwide. This research programme influenced policies and practices within our participating schools. We also developed reports specifically for Heads of Schools, whereby we presented our findings to them pre-publication in an easily digestible format in the hope of making a direct difference in the institutions from which our participants came. On a larger scale, this research programme also influenced policymakers internationally, as evidenced by citations in various policy documents focusing on professionalism, safe practice, and 'speaking up' [32, 33]. Finally, the research programme has influenced public awareness of healthcare professionalism through significant media engagement including international print news, and national TV and radio. The key beneficiaries of this research programme therefore include students, educators, and curriculum developers, as well as policymakers, clinicians, and patients/the public.

WIL dignity: In addition to this project yielding various research-related benefits (e.g., conference presentations, journal articles, university-based seminars, grants), our research impacted firstly on educational practice through the development and implementation of an open-access online resource for students and WIL supervisors based on the research. Entitled: 'Dignity during work-integrated learning: Your right and your responsibility' (see: https://www.monash.edu/learning-teaching/programs-for-students/wil-at-monash/dignity-module), we launched this online resource through an end-user engagement event including multiple different stakeholders (e.g., educators, students, programme developers, WIL coordinators) across the university. This launch triggered changes in clinical placement policies/procedures within the Faculty of Medicine, Nursing & Health Sciences at Monash University, Australia, making the resource mandatory for students to complete as part of their placement orientation for various programmes. Designed to promote students' and supervisors' understandings of workplace dignity, as well as improving their dignity behaviours during WIL, the key beneficiaries for this impact include WIL students, WIL supervisors, and university-based WIL coordinators.

HPER priorities: As well as this programme having positive research-related impacts (e.g., numerous publications, conference keynotes, grants), these studies have impacted institutional (e.g., Faculty of Medicine, Nursing & Health Sciences at Monash University; Chang Gung Memorial Hospital, Taiwan) or national policies and procedures for HPER grants (e.g., Scottish Medical Education Research Consortium). The research findings helped to define the scope of awards to direct the allocation of limited resources towards HPER priorities against the backdrop of resource-constrained environments. This served to benefit a multiplicity of HPER end-users (e.g., students, educators, curriculum developers) because HPER funding was directed towards studies in priority areas, so identified as most relevant and impactful (thus maximising research benefits) and away from those least relevant and impactful (thereby minimising research waste). Furthermore, the research findings yielded other practice-related impacts including improvements to national or institutional research infrastructure through the development of research networks around priority areas, enabling both researchers and end-users (e.g., educators, policymakers, clinicians) to come together in like-minded communities of practice. For example, in Taiwan, researchers belong to specific themed networks, with the annual conference being led by each one in turn.

Some scholars prefer to use the word stakeholders rather than beneficiaries, because certain people or organisations might be disadvantaged by research outcomes [2, 34]. While it is important to be mindful of the possible negative impacts of your research on stakeholders, we employ the term beneficiaries throughout this chapter because our focus is on the positive impacts from research, plus we remain consistent with REF terminology [26]. In their analysis of highly rated education impact case studies from the REF 2014, Laing et al. [22] identified a wide range of key beneficiaries of education research including students, educators, policymakers, non-government organisations, the labour market, and society. Hayes and Doherty [35 p. 123] described end-users of educational research as those: 'people and groups who are interested in the outcomes of educational research'. Before moving on to the next section, pause and reflect on the beneficiaries and impacts you might have for the HPER project you have in mind (see Box 12.4).

Box 12.4   Pause and reflect: Thinking about possible impacts from your research

Think about an HPER project that you are currently conducting or planning to conduct.

- Who might benefit from the findings of your research at individual, interactional, and/or organisational levels?
- What kinds of impact could you expect to achieve from this project?
- What reach/significance of impact do you think is possible to achieve?
- Over what time period do you think these impacts could happen?
- Revisit this pause and reflect box once you have read other sections in Chapter 12, and further developed your research impact ideas.

12.3 PHILOSOPHICAL UNDERPINNINGS OF DIFFERENT APPROACHES TO RESEARCH IMPACT

We have argued earlier in this book (see Chapter 2 and the philosophical underpinning sections of Chapters 5–9) that it is important for you to understand the philosophical foundations of different research approaches. In this section, we outline the different philosophies underpinning research impact: indeed, how you think about and approach research impact (e.g., planning for and assessing impact) will be inevitably shaped by your assumptions about the nature of reality (ontology), knowing (epistemology), and values (axiology) [4, 34]. So, thinking about chapters in Part II of this book, we discuss here the philosophical foundations of scientific, realist, interpretivist, critical, and pragmatic approaches to impact [4, 34].

12.3.1 Scientific Approaches to Research Impact

As discussed in Chapter 5, scientific approaches with positivist/post-positivist perspectives aim to explain/predict regularities in the natural world based on relationships between variables and cause–effect inferences. Commonly employing scientific methodologies including quantitative data collection and analyses, they value empiricism, facts, objectivity, and dualism. Therefore, the mechanisms through which impact is thought to be achieved from this scientific standpoint are direct/linear – that research causes impact – with experimental and statistical methods employed to evidence causality [4, 34]. Within this approach, logic models, such as those depicting inputs ⇒ activities ⇒ outputs ⇒ outcomes ⇒ impacts [36], can help to monitor and evidence how research findings are communicated, taken up, and used for benefits beyond academia [4]. Examples of the types of impact evidence relevant to HPER within this scientific approach might include identifying: (1) improvements in educational and/or healthcare practice based on research findings (e.g., as measured by student evaluation of teaching); (2) improvements in student learning based on improved evidence-based pedagogies (e.g., as measured by student assessment outcomes); or (3) institution-wide economic benefits through implementing cost-effective pedagogies based on research (e.g., as measured by budgetary dollars saved) [34]. See Box 12.5 for an overview of the philosophical approaches to impact taken by the chapter case studies.

12.3.2 Realist Approaches to Research Impact

As outlined in Chapter 6, realist approaches aim to identify what works (or does not work) for whom, under what circumstances, and why. So, realist research unpacks mechanisms that generate outcomes, and the contexts triggering those mechanisms; so-called context–mechanism–outcome configurations (CMOCs). Commonly employing naturalistic mixed methods combining quantitative and qualitative data, including realist logic to build and test programme theory, they value empiricism, complexity, theory, and context. The mechanisms through which impact is thought to be achieved from a realist standpoint are complex and interactive (e.g., via interaction between the resources available for implementing research and the reasoning of programme stakeholders such as practitioners and policymakers) [4]. Aligned with this approach, realist impact studies can examine the variability in impact outcomes for different programme stakeholders in different circumstances through exploring CMOCs [4]. Examples of the types of impact evidence relevant to HPER within this realist approach might include identifying: (1) improvements in educational practice through particular mechanisms within a specific context (e.g., workplace learning) based on research findings; (2) improvements in the learning outcomes through certain mechanisms for a specific type of learner (e.g., marginalised group) based on evidence-based pedagogies; and (3) changes to institutional policy through certain mechanisms for a particular healthcare discipline (e.g., medicine) based on research.

Box 12.5   Case studies: An overview of their philosophical approaches to impact

<u>Healthcare professionalism</u>: The philosophical approach used here could be described as primarily scientific. In this sense, we felt that through disseminating our findings directly to participating schools, as well as latterly through our textbook, and engagement with advisory and regulatory healthcare bodies and the mainstream media, we expected to *directly* improve professionalism practice, and be able to 'measure' this in some way. For example: (1) with our textbook, we could track the number of sales/downloads (i.e., over 25000 full-text downloads and over 1400 hard copies sold by September 2022), as well as citations on reading lists; (2) regarding claims to changing practice, we could count the number of healthcare bodies we engaged with and citations in their policy documents; (3) with our media engagement, we could track how many national news outlets our work appeared in and our total 'audience reach' (i.e., 14819085 readers/viewers/listeners); and (4) after receiving the Heads of Schools reports, we asked them directly what (if anything) they had changed in their schools as a result of our work.

<u>WIL dignity</u>: The philosophical approach to impact for this project could be described as critical for two reasons. Firstly, our understanding of the mechanisms through which impact could be achieved was through developing partnerships with key stakeholders, especially WIL students, supervisors, and coordinators, as well as attending to power dynamics and asymmetries between these stakeholders [16]. Our impact journey began from the very start of our research with the narrative enquiry designed to enable the later development of the educational resource, serving to influence students' and WIL supervisors' actions to promote dignity during WIL [34, 37]. Although we did not take a participatory approach to the research itself, we drew directly on WIL students' and supervisors' experiences to develop the educational resource [37], we invited WIL students, supervisors, and coordinators to the launch of the resource, and many of the impact evaluators were WIL supervisors (and one was a WIL student). Secondly, we gathered multiple sources of evaluation data to develop a compelling impact story for a Faculty Diversity & Inclusion Award in 2020 (including qualitative interviews and focus groups, solicited emails, and testimonials).

<u>HPER priorities</u>: The philosophical approach to impact for this research programme could be described as scientific for two reasons. Firstly, our understanding of impact for this research programme was direct/linear causality. Indeed, at all steps of this scientific logic model (inputs $\Rightarrow$ activities $\Rightarrow$ outputs $\Rightarrow$ outcomes $\Rightarrow$ impacts), we either saw ourselves as fully controlling the process, or we saw that the pathway was under our direct (outcomes) or indirect influence (impacts) [36]. Secondly, our treatment of impact was largely quantitative. We were, for example, easily able to 'measure' direct and proximate research outcomes and impacts in terms of numbers (see details later).

12.3.3   Interpretivist Approaches to Research Impact

As discussed in Chapter 7, interpretivist approaches aim to understand social phenomena such as individuals' views and experiences, privileging interpretations of phenomena taking account of time and place. Commonly employing qualitative methodologies and methods, they value language, dialogue, subjectivity, and context. Therefore, the mechanisms through which impacts are believed to occur from this interpretivist standpoint are primarily indirect through social interaction between researchers–users, and their consequent enlightenment or changed understandings [4]. This interpretivist approach highlights the unpredictability of research impacts, with interpretivist impact studies focusing on social interaction [4]. So, research–impact causation is somewhat inferred through the building of impact case studies [26], or impact stories [24], which attempt to triangulate multiple textual data sources (e.g., testimonials, social media analysis) to create compelling arguments for research impact [34]. Examples of the types of impact evidence relevant to HPER within this interpretivist approach might include identifying: (1) improvements in educational practice based on research findings (e.g., as evidenced by educational practitioners' social media activity); (2) improvements in student learning based on improved evidence-based pedagogies (e.g., as indicated through students' testimonials); or (3) changes to the general public's awareness and understandings of HPE based on research (e.g., as evidenced by analysis of media coverage of research) [34].

12.3.4   Critical and Pragmatic Approaches to Research Impact

As outlined in Chapters 8 and 9, critical and pragmatic approaches aim to facilitate change, and for critical approaches especially for disempowered/marginalised groups, which serve to contest conventional power relations and established ways of thinking and doing [38]. Both approaches can employ participatory methodologies including qualitative data collection and analysis; valuing improving the human experience, democracy, and change. Therefore, the mechanisms through which impacts are thought to be achieved often include building partnerships and activism [4]. Critical approaches especially can highlight the political aspects of research impacts with impacts on stakeholders' power relations, thereby sometimes challenging the status quo [4, 38]. Like interpretivist approaches to impact (discussed in section 12.3.3), research–impact causation in critical and pragmatic approaches is inferred through impact case studies/stories [24, 26], which triangulate textual data sources (e.g., through participatory monitoring, action research, or empowerment evaluation) [34]. Examples of the types of impact evidence relevant to HPER within these critical and pragmatic approaches might include identifying: (1) improvements in educational practice based on research findings (e.g., as evidenced through educational practitioners' action research); (2) improvements in student learning based on improved evidence-based pedagogies (e.g., as indicated by students' co-production of evidence-based pedagogies); or (3) changes to healthcare consumers' thinking about health professions education based on research (e.g., as evidenced by consumers' capacity-building as co-researchers) [34, 37]. Before moving on to the next section, pause and reflect on the philosophies underpinning your approach to impact (see Box 12.6).

Box 12.6   Pause and reflect: Your philosophies and pathways to research impact

- Thinking about the same HPER project as that used for Box 12.4, what are the philosophical underpinnings of your approach to research impact and why?
- Through what mechanisms do you think your impacts will be achieved?
- How will you assess your impacts based on this philosophical approach?
- What might your pathway to impact look like? Revisit this question once you have read section 12.4.

12.4   UNPACKING IMPACT PATHWAYS IN HPER

Scientific approaches imply that impact is generated through a direct/linear causal pathway from A (research) to B (impact). Although these scientific logic models [36] (e.g., inputs ⇒ activities ⇒ outputs ⇒ outcomes ⇒ impacts) can help researchers develop impact plans, applying such impact pathways to real impact studies demonstrates that: 'generating and realising impact is not a linear process and it is never complete, and in many aspects it cannot be planned ... Rather, the pathway has many highways, secondary roads, intersections, some dead ends or cul-de-sacs and many unexpected detours of interest along the way' [36 p. 6]. It comes as no surprise therefore that educational scholars have talked for decades about the complexity, non-linearity, and general messiness of impact pathways for educational research, employing words like: contested, convoluted, diffuse, haphazard, indirect, informal, invisible, long-term, mediated, multidirectional, obstructed, slow, and uneven to describe impact pathways [22, 23, 39–43].

To our knowledge, no studies to date have examined impact pathways in HPER. However, several studies have explored impact pathways for educational research by analysing highly rated impact case studies in the education unit of assessment for REF 2014 in the UK [22, 40]. The qualitative analysis of Cain and Allen [40] included 65 impact case studies assessed as having outstanding (4 star) or very considerable impacts (3 star) from 20 universities, whereas the qualitative analysis conducted by Laing et al. [22] included 85 highly rated (4 or 3 star) impact case studies from 21 universities (see section 12.6 for more details on impact assessment for REF 2014 and REF 2021). Although Cain and Allen [40] focused on the research to practice pathway, suggesting that this was messy, complex, and iterative, they found that most impact case studies reviewed included four activities serving to mediate the research–practice pathway [40]. Firstly, most case studies demonstrated that the underlying research discovered problems with educational practice, thereby serving an evaluative function. Secondly, the case studies demonstrated that research was disseminated beyond the research community to policymakers and/or practitioners, with policy often mediating the research–practice pathway. Common vehicles of dissemination to policymakers were direct and included reports and briefings, expert opinions, or consultancies. Dissemination to practitioners however was more diffuse involving intermediaries like subject associations or collaborative networks, including practitioner-orientated publications, conferences, and seminars. Thirdly, the case studies demonstrated that research was incorporated into educational programmes, resources (e.g., textbooks, toolkits, software), and the professional development of teachers (e.g., initial teacher education or continuing professional development). Finally, most case studies demonstrated changes in thinking and practice (e.g., curriculum, pedagogy, assessments).

Laing et al. [22] identified various national and international impacts from educational research including institutional changes and policy changes, as well as academics holding influential positions. As mentioned above, principal beneficiaries included policymakers, learners, educational practitioners, non-governmental organisations, labour markets, and society. Consistent with Cain and Allen [40], they identified various pathways to impact including through reports or briefings, training materials, workshops, online resources, purchasable products, and national standards. And such pathways were typically evidenced through social media outputs, web downloads, resource-uptake percentage, workshop attendance, quality marks, and testimonials about policy and practice changes. Interestingly, 65% of impacts resulted from research conducted more than 11 years previously, demonstrating that research impact pathways for educational research are often long-term, non-direct, and slow. Furthermore, most case studies were built around underpinning mixed methods or quantitative research serving to evaluate educational interventions to influence curriculum and practitioner or policy changes, or improve student outcomes [22].

Most recently, Cain et al. [44] have proposed how research can inform teachers and teaching through: (1) bounded decision-making, where research evidence is understood against the backdrop of practitioners' assumptions and discussed within their social contexts to bring about decisions; (2) practitioners' reflection, affecting their thinking and leading to changes in professionalism; and (3) organisational learning, where research is part of the fabric of informal and formal professional conversations within organisations. However, they also suggest that educational research can influence practice changes without necessarily influencing practitioners' thinking (e.g., by changing policies, resources, and services with practitioners ignorant of how research contributes to those changes). Although these impact pathway studies are based on educational research rather than HPER specifically, they resonate with our experiences of impact pathways in HPER (see Box 12.7).

Box 12.7   Case studies: An overview of their impact pathways

Healthcare professionalism: We made no overt attempts to plan for impact at the outset of our research programme. Instead, our impact plans developed reactively as the work progressed, and sometimes were triggered by outside events. For example, our media engagement work was largely activated by us reading/hearing other news reporting professionalism failings across UK hospitals that resonated with our research findings. So, we developed some press releases for some of our published papers, thereby actively engaging with the media. Prompted by our desire to develop a REF 2014 impact case study, we planned for impact in earnest following our two UK-wide questionnaire studies with medical and other healthcare students by purposively communicating findings with the heads of participating schools and then following up with them six months later, asking them if they had made changes based on our research [12]. We also started gathering evidence to measure impacts such as citations in regulatory/advisory body reports, as well as seeking out opportunities for commissioned research. Probably our most conscious effort at maximising impact was our writing of our healthcare professionalism textbook for students and healthcare educators [5]. While we primarily took a scientific approach to measuring impacts (see Box 12.5), we would nevertheless describe our impact pathway as rather convoluted, diffuse, haphazard, indirect, complex, and long-term.

WIL dignity: We planned our research impact at the outset in line with linear pathways typically espoused by scientific approaches. While this planned impact pathway was linear and reasonably proximate, we still foregrounded a critical research impact approach (as discussed earlier). For example, at all stages of the research impact pathway we focused on partnerships with various key stakeholders including groups considered to be marginalised/powerless (e.g., WIL students, WIL supervisors). We especially facilitated collaboration throughout the development, launch, and evaluation of our research-based educational resource to maximise its positive impacts, with this collaborative approach ultimately influencing student and supervisor uptake and use of the research-based resource [45], thereby impacting their WIL dignity attitudes, behaviours, and experiences.

HPER priorities: We planned our research impact from the outset aligned with scientific impact pathways [36 p. 2], including: (1) research inputs (e.g., personnel, funding), (2) research activities (e.g., data collection and analysis involving multiple stakeholders), and (3) research outputs (e.g., reports to funders, journal articles, conference presentations), alongside intended results from those outputs involving: (4) research outcomes (e.g., policy changes to funding awards, development of thematic research networks), and (5) research impacts (e.g., improved collaborative research environment, better decision-making about funding allocation in resource-constrained environment). As suggested by Greenhalgh and Fahy [46], research findings can be taken up directly (both linearly and proximately), especially in conditions such as ours. For example, we had straightforward research findings that aligned with local opinion leaders, the priority setting exercise concorded with existing motivations to change policies/guidelines, and key stakeholders were driven to implement study findings to simultaneously reduce research waste and maximise research benefits.

12.5 FACILITATORS AND BARRIERS TO ENHANCING RESEARCH IMPACT

When you are planning your research impacts, it is helpful that you attune to possible enablers and barriers, to capitalise on the former and minimise the latter. Fortunately, many scholars have already outlined common enablers and barriers to research impacts at several levels: (1) individual, such as researchers or end-users of research; (2) relational, such as researcher–user relationships; and (3) organisational, such as institutions producing research (e.g., higher education institutions) or those consuming research (e.g., clinical workplaces) [1, 21–23, 35, 37, 40, 43, 46–54]. While some of these enablers and barriers will feel very much under your control as a researcher (e.g., whether you publish in an open-access journal or not) and others will feel outside of your direct control (e.g., the climate of an organisation consuming your research), it is still important to be aware of these potential uncontrollables, as there may be opportunities to minimise barriers, or at the very least understand why your research might not be achieving the impacts you were hoping for. See Box 12.8 for a summary of the enablers and barriers for the case studies.

> **Box 12.8   Case studies: An overview of their impact facilitators/barriers**
>
> Healthcare professionalism: Key facilitators for our impact at the individual level involved us doing research supported by funders with high expectations for educational impacts (e.g., the Association for the Study of Medical Education, Advance HE), disseminating some of our research through open-access sources [12], and in practitioner-orientated journals (e.g., *Nursing Standard*), as well as strategic endurance in terms of strong and supportive working relationships between us. At a relational level, we worked hard to interact directly with research users (e.g., Heads of Schools) by seeking permission from them to conduct research within their schools, sharing reports with them, and following up on any impacts. And at the organisational level, our research impacts were facilitated through, for example, support, advice, and training from our respective university media offices who helped us write press releases and advised us on our interactions with the media (in terms of radio and TV interviews). While we experienced barriers to research impact at the level of the individual, namely lack of time for impact work, and some user resistance to our research findings (e.g., 'that doesn't happen in my school'), our barriers were mostly organisational given the sensitivities around the professionalism lapses we reported in our work. This often required careful negotiations with individuals and our institutions about how best to disseminate our findings beyond academia.
>
> WIL dignity: The key facilitators of research impact at the individual level included us being commissioned to do the research [46], and the research-based educational resource being developed by practitioners including educational designers [21, 46]. The relational level enablers included influential stakeholders being fully on board with the educational research and development. Team members repeatedly met with WIL stakeholders throughout the project to maximise resource uptake, use, and impacts [45]. Organisational enablers of impact included impact resources such as time and funding to support impact work (e.g., impact events such as our resource launch). Furthermore, many of our research team members were teaching and research academics, so capitalised on their educator and educational leadership roles to facilitate impacts. However, key barriers included the time required by WIL supervisors to engage with the educational resource (individual level), the lack of direct links to workplace-based WIL supervisors from wide-ranging disciplines beyond those of the team (relational level), and similarly, limited capacity to influence organisational uptake beyond the university, where WIL priorities and evidence-based educational practice cultures may have been different (particularly during the pandemic).
>
> HPER priorities: The key facilitators of research impact at the individual level included us doing commissioned and policy-related research, and the end-users possessing well-developed research capabilities and being situated within communities of enquiry valuing evidence. At the relational level, key enablers included the priority setting exercises being conducted as part of producer–user partnerships through organisational entities (e.g., Scottish Medical Education Research Consortium (SMERC), Monash Centre for Scholarship in Health Education (MCSHE), Chang Gung Medical Education Research Centre (CG-MERC)), and us being funded by internal or external stakeholders. At the organisational level, enablers included us having workload time, administrative support, and funding for

impact events within our organisations, as well as organisational cultures valuing research as part of quality improvement processes. Key barriers to us maximising the significance and reach of our impacts at the individual level, however, included some of our papers being published in closed sources, and some educational practitioners being resistant to change their scholarly activity based on our findings. At the relational level, we experienced some tensions between researchers and users, e.g., policymakers being driven by relevance, and researchers being curiosity-driven. Finally, barriers at the organisational level included us having limited resources to maximise the significance and reach of the findings outside of our immediate organisations.

12.5.1 Individual Facilitators and Barriers

If we consider facilitators and barriers relating to researchers first, we know that researchers can enable impact in various ways such as: conducting commissioned research by industry or government; conducting applied or evaluative research; developing guidelines from best-evidence syntheses; actively disseminating research beyond academia (e.g., practitioner-orientated journals and conferences) via open access; writing clearly for non-academic audiences such as employing translational visual abstracts; and finally through strategic endurance, that is, by relentlessly plugging away at impacts. Barriers at the individual level are often the mirror image of these enablers, such as doing basic or conceptual research inapplicable to real-world settings, publishing in closed sources, and publishing poor-quality research with inconclusive results. Regarding research users, impacts can be enabled through users developing their research capabilities, as well as them developing user communities valuing evidence. However, barriers for research users can include work overload, poor receptivity to research, and resistance to change policies and/or practices based on evidence, especially if existing policies or practices have purportedly served them well previously [1, 21, 22, 35, 40, 46–48, 50–52, 54, 55].

12.5.2 Relational Facilitators and Barriers

Research impacts can be enabled through researcher–user partnerships, either through researcher–user collaborative research teams as in participatory research designs (such as co-production and co-impact: see Chapter 8) [37], or partnerships through co-membership of advisory or regulatory bodies, think tanks, and/or committees, especially where different stakeholders share common understandings about research and its purposes, and understand and respect diversity [40]. Indeed, research enablers can involve intermediaries who broker researcher–user relationships such as associations, networks and media, and/or researchers engaging with such external stakeholders to secure impact resources. At this relational level, the key barrier outlined in the literature concerns the tensions between researchers and users because of their different understandings of knowledge or the purposes of research. For example, researchers may be primarily curiosity-driven, but educational practitioners may be mostly interested in the relevance of research to practice. Furthermore, researchers may be thinking about the relevance of their work in the long-term, whereas policymakers might be focusing on its short-term relevance [21, 22, 37, 46, 47, 50, 54–56].

12.5.3 Organisational Facilitators and Barriers

If we consider facilitators and barriers at the level of research-producing organisations first, the literature suggests that research impacts can be enabled through good institutional research impact leadership and strategy, including: (1) academics having sufficient access to organisational resources for impact including sufficient workload for impact activity, administrative support for impact activity, funding for impact events, impact training, and/or institutional knowledge brokers; and (2) institutional incentives for researchers to engage in impact including impact activity being rewarded as part of annual appraisals and/or promotions, as well as through institutional research impact awards. The mirror image of these enablers can be seen as organisational barriers for research impact within research-producing institutions (i.e., limited impact resources or incentives). Jones [55] also highlights the increased bifurcation of researcher and educator roles in universities leading to challenges securing educational research impacts. At the level of the research-using organisations, key enablers of research impacts include having evidence-based educational cultures accepting of evidence as part of quality improvement cultures, whereas barriers might include organisational constraints on policymakers such as research findings being inconsistent with dominant policy agendas, or political short-termism (with a lack of timeliness of research) [21–23, 43, 46, 47, 49, 50, 52–55].

While many different enablers and barriers to research impact exist at these three levels, the literature suggests that relational enablers are probably the most compelling (e.g., researchers developing solid and meaningful partnerships with users built on repeated interactions and trust) [21, 46, 47, 57]. This could include researchers' active engagement in professional networks supported by boundary organisations (e.g., professional associations or knowledge exchange organisations), or users being closely associated with research teams in the co-design and co-production of research and its co-impact (see Chapter 8 for more details about approaches to co-design) [21, 37, 53]. Before moving on to the next section, stop and do the activity in Box 12.9.

Box 12.9   Stop and do: Thinking about facilitators and barriers of research impact

Thinking about the same HPER project as that used for Box 12.4, think about the potential facilitators and barriers influencing potential research impacts:

- Identify 3–5 facilitators and barriers most relevant to your project.
- What can you do in the coming weeks and months to trigger these facilitators and minimise the barriers?
- How might you especially trigger relational enablers and minimise relational barriers? Which key stakeholders should you prioritise developing partnerships with?
- Talk to your research collaborators about your ideas, as well as thinking through what impact resources you might need throughout your project.

12.6   ASSESSING IMPACTS

As discussed earlier in section 12.3, there are different philosophical approaches to impact, meaning that different ways of understanding and assessing impact exist. While scientific and realist approaches typically examine causality through quantitative or mixed methods respectively, interpretivist, critical, and pragmatic approaches mostly infer causality through qualitative methods that serve to triangulate multiple textual data sources to develop compelling impact case studies. Interestingly, Greenhalgh et al. [4] suggested that many approaches to evidencing impact combine a scientific logic model illustrating any direct and proximal links between inputs–activities–outputs–outcomes–impacts, alongside a case study approach to depict indirect and distal links. Therefore, when you think about how to assess your research impacts, it is worth considering multiple sources of corroborative evidence (quantitative, qualitative, or both), while being mindful of the internal coherence of that evidence with your philosophical approach to impact. As discussed above, many scholars have contested simple cause–effect claims about education research and impact [42], as well as highlighting the general invisibility of impact pathways for educational research [40]. Furthermore, numerous scholars have flagged the difficulties of attributing impacts to research findings with any great certainty [4]. It is outside the scope of this chapter to outline the diversity of research impact assessment frameworks from the broader literature, so interested readers are directed elsewhere [3, 4, 34]. Instead, we focus here on impact case studies/stories as these are commonly employed for educational research [24], and often include a multiplicity of evidence sources. For example, educational scholars [22, 40] have identified a raft of metric and qualitative data sources employed as impact evidence in highly rated REF 2014 case studies for education (see the REF website: https://www.ref.ac.uk/2014). These included: traditional media outputs (e.g., newspapers, TV, radio), social media outputs (e.g., tweets, blogs, Facebook posts), use of websites and web downloads, resource uptake percentages, workshop attendance, learner outcomes, organisational outcomes, quality marks, and testimonials of policy/practice change [22, 40]. See Box 12.10 for an overview of how impacts were assessed for the case studies.

Box 12.10   Case studies: An overview of their impact assessment

Healthcare professionalism: As mentioned in Box 12.5, we assessed impacts in many ways aligned with a scientific approach that were largely quantitative (e.g., number of book sales/downloads, number of policy citations, media audience reach). Furthermore, we evaluated school impacts by asking Heads of Schools to whom we had sent our report what they had changed as a direct result of our report. We also collated any incoming evidence when we were informed of how our work changed curricula or continuous professional development programmes. We did further work ourselves in terms of Internet searches to see where our work was being discussed beyond academia, including examining our altmetric scores for publications. However, more aligned with an interpretivist approach to impact, we collated the different data sources to develop an impact case study for consideration by one of our institutions for UK REF 2014.

WIL dignity: We formally evaluated the WIL dignity educational resource via individual and group interviews with ten students and nine supervisors who had worked through the resource. We explored participants' perspectives of the usability and implementation of the resource, as well as their motivations to engage with the resource. In collating a faculty application for a Diversity & Inclusion award (and in essence, a narrative impact story), we also collated unsolicited emails we had received from end-users about the impacts of the resource, as well as seeking out testimonials from key WIL stakeholders attending our launch about the

(continued)

(continued)

perceived value of the resource in terms of effecting dignity during WIL. Through our formal evaluation and these informal conversations, we also became aware of the uptake and use of the resource in various programmes across the university.

HPER priorities: We assessed our direct and proximate research outcomes quantitatively (e.g., number of grants submitted/awarded in which priority areas, number of educational practitioners and researchers joining thematic networks), plus our more indirect and distal impacts through formal evaluations. For example, at MCSHE we conducted quantitative evaluation of end-of-award reports, plus quantitative evaluation of our bi-annual MCSHE learning and teaching research grant showcase. In Taiwan, the priority-setting work was included in key performance indicators that focused on membership numbers, research meetings (including conferences), invited guests, and grant applications.

Altmetrics have been identified as an important alternative to traditional citation-based metrics that assess the impacts of research on researchers/research [58]. Since they count citations in non-academic sources such as social media, they measure attention rather than impact per se [24]. Therefore, Friesen et al. [24] talk about the importance of so-called grey metrics for assessing research impacts in HPER. Including non-conventional citations (e.g., citations in policy reports, educational materials, or practitioner-orientated websites), informal conversations with end-users about their uptake and use of your research, or invitations to consult based on your research expertise, grey metrics are unindexed and/or informal citations that are difficult to track [24]. Although these sources of evidence can be described as titbits of impact information, taken together they can be employed to create a compelling story for research impact, such as those submitted to the UK REF in 2014 or 2021 (see REF website to access impact case studies from REF 2014: https://www.ref.ac.uk/2014 and REF 2021: https://www.ref.ac.uk). Here, researchers could illustrate their research impacts in a 4-page impact case study that summarised: (1) their impacts; (2) underpinning research; (3) references to their research; as well as providing (4) narrative details of their impacts; and (5) sources to corroborate impacts [59]. These impact case studies were assessed by the education panel for REF 2014 including expert peer reviewers as well as research users. They consider both the reach (spread/depth of influence on beneficiaries) and significance (intensity of influence) of impacts, assessing them according to a 5-point scale: 4* (outstanding), 3* (very considerable), 2* (considerable), 1* (recognised but modest) or unclassified (little or no reach or significance) [40]. As outlined above, such impact cases/stories, including diverse metrics combined into a narrative account, can illustrate how your research has been influential beyond academia [24]. Before moving on to the next section of this chapter, we encourage you to tackle Box 12.11 to appraise an impact case study.

Box 12.11   Stop and do: Appraising an impact case study

- Read the brief impact story in Box 1 of Friesen et al. [24 p. 960] titled: "Relationships of Power" Article Grows "Louder Than Words".
- What types of impact did the researchers generate from the underpinning research and who were the beneficiaries?
- Thinking about the research impact pathway outlined in Fryirs et al. [36], [i.e., inputs (e.g., funding) ⇒ activities (e.g., data collection) ⇒ outputs (e.g.,

journal article) $\Rightarrow$ outcomes (e.g., educational resource) $\Rightarrow$ impacts (e.g., improved student learning)], what (if any) impact pathways are visible in this case study?

- What sources of evidence did the authors draw on to demonstrate impacts, and over what time period?
- Thinking about the REF criteria for assessing impact, how would you rate the case study in terms of its reach and significance?
- What have you learnt from critically appraising this HPER impact case study that you can apply to your own research? Try writing your own impact story following the approach of Friesen et al. [24]. Share it with your collaborators and get feedback.

12.7 CHAPTER SUMMARY

In this chapter, we have outlined different ways of understanding research impact, diverse types of impact in HPER (e.g., policy and practice impacts), and varied beneficiaries (e.g., students, educators, policymakers). We have discussed different philosophical approaches to impact (scientific, realist, interpretivist, critical, and pragmatic) that serve to understand and assess impacts in different ways. We have unpacked impact pathways in HPER; while such HPER impacts are typically complex, non-linear, diffuse, and long-term, we can however still draw on scientific logic models to facilitate our planning of impact. We have outlined numerous enablers and barriers to research impact at multiple levels: individual (e.g., researchers conducting applied/evaluative research), relational (e.g., strong researcher–user partnerships), and organisational levels (e.g., available impact resources). We have also outlined diverse ways of assessing HPER impacts employing both quantitative and qualitative methods to develop compelling impact case studies/stories. The current impact agenda in higher education is certainly captivating – what researcher does not want to make a positive difference through their research? What organisation does not want to maximise limited resources to support research benefiting practice, policy, or society? However, we do urge you to develop your awareness of strident criticisms in the literature about this impact agenda – criticised for straitjacketing academic freedom, and disadvantaging certain types of research (e.g., basic, conceptual, blue-skies), methodologies (e.g., qualitative), and disciplines (e.g., humanities, arts, social sciences), many fear that the impact agenda will steer researchers towards conducting narrow types of research (such as applied, evaluative, and/or quantitative research), where it is easier to demonstrate direct and proximal impacts [22, 46, 60–62]. Indeed, this could reduce the diversity and vibrancy of the higher education research landscape [22]. We also encourage you to be continuously mindful of any negative impacts of your research on stakeholders. While research impacts are more likely to accrue from programmatic research rather than one-off studies [21, 22], we have included one case study in this chapter (WIL dignity) exploring the impacts that are possible from stand-alone HPER. We now encourage you to apply your learnings from this chapter to develop strategies to enhance impact from your own HPER. We invite you to expand your learning about impact through reading the references in Box 12.12.

> **Box 12.12   Recommended reading for HPER impact**
>
> Friesen F, Baker LR, Ziegler C, et al. Approaching impact meaningfully in medical education research. *Acad Med*. 2019;94(7):955–961 [24].
>
> Greenhalgh T, Rafferty J, Hanney S, et al. Research impact: a narrative review. *BMC Med*. 2016;14:78 [4].
>
> Reed MS, Bryce R, Machen R. Pathways to policy impact: a new approach for planning and evidencing research impact. *Evid Policy*. 2018;14(3):431–458 [57].
>
> Research Excellence Framework (REF). Annex A: Examples of impacts and indicators. In Panel criteria and working methods. UKRI; 2019:77–91. https://www.ref.ac.uk/publications-and-reports/panel-criteria-and-working-methods-201902 (accessed 30 Mar 2023) [26].

REFERENCES

1. Fleming JI, Wilson SE, Hart SA, et al. Open accessibility in education research: enhancing the credibility, equity, impact, and efficiency of research. *Educ Psychol*. 2021;56(2):110–121.

2. Reed MS. *The Research Impact Handbook*, 2nd ed. Aberdeenshire: Fast Track Impact; 2018.

3. Rivera SC, Kyte DG, Aiyegbusi OL, et al. Assessing the impact of healthcare research: a systematic review of methodological frameworks. *PLoS Med*. 2017;14(8):e1002370.

4. Greenhalgh T, Rafferty J, Hanney S, et al. Research impact: a narrative review. *BMC Med*. 2016;14:78.

5. Monrouxe LV, Rees CE. *Healthcare Professionalism: Improving Practice through Reflections on Workplace Dilemmas*. Chichester: Wiley Blackwell; 2017.

6. King O, Davis C, Clemans A, et al. Dignity during work-integrated learning: what does it mean for supervisors and students? *Stud High Educ*. 2021;46(4):721–736.

7. Gugel A, Babovič M, Monrouxe LV. Multi-phase healthcare professions education research priority setting in Taiwan. *Med Educ*. 2019;53(11):1159–1160.

8. Palermo C, King O, Brock T, et al. Setting priorities for health education research: a mixed methods study. *Med Teach*. 2019;41(9):1029–1038.

9. Rees CE, Monrouxe LV, Ternan E, et al. Workplace abuse narratives from dentistry, nursing, pharmacy and physiotherapy students: a multi-school qualitative study. *European J Dent Educ*. 2015;19(2):95–106.

10. Monrouxe LV, Rees CE, Endacott R, et al. 'Even now it makes me angry': healthcare students' professionalism dilemma narratives. *Med Educ*. 2014;48(5):502–517.

11. Rees CE, Monrouxe LV, McDonald LA. Narrative, emotion and action: analysing 'most memorable' professionalism dilemmas. *Med Educ*. 2013;47(1):80–96.

12. Monrouxe LV, Rees CE, Dennis I, et al. Professionalism dilemmas, moral distress and the healthcare student: insights from two online UK-wide questionnaire studies. *BMJ Open*. 2015;5(5):e007518.

13. Rees CE, Monrouxe LV. Medical students learning intimate examinations without valid consent: a multi-centre study. *Med Educ*. 2011;45(3):261–272.

14. Shaw MK, Rees CE, Anderson NB, et al. Professionalism lapses and hierarchies: a qualitative analysis of medical students' narrated acts of resistance. *Soc Sci Med*. 2018;219:45–53.

15. Davis C, King OA, Clemans A, et al. Student dignity during work-integrated learning: a qualitative study exploring student and supervisors' perspectives. *Adv Health Sci Educ.* 2020;25(1):149–172.

16. Rees CE, Davis C, King OA, et al. Power and resistance in feedback during work-integrated learning: contesting traditional student-supervisor asymmetries. *Assess Eval Higher Educ.* 2020;45(8):1136–1154.

17. Dennis AA, Cleland JA, Johnston P, et al. Exploring stakeholders' views of medical education research priorities: a national survey. *Med Educ.* 2014;48(11):1078–1091.

18. Ajjawi R, Barton KL, Dennis AA, et al. Developing a national dental education research strategy: priorities, barriers and enablers. *BMJ Open.* 2017;7(3):e013129.

19. Monrouxe LV, Liu GR-J, Yau SY, et al. A scoping review examining funding trends in health care professions education research from Taiwan (2006–2017). *Nurs Outlook.* 2020;68(4):417–429.

20. Yau S-Y, Babovič M, Liu GR-J, et al. Differing viewpoints around healthcare professions' education research priorities: a Q-methodology approach. *Adv Health Sci Educ.* 2021;26(3):975–999.

21. Gorard S, See BH, Siddiqui N. What is the evidence on the best way to get evidence into use in education? *Rev Educ.* 2020;8(2):570–610.

22. Laing K, Smith LM, Todd L. The impact agenda and critical social research in education: hitting the target but missing the spot? *Policy Futures Educ.* 2018;16(2):169–184.

23. Read R, Cooper A, Edelstein H, et al. Knowledge mobilisation and utilisation. In Levin B, Qi J, Edelstein H, et al., eds. *The Impact of Research in Education: An International Perspective.* Bristol: Policy Press; 2013: 23–40.

24. Friesen F, Baker LR, Ziegler C, et al. Approaching impact meaningfully in medical education research. *Acad Med.* 2019;94(7):955–961.

25. Research Excellence Framework (REF). UKRI. 2022. https://www.ref.ac.uk (accessed 15 November 2022).

26. Research Excellence Framework (REF). Annex A: Examples of impacts and indicators. In Panel criteria and working methods (2019/02). UKRI; 2019; 77–91. https://ref.ac.uk/publications-and-reports/panel-criteria-and-working-methods-201902 (accessed 15 November 2022).

27. Lo K, Waterland J, Todd P, et al. Group interventions to promote mental health in health professional education: a systematic review and meta-analysis of randomised controlled trials. *Adv Health Sci Educ.* 2018;23(2):413–447.

28. Brottman MR, Char DM, Hattori RA, et al. Toward cultural competency in health care: a scoping review of the diversity and inclusion education literature. *Acad Med.* 2020;95(5):803–813.

29. Foo J, Cook DA, Walsh K, et al. Cost evaluations in health professions education: a systematic review of methods and reporting quality. *Med Educ.* 2019;53(12):1196–1208.

30. Monrouxe LV, Grundy L, Mann M, et al. How prepared are UK medical graduates for practice? A rapid review of the literature 2009–2014. *BMJ Open.* 2017;7(1):e013656.

31. Rowland P, Anderson M, Kumagai AK, et al. Patient involvement in health professionals' education: a meta-narrative review. *Adv Health Sci Educ.* 2019;24(3):595–617.

32. General Medical Council. *Be Prepared: Are New Doctors Safe to Practise?* London: GMC; 2014.

33. Medical Deans Australia and New Zealand. Professionalism and professional identity of our future doctors. MDANZ; 2021. https://medicaldeans.org.au/resource/professionalism-and-professional-identity-of-our-future-doctors (accessed 15 November 2022).

34. Reed MS, Ferré M, Martin-Ortega J, et al. Evaluating impact from research: a methodological framework. *Res Policy*. 2021;50(4):104147.

35. Hayes D, Doherty C. Valuing epistemic diversity in educational research: an agenda for improving research impact and initial teacher education. *Aust Educ Res*. 2017;44(2):123–139.

36. Fryirs KA, Brierley GJ, Dixon T. Engaging with research impact assessment for an environmental science case study. *Nat Commun*. 2019;10(1):4542.

37. Banks S, Herrington T, Carter K. Pathways to co-impact: action research and community organising. *Educ Action Res*. 2017;25(4):541–559.

38. Kaushik V, Walsh CA. Pragmatism as a research paradigm and its implications for social work research. *Soc Sci*. 2019;8(9):255.

39. Bates R. Does educational research have any impact on educational policy and practice. *J Educ Stud*. 2002;24(2):1–9.

40. Cain T, Allan D. The invisible impact of educational research. *Oxf Rev Educ*. 2017;43(6):718–732.

41. Santen SA, Deiorio NM, Gruppen LD. Medical education research in the context of translational science. *Acad Emerg Med*. 2012;19(12):1323–1327.

42. Taber KS. The impact of chemistry education research on practice: a cautionary tale. *Chem Educ Res Pract*. 2014;15(4):410–416.

43. Watson L. Developing indicators for a new ERA: should we measure the policy impact of educational research? *Aust J Educ*. 2008;52(2):117–128.

44. Cain T, Brindley S, Brown C, et al. Bounded decision-making, teachers' reflection and organisational learning: how research can inform teachers and teaching. *Br Educ Res J*. 2019;45(5):1072–1087.

45. Morton BM. Barriers to academic achievement for foster youth: the study behind the statistics. *J Res Child Educ*. 2015;29(4):476–491.

46. Greenhalgh T, Fahy N. Research impact in the community-based health sciences: an analysis of 162 case studies from the 2014 UK Research Excellence Framework. *BMC Med*. 2015;13(1):232.

47. Ion G, Stingu M, Marin E. How can researchers facilitate the utilization of research by policy-makers and practitioners in education? *Res Pap Educ*. 2019;34(4):483–498.

48. Maggio LA, Leroux TC, Meyer HS, et al. #MedEd: exploring the relationship between altmetrics and traditional measures of dissemination in health professions education. *Perspect Med Educ*. 2018;7(4):239–247.

49. Nutley S. Reflections on the mobilisation of education research. In Levin B, Qi J, Edelstein H, et al., eds. *The Impact of Research in Education: An International Perspective*. Bristol: Policy Press; 2013: 243–262.

50. Onyura B, Legare F, Baker L, et al. Affordances of knowledge translation in medical education: a qualitative exploration of empirical knowledge use among medical educators. *Acad Med*. 2015;90(4):518–524.

51. Rodrigues J. Get more eyes on your work: visual approaches for dissemination and translation of education research. *Educ Res*. 2021;50(9):657–663.

52. Qi J, Levin B. Introduction and overview. In Levin B, Qi J, Edelstein H, et al., eds. *The Impact of Research in Education: An International Perspective*. Bristol: Policy Press; 2013: 1–21.

53. Reed RL, McIntyre E, Jackson-Bowers E, et al. Pathways to research impact in primary healthcare: what do Australian primary healthcare researchers believe works best to facilitate the use of their research findings? *Health Res Policy Syst.* 2017;15(1):17.

54. Smith K, Fernie S, Pilcher N. Aligning the times: exploring the convergence of researchers, policy makers and research evidence in higher education policy making. *Res Educ.* 2021;110(1):38–57.

55. Jones M. Mentoring and coaching in education practitioners' professional learning. *Int J Mentor Coach Educ.* 2015;4(4):293–302.

56. Wilson M. Quality educational research outputs and significance of impact: enduring dilemma or stimulus to learning transformations between multiple communities of practice? Hilary Place Papers: University of Leeds; 2013.

57. Reed MS, Bryce R, Machen R. Pathways to policy impact: a new approach for planning and evidencing research impact. *Evid Policy.* 2018;14(3):431–458.

58. Maggio LA, Meyer HS, Artino AR. Beyond citation rates: a real-time impact analysis of health professions education research using altmetrics. *Acad Med.* 2017;92(10):1449–1455.

59. Research Excellence Framework (REF). Assessment framework and guidance on submissions. UKRI; 2011. https://www.ref.ac.uk/2014/media/ref/content/pub/assessmentframeworkandguidanceonsubmissions/GOS%20including%20addendum.pdf (accessed 15 November 2022).

60. Patterson J. Punch drunk on research impact: a critical analysis of textual power politics. *Power Educ.* 2013;5(1):76–86.

61. Reichard B, Reed MS, Chubb J, et al. Writing impact case studies: a comparative study of high-scoring and low-scoring case studies from REF2014. *Palgrave Commun.* 2020;6(1):31.

62. Gunn A, Mintrom M. Higher education policy changes in Europe: academic research funding and the impact agenda. *Eur Educ.* 2016;48(4):241–257.

CHAPTER 13

Concluding Foundations of Health Professions Education Research

Lynn V. Monrouxe[1] and Charlotte E. Rees[2,3]

[1] The University of Sydney, Camperdown, New South Wales, Australia
[2] The University of Newcastle, Callaghan, New South Wales, Australia
[3] Monash University, Clayton, Victoria, Australia

> All scientists choose, adapt, and create tools appropriate to their reading of problems and opportunities in their fields. In turn, new or adapted tools can change the questions asked and the answers given, leading to new research cycles. The dialectic between the evolution of tools and the refinement of problems characterizes growth in a field. [1 p. 35]

Whether you identify with the term scientist or not, the evolution highlighted in this opening quotation is relevant to all research domains, being equally pertinent for health professions education research (HPER) as it is for any other research field. When a field is growing, it inevitably moves from one place to another. Continuing with the journey metaphor introduced in Chapter 1, you are now nearing the end of your travels with us, especially if you have read this book cover-to-cover. Here, like any expedition, we enter the evaluation phase of our book-writing journey as we look back on our original goals: facilitating the development of your research capabilities, alongside the quality and impact of your research. In doing so, we reflect on lessons learnt from our experiences writing this book, as we summarise key matters that cross-cut the twelve chapters and three parts of the book. We structure our concluding remarks focusing initially on three cross-cutting matters: research (section 13.1), relational (section 13.2), and self (section 13.3). In section 13.4, we complete the chapter by contemplating what next for future HPER innovations, before providing our closing remarks in section 13.5.

Foundations of Health Professions Education Research: Principles, Perspectives and Practices,
First Edition. Edited by Charlotte E. Rees, Lynn V. Monrouxe, Bridget C. O'Brien, Lisi J. Gordon, and Claire Palermo.
© 2023 John Wiley & Sons Ltd. Published 2023 by John Wiley & Sons Ltd.

13.1 CROSS-CUTTING RESEARCH MATTERS

One of the most noticeable aspects of HPER, and education research more generally, is the breadth of disciplines drawn upon methodologically and theoretically. This disciplinary breadth is both enriching and challenging for early, mid-career, and senior researchers alike, as we try to comprehend the background and applicability of the multiplicity of approaches available to us [2–6]. Enriching, as our eyes are opened to new, and sometimes radical, ways of scholarly thinking and acting. This breadth is also challenging due to the variable use of terminology, with a lack of consensus on a single methodology or method for many of the research approaches.

13.1.1 Variable Terminology

Firstly, the polysemous nature (multiple meanings) of words, labels, and phrases used in HPER can be challenging, even for seasoned researchers. This is because variation in meaning can be subtle at times. Other times, shifts in meaning come about due to the research approach, discipline, and context (including time) in which language is used. Thus, you will notice that we use similar words across the chapters, yet sometimes meaning is different (as illustrated in our book glossary). One of the most striking examples of polysemy is the word 'theory' (see Chapter 2). Theory can be appropriated for a wide range of constructs and at different levels of abstraction, which are not always easily reconcilable [4]. Indeed, the use of theory is ubiquitous in research and prolific across the entirety of our book, not just Chapter 2. We talk of grand theory, programme theory, evidence-based theory, theory-driven, theory-based, social theory, grounded theory, critical theory, activity theory, and so on. But what we mean in each instance can differ. Sometimes subtly, sometimes quite radically. Another example is 'abduction' (see Chapters 2, 6, 7, and 9). For interpretivists, abduction often points to the movement between data and known theories to generate new insights. For pragmatists, abduction is commonly associated with reasoning: the researcher moves to-and-fro between induction (inferred via observing) and deduction (inferred via verification). Both meanings are related, but the resulting actions can be quite different.

A third example is causation (see Chapters 5 and 6). Causation varies greatly depending on your research approach, with implications on the claims you can legitimately make. Thus, causality within scientific approaches asserts a constant conjunction between two variables, with one being the causative factor (independent variable) of the other (dependent variable). Furthermore, in scientific approaches, once a causative relationship is established, it is deemed true for most people (i.e., context independent). Scientists make this assumption based on the random assignment of participants to treatment and control groups, and the presence of statistically significant probability. Contrastingly, the concept of generative causality comes into play in realist approaches to explain why things happen: 'the events we observe and experience are generated through the complex interactions of generative mechanisms (or systems) that have causal powers or tendencies' [7 p. 172]. Further, such causal mechanisms are situated in complex systems, privilege context through a detailed description of it, reside at the individual (scientific realism) or structural (critical realism) levels, and are non-material (e.g., social systems, institutes, beliefs, motivations). However, interpretivist approaches tend to shun the idea of causality in the unidirectional scientific sense. Here, explanations comprise multiple viewpoints, each being equally credible and non-generalisable (although transferable knowledge can occur). Nevertheless, depending on the specific interpretivist methodology, the issue of causality might still be invoked as a way of understanding participants' perspectives of their own social worlds and their roles within [8].

Given this linguistic diversity, such richness requires careful attention when thinking about, working within, and disseminating your research. A key take-home message is that you should become acquainted with different approaches to research and their associated ontological, epistemological, and axiological assumptions (as discussed in Chapter 2, and across Part II). This will facilitate your appreciation of what comprises data, the different ways of working with data, the claims you can make from your data and analysis, and how you conceptualise and ensure quality. Furthermore, when communicating your research, make sure to clarify what you mean when you use a word that has the potential to hold multiple meanings. Also, if your approach is not dominant in your area, consider contrasting your understanding with more dominant understandings (so the reader avoids incorrect assumptions). Ultimately, clarity within your own understanding of polysemous words will strengthen your work and others' understandings and evaluations of it.

13.1.2   No Agreed Single-way within Research Approaches

The variable ways in which philosophical positions can be actualised also adds confusion. Such variability probably relates to how research is socially constructed in and through different disciplinary groups contributing to methodological advances. As such, shifts within research approaches occur over time, as illustrated in the perspectives presented in Part II of our book. Thus, within scientific approaches, we present positivist and post-positivist scientific approaches: the former adopting a singular, rigorous focus on logical inference based on empirical evidence seeking to objectively verify an *a priori* hypothesis; the latter drawing on Popper's notion of falsification (that is, disproving the null hypothesis) [9]. Post-positivism developed from positivism, with both approaches building theory through hypothesis generation and systematic testing, but having different viewpoints on the social world [9]. Similarly, in Chapter 6 we present scientific and critical realist approaches to programme evaluation (with proponents of each approach critiquing the other – critical realists critiquing scientific realism, and scientific realists critiquing critical realism) [10, 11]. Furthermore, when we reflect on differences between scientific and critical realist approaches to programme evaluation, we know first-hand how this might cause confusion: even in our own work we reveal how we approached this work from scientific realist perspectives, only to later realise we are taking critical realist perspectives (see Chapter 6, Box 6.3) [12]. Our third example of variability in approaches is discussed in Chapter 9 (i.e., grounded theory). With its origins in post-positivism (so-called classic grounded theory), there have been shifts over time towards adopting more interpretivist philosophical approaches (see Chapter 2, section 2.3.3) [13]. Despite this transition, Charmaz (a proponent of constructivist grounded theory) identifies the methodology as being pragmatic (hence we focus on grounded theory in Chapter 9, see section 9.3.3) [14].

Such fluidity around the varied, and occasionally subtle, natures of research perspectives can sometimes lead to confusion in distinguishing between different approaches. This is particularly the case when the research procedures undertaken across different perspectives share core features. For example, positivists and post-positivists advocate experimental methods, scientific and critical realists examine generative mechanisms underlying outcomes, and classic and constructivist grounded theorists undertake coding, memo-writing, and constant comparative techniques. Additionally, there is a tendency for differences to be polarised by advocates of any given approach, leading to an 'either–or' understanding. However, shifts over time have been relatively gradual; developed through wider debates around the nature of knowledge, knowing, and the role of researchers. These discussions – with multiple conflicting opinions and practices – will continue across your research career (as they have done throughout ours). We believe this is where our book can assist you. Chapter 2 provides you with an overview of different approaches to theory, including their underlying philosophical considerations (see Table 2.1). These are further delineated across Part II. We urge you to familiarise yourself with debates relating to your chosen approach, and then to read more widely (there are lots of methodology journals); even going back to original articles to understand perspectives in context. Try to approach your reading critically and reflexively, considering explicit and implicit rationales and claims. Ultimately, there are no absolute right or wrong versions of each approach. We therefore urge you to strive for clarity regarding which approach you are adopting (and why), including the nuances within your chosen approach based on the latest methodology writings, and communicate this clearly: within your team, through ethics processes, and as you prepare for and disseminate your work.

13.2 CROSS-CUTTING RELATIONAL MATTERS

We now consider relational matters identified across the book, focusing on three levels: relationships within your research team, research–researcher relationships, and your relationships with the wider HPER community.

13.2.1 Relationships within the Research Team

Across our book, we examine wide-ranging research practices, including considerations around team relationships. For example, in Chapters 3 and 5 respectively, we touch on team challenges when differences of opinion exist regarding authorship practices or philosophical clarity. In Chapter 7, we discuss the utility of engaging in team reflexivity to enhance research quality. In Chapter 8, our colleagues outline the importance of including consumers as team members to redress power imbalances. And finally, in Chapter 9, our colleagues illustrate the importance of team understandings when using diverse perspectives. We have not yet addressed relational issues pertaining to early career researchers (ECRs) doing team-based research with more senior researchers. So, here we provide some commentary to support ECRs.

It is commonplace for senior mentors to encourage ECRs to join larger, often more established teams, with cultural diversity frequently promoted. This practice is advocated as mutually beneficial for the wider team, as well as ECRs. Certainly, our book was formed on this basis: the five editors knew each other, most having worked together previously, and the diverse range of international ECRs were individually known to us or came recommended by HPER colleagues. Nevertheless, as an ECR, becoming involved with relatively unfamiliar research teams can have positive and negative implications. On the positive side, there is potential to develop new collaborations and to showcase personal knowledge and skills. Conversely, power relations within the team can lead to teamwork struggles around negotiating research approaches, processes, workload, and adequate recognition [15]. While many senior researchers try to build egalitarian teams, research projects always run the risk of traditional hierarchies involving (often unintentional) asymmetric power relationships. This risks ECRs being disempowered and overruled by seniors in decision-making conversations where they are given greater workloads with inadequate recognition. Often with short-term contracts, and working long hours, ECRs are eager for job security through continuing rather than fixed-term or casual appointments [15]. While power is dynamically relational, as senior researchers, we should be continuously mindful that ECRs are typically vulnerable in teams.

13.2.2   Research–researcher Relationships

Your role as a researcher in conducting research is also an important consideration. The research–researcher relationship includes issues of researcher as insider, outsider, or alongsider (see Chapter 2, Table 2.1), and researcher as analytical expert, knowledge co-constructor, or facilitator of co-design with participants. Essentially, these research–researcher relationships are influenced by foundational issues of objectivity or subjectivity, and researcher bias or reflexivity. Thus, Chapter 5 touches on researcher bias and minimising this through objective measurements. Chapter 6 alludes to objective reality while simultaneously recognising subjectivist accounts when considering critical realist evaluation. Chapters 7 and 8 accept knowledge as subjective and privilege researcher reflexivity, and Chapter 9 considers both objectivity and subjectivity (e.g., when discussing action research, considerations include integrating objective, intersubjective, and subjective positions).

We acknowledge that the nuances between these different researcher positions *vis-à-vis* knowledge and power are complex, and are therefore difficult to negotiate as novice researchers. When coming from a traditional scientific background (e.g., as a clinician) which attempts to minimise the role of the researcher on the research, novice health professions education (HPE) researchers may find it particularly difficult to adjust to their position in qualitative research, which conducts research from the inside (see Chapter 2, Table 2.1). As experienced researchers, even we have succumbed to 'scientific hangovers' in our qualitative research from our original scientific research training. For example, I (Lynn) was partly drawn to the longitudinal audio diary method to investigate medical students' professional identity development because I thought I could remove myself from the research process, thereby minimising my influence on what participants said and how they said it [16]. Only later, when analysing the data, did I realise that I was very much present in participants' talk, despite being physically absent: 'the relationship between myself and individual participants was beginning to develop: many recordings continued to begin with a hello, but then often went into a recognition of time passing, and the diary entries had the feeling that I was about to "catch-up" on their news and events' [16 p. 86]. Whether you consider this presence a case of the researcher skewing the data or as co-constructing knowledge through the research processes will depend on your beliefs about the nature of reality and knowing. Regardless of your philosophical approach, establishing, developing, sustaining, and ending relationships with your participants and the community involved in your research is a key consideration regarding the research–researcher relationship, especially when undertaking longitudinal or participatory methods [16–19]. Each of these phases requires sensitivity towards research questions being explored, and your methodology, alongside your relationships with co-researchers and participants, including your ethical stance, and how you might disseminate your work [20].

13.2.3   Relationships with the Wider HPER Community

As an ECR, you are not only part of a research team, but you are also becoming a member of an international community of HPER scholars. As you develop your research capabilities, we urge you to critically evaluate your practices, considering better ways of doing research and taking responsibility for pushing the field forward. We therefore encourage you to share your experiences and have the courage to explore new and thoughtful ways of researching based on the foundations provided in this book. We believe that critical thinking – based on experience and theory – is key to creativity and innovation in HPER. Indeed, we seek to innovate through our own research, sometimes by developing entirely new ways of analysing data (e.g., momentum analysis) [21], or bringing methods and analytical lenses originating outside HPER into the field (e.g., dramaturgy analysis, metaphor analysis, laughter analysis, linguistic enquiry word count analysis) [16, 22–25]. These novel approaches, adopted from social sciences more broadly, have enabled us to examine innovative questions (see Box 13.1). Furthermore, we developed these novel explorations during our early to mid-career phases. Indeed, we might argue that early in your career is the optimal time to dabble with methodological innovation, as attested by numerous ECR book contributors sharing case studies across this book, including many examples of innovation (e.g., realist economic evaluation (see Chapter 6) [26], poetic inquiry (see Chapter 7) [27], co-design with mental health consumers and decolonising methodologies (see Chapter 8) [19, 28]). Reflecting on Rachel Ellaway's message in the Foreword, we urge you to become HPER's next generation, reinventing the foundations, forming: 'a standing wave defined both by tradition and the changing perspectives of the scholars in the field over time'.

Box 13.1 Novel analytic approaches to examine innovative questions

- What topics are under discussion when focus groups participants' talk gets animated? (i.e., momentum analysis) [21].
- How are patient roles in bedside teaching constructed through talk and action? (i.e., dramaturgy analysis) [29].
- What metaphoric talk is used to describe student/doctor–patient relationships? (i.e., metaphor analysis) [25].
- How is laughter used in the construction of power during workplace learning? (i.e., laughter analysis) [23].
- What is the relationship between healthcare students' negative emotion talk and their professionalism dilemma narratives? (i.e., linguistic enquiry word count analysis) [30, 31].

13.3 CROSS-CUTTING MATTERS OF THE SELF

We now turn to matters of the self, with research and relational matters inevitably impacting on your researcher identity development. We begin this section by asking you to reflect on what comes to mind when you think about yourself as a researcher: what do you think, feel, or want to say about your researcher identity? Look at Box 13.2 for quotations provided by doctoral students talking about their researcher identities who are: 'at the peak of their epistemological and ontological growth' [32 p. 806]. Are you a wanderer, a chameleon, a warrior, or something else entirely? Your response to this question will be influenced by various personal characteristics, including your age, gender, nationality, race/ethnicity, social class, and research experience [32–35]. Your response could also be influenced by broader contexts in which you are situated, including your familial and professional (or work) activities [35]. Indeed, all these factors intersect as you consider who you are as a researcher [36, 37].

Box 13.2   Researcher as wanderer, chameleon, and warrior

The following metaphors have been identified by researchers interviewing doctoral students of colour who were: 'at the peak of their epistemological and ontological growth' [32 p. 806]. Perhaps their experiences resonate with you?

- **The wanderer:** 'Once exposed, my research agenda has become my research identity. I have not become someone I was not, but was able to understand who I am through an exercise in navigating who I was.' [32 p. 806]

- **The chameleon:** 'What I have become is an amalgamation of my unique past and present experiences that now translates into a knowledge that includes the articulation of research traditions, like critical theories and a commitment to social justice. Am I still a chameleon? Yes – I believe I am still adapting a little, hiding a little, and revealing a little as I grow as a researcher.' [32 p. 807]

- **The warrior:** 'The presence of war or struggle has generated the agitation that I needed to resist being moulded into an imitation of a predetermined paradigm as an educational researcher. It has allowed me to refine and strengthen those skills and talents that I already possessed, as well as to discover myself within the research process, which has generated peace for me.' [32 p. 807]

Your researcher identity evolves as your capability and confidence improves, and you enact your sense of autonomy and agency [35]. Furthermore, feedback, validation, reflection, and supportive relationships can facilitate this process of identity development, while any dissonance between your intersecting identities (as well as comparing yourself with idealised versions of what it means to be a scholar) are potential catalysts for identity disturbances [35]. Here, the issue of imposter syndrome could come into play, whereby learning to research, and developing your own researcher identity might feel like: 'a precarious adventure' [38 p. 380]. In terms of specific qualities, becoming a researcher requires you to develop a range of researcher characteristics, including: 'good people skills; resilience, patience, and persistence in the face of ambiguity and slow progress; and versatility, flexibility, and meticulousness in carrying out the details of the project' [39 p. 391]. The degree to which you identify with these characteristics can also affect how you feel about yourself as a researcher. This brings us to consider researcher qualities as you engage with this book (discussed in sections 13.1 and 13.2).

Regarding research matters, given the variability in terminology, alongside multiple and contested ways of doing any single research approach, we believe that ECRs should develop their tolerance of uncertainty. Indeed, uncertainty tolerance is linked with your own beliefs about the nature of knowledge and knowing (your personal epistemology). Such beliefs mediate how we make sense of the world, including the research world [40, 41]. Those researching personal epistemologies generally agree there are four core assumptions, each on a scale from simple (relatively black and white thinking) to complex, comprising: (a) the relative certainty (and uncertainty) of knowledge; (b) its source (external or internally constructed); (c) whether there are general facts or whether knowledge is context dependent; and (d) how knowledge is justified (by appeal to authority or by argument and evidence). Our personal epistemology can shift back and forth in terms of sophistication across these scales with each being contextually bound. Due to such complexity, these can be thought of as our epistemological resources that we draw upon as and when required [42]. The most sophisticated level of epistemological resources can afford you phronesis: a practical wisdom facilitating your ability to deal with uncertainty and understanding the contextual nature of the social world [43]. Interestingly, it has been argued that engaging in epistemic reflexivity can increase sophistication in terms of personal ways of knowing [44]. Such reflexivity involves critical thinking around your own epistemological assumptions, evaluating them from multiple perspectives, resulting in a greater tolerance of uncertainty. Epistemic reflexivity and awareness also make you a better, more ethical peer reviewer by helping to identify how assumptions influence judgement and interpretations of others' work. By recognising this influence, we can ensure we select criteria that align with the researchers' approach rather than our own inclinations and preferences.

Concerning relational matters, the issue of reflexivity comes into play. As highlighted in section 13.2.2, research–researcher relationships are central to research quality. We have already suggested in Part II (Chapters 7 and 8) that over time, your goal should be to embody research quality through engaging in the process of researcher and team reflexivity [45]. Having this sense of critical self-awareness when undertaking research is important for the embodiment of your researcher identity, especially in your role as knowledge producer [46]. Critical self-awareness is also important for researcher reflexivity, which has been metaphorically described as: 'entering a hall of mirrors that illuminates a social phenomenon from many angles' [47 p. 233], and even engaging in a: 'prismatic dialogue ... to refract and diffract [a variety of perspectives]' [45 p. 220]. Thus, reflexivity emphasises exploring your presence within the research process as a way to develop researcher relationships and improve your research quality [48]. For this to lend credibility to your research, such reflexivity must not be undertaken as a: 'rhetorical flourish' [47 p. 233]. Rather, it requires critique around your involvement in reflexive activities, especially within researcher relationships, and taking responsibility for knowledge changing due to our research practices, including your own creativity (see section 13.2.3) [49].

13.4 FUTURE DIRECTIONS

What of the future of HPER? While some might argue we need a crystal ball to forecast what comes next, perhaps we should start with a mirror. Reflecting the here and now as we write this chapter, this book has been written during a time of global turmoil. Such turmoil reminds us of the instability and impermanence of concepts, constructs, and methodologies, alongside the importance of strong foundations (see Foreword). So, what is lacking? Where are the absences? What are our research blind spots? And as we gaze into the crystal ball, we are hopeful that you, the future of HPER, are bold enough to advance the ever-shifting boundaries of this field – both theoretically and methodologically.

13.4.1 The Mirror

In Chapter 1, we reflected on the past decades in HPER, identifying two key trends: the exponential growth of knowledge syntheses and a general turn from positivist to constructionist and critical approaches. Here, we deploy our metaphorical mirror, looking back over the book to reflect on the state of HPER currently in terms of what appears to be absent. We also consider emerging research approaches with wider applications.

In their review of teacher education research, Mayer and Oancea [50] lament the scarcity of multi-site, comparative, longitudinal, and policy-orientated work. We can easily make the same observations for HPER, with its plethora of small, single-site, cross-sectional studies. Furthermore, such studies in HPER often stand in isolation, tending not to be part of a wider body of previously situated literature building on each other. Part of this problem reflects the paucity of funding available for HPER [51], making it harder to commit to sustained levels of research over longer time periods. However, this can be mitigated by developing larger, multi-site, interdisciplinary teams undertaking careful planning of multiple smaller-scale, but related, studies that are theoretically linked with overarching research frameworks, goals, purposes, objectives, and research questions. This enables the systematic development of a strong knowledge base, without relying on external funding. Furthermore, pragmatic and realist approaches (including realist economic research) sit well within this remit as the use of mixed methods and unpacking what works, for whom, and why are central to this vision.

Regarding interpretivist research approaches, the import of humanities and its associated sensibilities seems to be having an influence on HPER, albeit slowly. For example, we highlighted poetic inquiry in Chapter 7, an approach paying careful attention to participants' language use to reflect on meaning and provide space for wonderment and surprise [27, 52]. This approach is just one from a wider, largely heterogeneous, body of work drawing on narrative, discursive, and visual enquiry, which serves to extend beyond merely what is said, as is common with qualitative HPER that typically constructs themes from the content of participants' talk in individual or group interviews [53, 54]. Furthermore, extending beyond exploring sociocultural interactions, as is typical in interpretivist approaches in HPER, to consider sociomaterial interactions will be increasingly important in future HPER [55]. Based on sound philosophical foundations, these research spaces are full of creativity and exploration, but not in thoughtless, ad hoc ways – a philosophical free-for-all, where anything goes.

Reflecting on critical approaches, with the strong impetus for diversity and inclusivity in HPE and HPER, we note that community participatory and Indigenous research methodologies are slowly emerging in HPER [56–57]. Indeed, an essential (but often missing) element within HPE is cultural safety. An important part of cultural safety in HPER includes how research is undertaken, alongside considering researcher–participant power dynamics. One of the greatest challenges facing participatory approaches in HPER is the time required for researchers and participants as researchers to develop meaningful relationships. This includes the development of mutual trust and respect, openness, and transparency; acceptance of cultural differences; attention to power imbalances; and developing appropriate methods for conflict resolution [60]. Additionally, an openness to different ethical standpoints, including Indigenous values, is important. Finally, being able to find appropriately diverse team membership can be challenging when the workforce lacks diversity (the very issue we seek to redress).

13.4.2 The Crystal Ball

While the mirror exposes the emergence of wide-ranging novel, person-centred, and imaginative research methodologies and methods as identified across our book, the crystal ball gazes forward, suggesting a technological future replete with computerised educational possibilities and big data affordances. We are indeed: 'moving towards the "datafication" of society, where devices to capture, collect, store and process data are becoming ever cheaper and faster, whilst the computational power is continuously increasing' [61 p. 71]. Twitter, Facebook, LinkedIn, Instagram, Sina Weibo, YouTube – information is omnipresent. Indeed, the ease of accessing, collecting, and analysing readily available data lends itself to considering research questions focusing on online and offline behaviours, as well as the organisation of courses and even the structure of institutions (e.g., universities, hospitals, private practices). Despite the backlash following the Cambridge Analytica controversy, with social media platforms strictly controlling access to data via application programming interfaces (APIs), the door has not completely shut on big data access for addressing critical research questions (although it has been severely hampered across a few key networks such as Twitter and Facebook) [62]. However, big data sources for HPER could be gleaned from various education platforms and systems (e.g., assessment scores, social media profiles, library use, learning management systems, massive open online courses, learning object repositories, and open educational resources) [63–65].

A consensus definition of big data is that it comprises sufficient high volume (i.e., high numbers) [66], velocity (i.e., generating/processing speed), and variety (i.e., structured/unstructured data generated by people or machines): 'to require specific Technology and Analytical Methods for its transformation into Value' [67 p. 131]. The core themes of big data comprise: information, technology, methods, and impact [67]. Big data in education can predict, cluster, and examine relationships and outliers, in addition to undertaking quantitative social network analyses [68]. Big educational data in the form of learning analytics can be used to examine a variety of aspects around: students' studying behaviours (with the aim of changing learning environments), students' competencies (to improve curricula), students' undesirable behaviours and affect (e.g., frustration, confusion, or boredom), predicting students' educational outcomes and completion (to inform training practices), and students' progression and retention [63–65]. Furthermore, advances in computer science methods means that we can rigorously and efficiently analyse unstructured big data (e.g., written and spoken words, pictures), alongside physiological automatic responses [69, 70]. These techniques allow us to access emotions, attitudes, thoughts, and behaviours on a grand scale; thereby opening up new questions we might ask of data.

However, the benefits of big data come with associated risks, including poor quality data, lack of governance frameworks, and wider ethical considerations [61, 71]. For example, within HPER, ongoing surveillance via continuous data collection and analysis might inhibit students' learning or lead to increased stress levels [61]. As technology develops to enable location tracking and biometric data (not just academic performance), there is also uncertainty around data ownership (does data belong to the individual, the institution, or the external organisation providing the data gathering/analytic tool?), consent (including withdrawal processes), and confidentiality [61, 64]. These can ultimately lead to problems pertaining to trust. Another concern is that they encourage data-driven, rather than knowledge-driven, approaches [72], some believing this could herald the end of theory [73]. Although the arguments around big data are many and varied, it is thought possible to: 'draw valuable insights from big data that are situated and reflexive' [72 p. 10]. Ultimately, with this era already upon us, ECRs in HPER wishing to engage in such developments will need even stronger foundational understandings of ontological, epistemological, methodological, and axiological issues in research, as well as advanced capabilities in ethics, research design, and data analytics.

13.5   CLOSING REMARKS

In this chapter, we have summarised key cross-cutting book themes relating to research, relationships, and the self, as well as contemplating what next for HPER. While we come to the end of this book, this is not the end of our journey, nor is it the end of yours. For us, we have learned much in the writing of this book, from our readings and from our collaborations with each other and our book contributors (ECR and senior researchers alike). We are committed to continuing our learning journeys in HPER. For you, finishing this book could represent just the start of your journey. We hope that through your reading and practical engagement with this book, whether you identify as a wanderer, chameleon, or warrior [32], you will feel a closer affinity to your developing researcher identity. We also hope that this book has stimulated your curiosity about HPE, as well as your desire to build new knowledge in HPER and translate that knowledge into improved educational policies and practices. Continuously curious, the research journey never really ends, so we urge you to create new knowledge and make a difference, but we also encourage you to create methodological and theoretical innovations in HPER. We challenge you to build on these foundations and advance the field of HPER into the future.

REFERENCES

1. Kelly AE, Lesh RA. Trends and shifts in research methods. In Kelly AE, Lesh RA, eds. *Handbook of Research Design in Mathematics and Science Education*. Mahwah, NJ: Lawrence Erlbaum Associates; 2000: 35–44.

2. Brennan J, Teichler U. The future of higher education and of higher education research. *High Educ.* 2008;56(3):259–264.

3. Tight M. Theory development and application in higher education research: the case of threshold concepts. In Huisman J, Tight M, eds. *Theory and Method in Higher Education Research II*. International Perspectives on Higher Education Research, vol. 10. Bingley: Emerald Group Publishing Limited; 2014: 249–267.

4. Tight M. Theory development and application in higher education research: tribes and territories. *High Educ Policy.* 2015;28(3):277–293.

5. Tight M. Theory development and application in higher education research: the case of academic drift. *J Educ Adm Hist.* 2015;47(1):84–99.

6. Tight M. Theory application in higher education research: the case of communities of practice. *Eur J High Educ.* 2015;5(2):111–126.

7. Mingers J, Standing C. Why things happen – developing the critical realist view of causal mechanisms. *Inf Organ.* 2017;27(3):171–189.

8. Orlikowski WJ, Baroudi JJ. Studying information technology in organizations: research approaches and assumptions. *Inf Syst Res.* 1991;2(1):1–28.

9. Hammersley M. From positivism to post-positivism: progress or digression? *Teoria Polityki.* 2019;3:175–188.

10. Porter S, O'Halloran P. The use and limitation of realistic evaluation as a tool for evidence-based practice: a critical realist perspective. *Nurs Inq.* 2012;19(1):18–28.

11. Riley S, Brooks J, Goodman S, et al. Celebrations amongst challenges: considering the past, present and future of the qualitative methods in psychology section of the British Psychology Society. *Qual Res Psych.* 2019;16(3):464–482.

12. Pawson R. *The Science of Evaluation: A Realist Manifesto*. London: SAGE; 2013.

13. O'Connor A, Carpenter B, Coughlan B. An exploration of key issues in the debate between classic and constructivist grounded theory. *Grounded Theory Rev: An Int J.* 2018;17(1):np.

14. Charmaz K. *Constructing Grounded Theory*, 2nd ed. Thousand Oaks, Calif.: SAGE; 2014.

15. Liinason M. Young blood: the social politics of research collaboration from the perspective of a young scholar. In Griffin G, Hamberg K, Lundgren B, eds. *The Social Politics of Research Collaboration*. New York and London: Routledge; 2013: 105–118.

16. Monrouxe LV. Solicited audio diaries in longitudinal narrative research: a view from inside. *Qual Res*. 2009;9(1):81–103.

17. Gordon L. Making space for relational reflexivity in longitudinal qualitative research. *Med Educ*. 2021;55(11):1223–1224.

18. Mertler CA. *The Wiley Handbook of Action Research in Education*. Hoboken, NJ: Wiley Blackwell; 2019.

19. Tuhiwai Smith L. *Decolonizing Methodologies: Research and Indigenous Peoples*. 3rd ed.London: Bloomsbury; 2021.

20. Stevenson FA, Gibson W, Pelletier C, et al. Reconsidering 'ethics' and 'quality' in healthcare research: the case for an iterative ethical paradigm. *BMC Med Ethics*. 2015;16(1):21.

21. Knight LV, Rees CE. "Enough is enough, I don't want any audience": exploring medical students' explanations of consent-related behaviours. *Adv Health Sci Educ*. 2008;13(4):407–426.

22. Rees CE, Ajjawi R, Monrouxe LV. The construction of power in family medicine bedside teaching: a video observation study. *Med Educ*. 2013;47(2):154–165.

23. Rees CE, Monrouxe LV. "I should be lucky ha ha ha ha": the construction of power, identity and gender through laughter within medical workplace learning encounters. *J Pragmat*. 2010;42(12):3384–3399.

24. Rees CE, Monrouxe LV, McDonald LA. 'My mentor kicked a dying woman's bed...' analysing UK nursing students' 'most memorable' professionalism dilemmas. *J Adv Nurs*. 2015;71(1):169–180.

25. Rees CE, Knight LV, Wilkinson CE. Doctors being up there and we being down here: a metaphorical analysis of talk about student/doctor-patient relationships. *Soc Sci Med*. 2007;65(4):725–737.

26. Rees CE, Nguyen VNB, Foo J, et al. Balancing the effectiveness and cost of online education: a preliminary realist economic evaluation. *Med Teach*. 2022;44(9):977–985.

27. Brown MEL, Proudfoot A, Mayat NY, et al. A phenomenological study of new doctors' transition to practice, utilising participant-voiced poetry. *Adv Health Sci Educ*. 2021;26(4):1229–1253.

28. Brand G, Sheers C, Wise S, et al. A research approach for co-designing education with healthcare consumers. *Med Educ*. 2021;55(5):574–581.

29. Monrouxe LV, Rees CE, Bradley P. The construction of patients' involvement in hospital bedside teaching encounters. *Qual Health Res*. 2009;19(7):918–930.

30. Monrouxe LV, Rees CE. "It's just a clash of cultures": emotional talk within medical students' narratives of professionalism dilemmas. *Adv Health Sci Educ*. 2012;17(5):671–701.

31. Rees CE, Monrouxe LV, McDonald LA. Narrative, emotion and action: analysing 'most memorable' professionalism dilemmas. *Med Educ*. 2013;47(1):80–96.

32. Murakami-Ramalho E, Piert J, Militello M. The wanderer, the chameleon, and the warrior: experiences of doctoral students of color developing a research identity in educational administration. *Qual Inq*. 2008;14(5):806–834.

33. Metz MH. Intellectual border crossing in graduate education: a report fom the field. *Educ Res*. 2001;30(5):1–7.

34. Murakami-Ramalho E, Militello M, Piert J. A view from within: how doctoral students in educational administration develop research knowledge and identity. *Stud High Educ*. 2013;38(2):256–271.

35. Choi YH, Bouwma-Gearhart J, Ermis G. Doctoral students' identity development as scholars in the education sciences: literature review and implications. *Int J Dr Stud.* 2021;16:89–125.

36. Monrouxe LV. When I say... intersectionality in medical education research. *Med Educ.* 2015;49(1):21–22.

37. Tsouroufli M, Rees CE, Monrouxe LV, et al. Gender, identities and intersectionality in medical education research. *Med Educ.* 2011;45(3):213–216.

38. Coryell JE, Wagner S, Clark MC, et al. Becoming real: adult student impressions of developing an educational researcher identity. *J Furth High Educ.* 2013;37(3):367–383.

39. Angen MJ. Evaluating interpretive inquiry: reviewing the validity debate and opening the dialogue. *Qual Health Res.* 2000;10(3):378–395.

40. Hofer B, Bendixen L. Personal epistemology: theory, research, and future directions. In Harris KR, Graham S, Urdan T, et al. eds. *APA Educational Psychology Handbook: Vol 1. Theories, Constructs, and Critical Issues.* Washington DC: American Psychological Association; 2012: 227–256.

41. Hofer BK, Pintrich PR. *Personal Epistemology: The Psychology of Beliefs about Knowledge and Knowing.* Mahwah, NJ: Lawrence Erlbaum Associates; 2002.

42. Hammer D, Elby A. On the form of a personal epistemology. In Hofer BK, Pintrich PR, eds. *Personal Epistemology: The Psychology of Beliefs about Knowledge and Knowing.* Mahwah, NJ: Lawrence Erlbaum Associates; 2002: 169–190.

43. Eastwood JL, Koppelman-White E, Mi M, et al. Epistemic cognition in medical education: a literature review. *Int J Med Educ.* 2017;8:1–12.

44. Feucht FC, Lunn Brownlee J, Schraw G. Moving beyond reflection: reflexivity and epistemic cognition in teaching and teacher education. *Educ Psychol.* 2017;52(4):234–241.

45. Vettraino E, Linds W, Downie H. Embodied reflexivity: discerning ethical practice through the six-part story method. *Reflective Pract.* 2019;20(2):218–233.

46. Albert M, Hodges B, Regehr G. Research in medical education: balancing service and science. *Adv Health Sci Educ.* 2007;12(1):103–115.

47. Riessman CK. Entering the hall of mirrors: reflexivity and narrative research. In De Fina A, Georgakopoulou A, eds. *The Handbook of Narrative Analysis.* Hoboken, NJ: John Wiley & Sons, Inc.; 2015: 219–238.

48. Barry CA, Britten N, Barber N, et al. Using reflexivity to optimize teamwork in qualitative research. *Qual Health Res.* 1999;9(1):26–44.

49. Keevers L, Treleaven L. Organizing practices of reflection: a practice-based study. *Manag Learn.* 2011;42(5):505–520.

50. Mayer D, Oancea A. Teacher education research, policy and practice: finding future research directions. *Oxf Rev Educ.* 2021;47(1):1–7.

51. Archer J, McManus C, Woolf K, et al. Without proper research funding, how can medical education be evidence based? *BMJ.* 2015;350:h3445.

52. Brown MEL, Kelly M, Finn GM. Thoughts that breathe, and words that burn: poetic inquiry within health professions education. *Perspect Med Educ.* 2021;10(5):257–264.

53. Nimmon L, Atherley A. Qualitative ego networks in health professions education: capturing the self in relation to others. *Med Educ.* 2022;56(1):71–81.

54. Rees C. Drawing on drawings: moving beyond text in health professions education research. *Perspect Med Educ.* 2018;7(3):166–173.

55. Fenwick T, Nimmo GR. Making visible what matters: sociomaterial approaches for research and practice in healthcare education. In Cleland J, Durning SJ, eds. *Researching Medical Education.* Chichester: Wiley Blackwell; 2015: 67–80.

56. Doran F, Wrigley B. Cultural safety: teachers' engagement with an Indigenous pedagogical method in undergraduate nursing education. *Contemp Nurse.* 2022;58(1):58–70.

57. Forsyth C, Irving M, Short S, et al. Students don't know what they don't know: dental and oral health students' perspectives on developing cultural competence regarding Indigenous peoples. *J Dent Educ.* 2019;83(6):679–686.

58. McKivett A, Hudson JN, McDermott D, et al. Two-eyed seeing: a useful gaze in Indigenous medical education research. *Med Educ.* 2020;54(3):217–224.

59. Wilson C, Heinrich L, Heidari P, et al. Action research to implement an Indigenous health curriculum framework. *Nurs Educ Today.* 2020;91:104464.

60. Brush BL, Mentz G, Jensen M, et al. Success in long-standing community-based participatory research (CBPR) partnerships: a scoping literature review. *Health Educ Behav.* 2019;47(4):556–568.

61. Da Bormida M. The Big Data world: benefits, threats and ethical challenges. In Iphofen R, O'Mathuna D, eds. *Ethical Issues in Covert, Security and Surveillance Research (Advances in Research Ethics and Integrity, Vol. 8).* Advances in Research Ethics and Integrity, Vol. 8. Bingley: Emerald Publishing Limited; 2021: 71–91.

62. Bruns A. After the 'APIcalypse': social media platforms and their fight against critical scholarly research. *Inf Commun Soc.* 2019;22(11):1544–1566.

63. Sun X, Fu Y, Zheng W, et al. Big educational data analytics, prediction and recommendation: a survey. *J Circuits Syst Comput.* 2022;31(9):2230007.

64. Reyes JA. The skinny on big data in education: learning analytics simplified. *TechTrends.* 2015;59(2):75–80.

65. Vaitsis C, Nilsson G, Zary N. Big data in medical informatics: improving education through visual analytics. *Stud Health Techno Inform.* 2014;205:1163–1167.

66. Miniwatts Marketing Group. Internet world stats: usage and population statistics. Miniwatts Marketing Group; 2022. https://www.internetworldstats.com/stats.htm (accessed 21 September 2022).

67. De Mauro A, Greco M, Grimaldi M. A formal definition of big data based on its essential features. *Libr Rev.* 2016;65(3):122–135.

68. Leppink J, Pérez-Fuster P. Social networks as an approach to systematic review. *Health Prof Educ.* 2019;5(3):218–224.

69. Schwaiger J, Hammerl T, Florian J, et al. UR: SMART–a tool for analyzing social media content. *Ind Syst E-Bus Manag.* 2021;19(4):1275–1320.

70. Carrion B, Onorati T, Díaz P, et al. A taxonomy generation tool for semantic visual analysis of large corpus of documents. *Multimed Tools Appl.* 2019;78(23):32919–32937.

71. Funk E, Riddell J, Ankel F, et al. Blockchain technology: a data framework to improve validity, trust, and accountability of information exchange in health professions education. *Acad Med.* 2018;93(12):1791–1794.

72. Kitchin R. Big Data, new epistemologies and paradigm shifts. *Dig Data Soc.* 2014;1(1):1–12.

73. Anderson C The end of theory: the data deluge makes the scientific method obsolete. *Wired*; 2008; 23 June. https://www.wired.com/2008/06/pb-theory (accessed 11 October 2022).

Afterword: Inspiring Early Career Researcher-led Developments in Health Professions Education Research into the Future

We are a group of six researchers in the earlier stages of our research careers, having completed our PhDs within the last two to ten years. Our levels of experience in health professions education research (HPER) range from novice to more experienced, but we have all contributed to designing, conducting, and disseminating various HPER projects. We are from diverse disciplinary backgrounds, including dietetics, education, nursing, physiotherapy, and podiatry. Our HPER interests and methodological experiences are also varied, as are our evolving researcher identities. Collectively, we have contributed to writing six chapters in this book, alongside peer-reviewing all book chapters. Given our proximity to the book's intended audience (i.e., early and mid-career education researchers), we now share some of our reflections and insights on the book, including how it might be used and its potential impacts.

What we really like about this book is that it provides a comprehensive overview of almost every aspect of HPER, logically sequenced from research idea inception through to evaluating research impact. It provides a common language and starting point from which health professions education (HPE) researchers from different disciplinary backgrounds can converse and collectively build their understanding. By weaving in real-life examples, the book brings to life numerous complex, frequently misunderstood, and often contentious concepts. The book is written in a way that is both accessible and honest, and directs you to additional resources and readings for more information. It frames research as a developmental process, presenting key concepts and guiding you (as early and mid-career researchers) to pause and reflect on how these may apply to your own research activities. We are excited by the diverse ways to conduct HPER and how the book highlights this. There is something for everyone, with many new learnings to be had.

The book is structured to provide a framework for designing high-quality HPER and covers a range of research approaches. It encourages you to consider the opportunities and challenges associated with each. It provides clear definitions of key concepts and examples to show real-world application, helping you to counter the

Foundations of Health Professions Education Research: Principles, Perspectives and Practices,
First Edition. Edited by Charlotte E. Rees, Lynn V. Monrouxe, Bridget C. O'Brien, Lisi J. Gordon, and Claire Palermo.
© 2023 John Wiley & Sons Ltd. Published 2023 by John Wiley & Sons Ltd.

ambiguities and frequent misinterpretations that can lead to feelings of being over-whelmed, particularly for more novice researchers. Each chapter provides a holistic and balanced view of key topics, prompting deeper thinking on aspects such as philosophical underpinnings and ethical issues. We believe this will inspire you as researchers to consider new ways to progress your work. The diversity of the authorship team in terms of nationality, personal characteristics, research and methodological interests, and experience has made for a rich and considered discussion of a variety of HPER principles, perspectives, and practices.

To make the most of this book, we encourage you to start slowly, particularly if you have little research experience. Pick the chapters that appear most relevant to your research or stage of your research journey. Accept that you may not understand everything on your first read, and be prepared to persist. Take notes and set aside time to pause and reflect when prompted to do so. Chat about your learnings with your peers, supervisor(s), or other research team members. Seek out others with experience in a particular approach if you or your research collaborators lack the expertise. Be open to considering alternative approaches and then read those chapters. Do not discount a chapter based on the title alone; embrace exploring new concepts. Give yourself time and space to reflect on the various approaches and in doing so develop an appreciation for their similarities and differences. Revisit chapters of the book throughout your research journey, particularly if you change tack or want to learn about a concept more deeply. Your existing knowledge and motivation to read the book will influence the gems that you will uncover while reading. The authors have been honest (and critical) in their recounting of research experiences and projects, and some of the examples may not reflect optimal contemporary HPER practice. So, consider the case studies critically and contemplate how else the authors might have approached their research.

You may use this book to reflect on or appraise existing HPER. You might like to establish a book club to tackle sections of the book. You could discuss the concepts, complete the activities, and consider how to use the different approaches to answer different research questions for a particular topic. Although the book is orientated towards early and mid-career researchers, it may be equally useful for more experienced researchers less familiar with particular approaches to HPER. The book can complement other sources of support and information for novice and experienced researchers alike.

We do acknowledge that the structure of the book suggests neat boundaries around the different approaches, which fails to recognise the blurriness of boundaries. HPER can be messy in real life, taking non-linear courses and involving methodological borrowing. Although the book covers a lot of foundational ground in terms of HPER principles, perspectives, and practices, there is potential for additional or more in-depth discussion of topics (e.g., advanced HPER approaches, data analysis techniques, novel research dissemination strategies such as podcasts and visual abstracts) to be addressed in future books or by other resources. There is also potential to develop and use alternate ways to present some of the key concepts in the book. For example, using visual illustrations to map different approaches, alongside explanations of each approach's philosophical stance. Focusing on a single research topic across different case studies may help to show how different approaches can be applied to explore the same topic from different angles and/or using different data collection and analysis methods.

As relatively novice HPE researchers, we experienced our very own Aha! moments as we contributed to the book. For instance, we realised the importance of internal coherence, and how it sets the foundation for all key decision-making during our research. We recognised that there are different levels of engagement with quality constructs: from superficial through to deep deliberation. We found that many of the case studies resonated with us, particularly the ethical dilemmas and challenges associated with different approaches. We realised that there are always things that could be done differently or better. We were surprised to note some similarities between the different approaches, despite their different philosophical underpinnings, such as for scientific and realist approaches. As we worked through the writing and reviewing of the chapters, we reflected that our current research activities could be enhanced by applying some of the key principles, perspectives, and practices discussed in this book. We also realised the importance of being explicit about the methodological approaches and concepts in our reporting, given HPER's ongoing evolution and the various ways in which concepts are viewed in HPER and wider research communities. We observed our senior HPER author colleagues engage in some enlightening conversations and debates about elements of content, and concepts, and this strengthened our confidence in voicing our thoughts and opinions. We were also encouraged by their openness to continual learning and different ways of doing things. Finally, we appreciated that many of the chapters are forward-thinking, helping to promote novel and important developments and innovations in HPER.

As novice researchers, it is our responsibility to not only build our research capabilities, but also consider how we can contribute to others' learning in the HPER community. Our senior HPER colleagues for this book have challenged us to embrace opportunities of driving methodological and theoretical developments in HPER into the future. And we invite you to join us. Inspired by Marcel Proust, we encourage you to open your eyes to new ways of seeing and doing in HPER.

My destination is no longer a place, rather a new way of seeing.
                                                            Marcel Proust

Olivia A. King, Louise Allen, Jonathan Foo,
Van N.B. Nguyen, Mahbub Sarkar, and Ella Ottrey
Monash University, Clayton, Victoria, Australia

Book Glossary

A

Abduction: (Chapters 6, 7 and 9) Abduction can mean different things depending on your research approach. From a realist approach (Chapter 6), it can describe: 'a way of thinking that occurs when a researcher starts with a problem and empirical evidence regarding it and then suggests a hypothesis of why this problem exists and how the empirical evidence can be explained' [2 p. 109]. From interpretivist and pragmatic approaches (Chapters 7 and 9), it can reflect a moving back and forth between inductive and deductive reasoning such that observations are used to generate theories and theories are evaluated through action [3]. It can also reflect an oscillation between theory ('in the clouds') and data ('on the ground') [4 p. 187], with this cycling back and forth between theory and data deepening understanding (Chapter 7) [5].

Abstraction: (Chapter 6) Associated with realist approaches, abstraction: '... involves re-describing that which is observed ... to describe the sequence of causation, or the relations between things, that gives rise to observed regularities in the pattern of events' [6 p. 13].

Academic freedom: (Chapters 2 and 3) The freedom of teachers, students, and academic institutions to pursue knowledge wherever it may lead, without undue or unreasonable interference; it 'protects the pursuit and dissemination of knowledge through free inquiry and ensures that university research and teaching is authoritative and unbiased' [7 p. 47].

Actionability: (Chapter 9) A form of enquiry based on participants' experiences and real-world problems that seeks to create or achieve outcomes (e.g., knowledge) with practical relevance and consequences, in contrast to other forms of enquiry that might serve to describe or explain observations [8, 9]. In action research, actionability is a key marker of quality described as: 'people's ability to use knowledge to produce the actions they want' [10 p. 583].

Altmetrics: (Chapters 11 and 12) Short for alternative metrics, altmetrics are: 'the collection of digital indicators related to scholarly work, with the indicators derived from activity and engagement among diverse stakeholders and scholarly outputs in the research ecosystem, including the public sphere' [11 p. 1149]. Altmetric scores essentially: 'quantify the digital attention an article receives in a multitude of online sources' [12 p. 131]. This includes blogs, news, public policy, and social media [12].

Anonymisation: (Chapter 3) A process to render personal data non-personal [13].

A posteriori (or post hoc) theory: (Chapter 2) In qualitative studies especially, it is commonplace for macro or micro theories to be used post data collection to help interpret data [1].

Applied research: (Chapter 12) Common in health professions education research, applied research is: 'targeted at solving well-defined, immediate problems' [14 p. 253].

A priori theory: (Chapter 2) Linked with a deductive approach, a priori theory is that which is explicitly/consciously in mind at the outset of a study, thereby shaping the research process.

Atheoretical: (Chapter 2) Work can be described as atheoretical when it lacks: 'explicit description, review or reexamination or modification of theories/concepts/models/paradigms in guiding the research or review concerned' [15 p. 244].

Authenticity: (Chapters 7 and 8) A quality marker in qualitative research approaches based on how well researchers harness diverse perspectives, and calls to action, of all participants during data collection and analysis [16, 17].

Autonomy: (Chapter 3) The capacity to make an informed, uncoerced decision [18].

Axiology: (Chapter 2) Relates to: 'the values and/or value judgements' shaping a chosen research approach [19 p. 688].

B

Beneficence: (Chapter 3) Providing benefits and balancing benefits against risks [18].

Beneficiaries: (Chapter 12) Any stakeholders who benefit from the research. See also *consumer engagement*.

Bias: (Chapters 3, 5 and 7) Can be seen as researcher practices or actions influencing research methods and thereby adversely affecting neutrality and objectivity [20].

C

Causality: (Chapters 5 and 6) Causality can have different meanings depending on the research approach. For example, scientific approaches (Chapter 5) identify cause–effect relationships between independent (e.g., A) and dependent (e.g., B) variables [21]. Causal inferences rely on association (e.g., A correlates with B), temporal precedence (A must precede B in time for A to cause B), and lack of confounders (B is caused by A rather than by C or D) [21]. However, unlike these scientific *constant conjunctions*, in realist approaches (Chapter 6): 'causation is understood in terms of how individuals construct causes and give them meaning – there may be multiple different understandings of different contextual conditions and of how interventions lead to outcomes ...' [22 p. 3]. With respect to this realist generative causation: 'actors have a potential for affecting change by their very nature' [23 p.81].

Codes of conduct: (Chapter 3) Sets of rules, principles, and standards outlining the responsibilities and moral/ethical expectations of individuals and/or organisations [24], which: 'differ in scope, form, and content' [25 p. 67].

Coercion: (Chapter 3) The practice of persuading someone to do something that they would otherwise not do, such as taking part in a research study, by using pressure [18].

Co-impact: (Chapter 12) '... an umbrella term referring to the generation of change as a result of individuals, groups and organisations working together' [26 p. 542].

Conceptual framework: (Chapters 2 and 10) Although variously defined, a conceptual framework can be seen as providing: 'the orientation to the study ... how the study contributes to the body of knowledge on the topic, how elements of the study align, and how the study design and methodology meet rigorous research standards' [27 p. 36]. More simply, it can be described as: 'a map of how previous research and literature work together to shape a research project' [28 p. 529].

Confirmability: (Chapters 2, 7 and 8) A marker of quality in qualitative approaches regarding whether findings and their interpretation clearly match the data from which they were derived [17].

Conflict of interest: (Chapter 3) Refers to situations in which financial or other personal considerations may compromise, or have the appearance of compromising, a researcher's professional judgement in conducting or reporting research [29, 30].

Confucianism: (Chapter 3) A Chinese philosophy focusing on the importance of personal ethics and morality [31].

Consent: (Chapter 3) Securing permission from someone about their willingness to participate in research [18]. This includes giving adequate information (informed consent) and participants having capacity (cognitive ability) to understand this information. The primary purpose of seeking informed consent is to respect the ethical principle of *autonomy*; that participants remain in control of their own lives [18, 32].

Constant conjunction: (Chapters 5 and 6) A Humean conception of causality in positivist experimental science (and thus closed systems), a constant conjunction assumes that: 'if one event is invariably followed closely by another event, then it can be concluded that the former is the cause of the latter' [33 p. 19].

Constructionism: (Chapters 2 and 7) Constructionism is about: 'knowledge being constructed through social interaction, especially language ... constructionism ... focuses on the interactional and structural processes in the construction of meaning' [34 p. 846]. Other tenets central to constructionism involve criticism of accepted ways of knowing, knowing influenced by place and time, and diverse constructions of the world affecting different actions [35]. See also *social constructionism*.

Constructivism: (Chapters 2 and 7) Constructivism asserts that a person: 'selects information, constructs hypotheses, and makes decisions, with the aim of integrating new experiences into his [*sic*] existing knowledge and experience' [36 p. 11]. Constructivists often make claims around knowledge being stored in our cognition (as mental models) and how this develops in stages over time (cognition precedes knowledge). See also *social constructivism* for a different perspective [36].

Constructivist grounded theory: (Chapters 2 and 9) A methodology based on pragmatic philosophy and constructivist perspectives of knowledge (as subjective, situated in context, and created through interaction). The methodology pays careful attention to research relationships, context, and use of data; it employs strategies such as coding, memo-writing, and theoretical sampling to develop an abstract understanding of social processes and phenomena [37].

Consumer engagement: (Chapter 12) Consumers are involved in research to ensure that it is: 'relevant and important to the needs of the people [the] research is about' [38 p. 17]. Consumers in HPER can comprise individuals (from a range of stakeholder groups) and/or organisations depending on research foci.

Context–mechanism–outcome configurations (CMOCs): (Chapter 6) In realist approaches, CMOCs refer to: '... the causal links between context, mechanism and outcome' [23 p. 83].

Contexts: (Chapter 6) In realist approaches, contexts are conceptualised as dynamic and relational features that shape mechanisms through which interventions work [22]. They: 'are not just things or people (material and social) but psychological, organisational, economic, technical and so on relationships (forces) that interact and influence each other' [22 p. 8].

Credibility: (Chapters 2, 7 and 8) A marker of quality in qualitative approaches, credibility reflects the eloquence of the findings in terms of representing participants' and researchers' multiple realities [17].

Critical action research: (Chapter 8) Critical action research challenges accepted research approaches and makes the assumption that knowledge is power that must be shared with others so that they can enact change [39].

Critical appraisal: (Chapter 4) The act of evaluating the quality of research, often based on criteria identified in tools developed for reviewing studies with specific methodologies or study designs [40, 41].

Critical consciousness: (Chapter 8) Shedding light on power structures and reflecting on situations to promote equity and social justice [42].

Critical discourse analysis: (Chapter 8) Critical discourse analysis '... allows for systematic examination of institutions and structures that inform the production and interpretation of language and identification of power imbalances within a socio-cultural context' [43 p. 2].

Critical enquiry: (Chapter 8) Critical enquiry '... addresses power, inequality and injustice ... embedded in a transformative paradigm that seeks to expose, oppose, and redress forms of oppression, inequality, and injustice' [44 p. 35].

Critical pedagogy: (Chapter 8) A teaching approach in which educators support students to critique structures of power and oppression within the act of learning and teaching [45].

Critical race theory: (Chapter 8) A theoretical approach that serves to shed light on race, racism, and power and their interconnections [46].

Critical realism: (Chapters 6 and 8) Critical realism 'views reality as complex and recognizes the role of both agency and structural factors in influencing human behaviour' [47 p. 168].

Critical theory: (Chapter 8) A term encompassing a range of: 'theories that include feminist, anti-racist, anti-colonialist, queer, and many other positionalities. Critical theory today represents a space that embraces vast social concerns and other conflict theories – that is, theories that stress intergroup struggles and anchor their analyses in people's everyday lives, often as they are determined by their ascribed characteristics, defined as individual traits over which one has no control.' [48 p. 842]

Crystallisation: (Chapter 7) Crystallisation can be seen as a marker of quality in qualitative research that focuses on comprehensiveness rather than its alternative *triangulation*, which instead focuses on convergence. Rather, crystallisation: 'offers an "infinite variety of shapes, substances, transmutations, multidimensionalities, and angles of approach" that can then provide a richly complex understanding of the topic' [49 p. 45].

D

Data falsification: (Chapter 3) This involves manipulating or falsifying research data or fabricating data with the intention of giving a false impression [30].

Deductive: (Chapter 2) A deductive approach sets out to test or verify a theory, with theory being the organising framework for the study influencing research questions/hypotheses, data collection, and analysis [28, 50]. Deductive use of theory is about interrogating data from a theoretical perspective [4], and while it is typically associated with objective quantitative methods, some qualitative methods also employ theory deductively [4, 50, 51].

Demi-regularities: (Chapter 6) A term often associated with realist approaches, demi-regularities can be described as: '... semi-predictable patterns between contexts, underlying generative mechanisms and outcomes, such that these patterns are generalizable' [22 p. 3].

Deontology: (Chapter 3) Ethical theories that place special emphasis on the relationship between duty and the morality of human actions. The term deontology is derived from the Greek deon 'duty' and logos 'science' [18].

Dependability: (Chapters 2, 7 and 8) A marker of quality in qualitative research approaches that relates to the *trustworthiness* of data [17].

Discourse: (Chapter 8) Discourse '... in the most general sense, is the study of language as it is used in society expressed either through conversations or in documents' [47 p. 217].

Dualism: (Chapters 2 and 5) Dualism involves the researcher keeping themselves separate from the study objects or participants in the belief of maintaining value-free neutrality and objectivity [21].

E

Empiricism: (Chapter 5) A theory that knowledge is based (wholly or primarily) on sensory experiences: 'the belief that people should rely on practical experience and experiments, rather than on theories, as a basis for knowledge' [52].

Entities: (Chapter 6) Relevant to realist approaches, entities: 'are things which "make a difference"... [and can be] material (e.g., water), immaterial (e.g., class) or both (e.g., contract) ... entities may also be real in different ways and at different levels' [6 p. 202].

Epistemology: (Chapter 2) This term refers to: 'the relationship between the knower (i.e., the scientist, the inquirer) and the known (i.e., reality, that which is knowable)' [19 p. 688].

Ethics: (Chapter 3) 'As a philosophical discipline of study, ethics is a systematic approach to understanding, analysing, and distinguishing matters of right and wrong, good and bad, and admirable and dishonorable as they relate to the well-being of and the relationships among sentient beings' [53 p. 23].

Experiment: (Chapter 5) An experiment has been defined as: 'research in which variables are systematically manipulated and their effects upon other variables observed' [54, 55 p. 546].

F

Framing: (Chapter 4) An element of quality that establishes the study's *conceptual framework*, problem statement, and research question [51].

G

Generalisability: (Chapters 2 and 5) A marker of quality in scientific approaches, generalisability involves claims about the extent to which study findings can be extrapolated from the study sample to a broader population across contexts and domains [20].

Generative mechanism: (Chapter 6) Aligned with realist approaches, a generative mechanism can be described as: 'a trans-empirical but real existing entity, explaining why observable events occur' [56 p. 60].

Ghost authorship: (Chapter 3) A situation where a significant contributor to an article is not listed as an author [57].

Gift authorship: (Chapter 3) A situation where a person who has made no, or insignificant, contribution to the research or publication is named as an author [30].

Grand theory: (Chapter 2) Grand theory is non-specific and abstract theory that has been described as: 'universal, societal level theories' such as *constructionism* [58 p. 5].

Grey metrics: (Chapter 12) '... a novel indicator of research impact ... Which can contribute to identifying meaningful research impact not currently captured ... [including] non-conventional citations, informal sharing of research findings, informal and formal consults, and communications indicating appreciation or applications related to one's research ... they may be difficult to track due to being informal and unindexed, and yet contribute crucial insights to how one's research is making an impact' [59 p. 956].

H

Human Research Ethics Committees (HRECs): See *Institutional Review Boards (IRBs)*.

I

Impact: (Chapters 4 and 12) An element of quality that discusses interpretations and implications in a way that has potential influence on education practice, policy, and theory [60].

Implementation science: (Chapter 12) This science '... is concerned with the theories, models and methods used in KT [knowledge translation] to inform and improve HPE [health professions education]' [61 p. 1160].

Inductive: (Chapters 2 and 7) An inductive approach sets out to develop theory that is grounded in data [4, 28, 50, 51]. Typically associated with qualitative research, it privileges subjectivity [50, 51].

Information power: (Chapter 7) An alternative to *saturation*, information power is a concept providing evidence that: 'samples are adequate ... in terms of being of sufficient size to allow transferability to other contexts ...' [49 p. 46]. Introduced by Malterud et al., information power considers sample size in qualitative research based on study aims, specificity of sample, theory usage, dialogue quality, and analysis strategy [62].

Institutional Review Boards (IRBs): (Chapter 3) Also known as *Human Research Ethics Committees (HRECs)*, IRBs are groups that are formally designated to review and monitor research involving human participants. They serve an important role in the protection of the rights and welfare of human research participants [63].

Intellectual freedom: (Chapter 3) Intellectual freedom is the right of every individual to both seek and receive information from all points of view without restriction.

Internal coherence: (Chapters 2 and 4) An element of quality that considers how well a study demonstrates alignment of ontology, epistemology, axiology, methodology, and methods [64]. Internal coherence can also refer to the alignment between multiple theories employed within research such as grand, macro and/or micro theories [65].

Interpretivism: (Chapters 2 and 7) Interpretivism '... looks for culturally derived and historically situated interpretations of the social life-world' [66 p. 67].

Intersubjectivity: (Chapter 9) Reality is neither completely objective nor completely subjective; intersubjectivity embraces the co-existence of a single reality (or truth) and individual interpretations of this reality [3].

Iterative: (Chapter 7) A systematic, repetitive, recursive process. In data analysis, this can mean that a section of qualitative data is selected, categorised/conceptualised, and coded/labelled; then another section of data undergoes the same process and so on. Iterative sampling can mean that more data are collected as researchers cycle back and forth between data collection and data evaluation/analysis to ensure sensitivity to data variabilities, enabling adequate addressing of study objectives [67].

J

Journal impact factor (JIF): (Chapter 11) A measure of quality ranking for a journal that considers the average number of citations received per article in the previous two years. To receive an impact factor rating, journals must have been publishing for at least three years [68].

Journal quartile: (Chapter 11) A measure of quality ranking of a journal based on impact factors for their field, which allows journals to be ranked from highest to lowest impact factor by field, with the highest 25% being in the top quartile (Q1) and so on. Sites such as Clarivate and Scimago rank journals by quartile [68, 69].

K

Knowledge brokers: (Chapter 12) Knowledge brokers can be seen as intermediary people or organisations: 'that link researchers with users of research as a means of both exchange and translation' [70 p. 2].

Knowledge exchange: (Chapter 12) Knowledge exchange implies: 'that knowledge moves in a non-linear fashion and can be altered or shaped into different forms as it passes from person to person' [71 p. 24].

Knowledge mobilisation: (Chapter 12) Knowledge mobilisation '... is about building stronger connections between research, policy and practice so that ... education practice can be based on reliable evidence rather than belief, ideology or whim' [72 p. 1].

Knowledge transfer: (Chapter 12) Knowledge transfer '... implies that knowledge is like an object that can be transferred in a linear fashion by simply handing from one person to another' [71 p. 24].

Knowledge translation: (Chapter 12) 'there is broad consensus that KT [knowledge translation] aims to optimise the adoption, appropriate adaptation, delivery, and sustainability of effective practices and policies within defined contexts' [61 p. 1160].

L

Least publishable units (LPUs): (Chapter 3) This is where an output includes: 'just enough contribution to be recognized as such in a single paper – just enough to be reluctantly accepted' [73 p. 281].

Lesson study: (Chapter 9) A study whereby teachers develop, teach, and observe a research lesson and examine its impact on student learning [74].

Lines of action: (Chapter 9) Behaviours or actions taken as part of the enquiry process [3]. Typically, this involves implementing interventions and observing the effects or collecting information through stories that describe perceptions of the world, then sharing the information [75 p. 1049].

M

Macro theory: (Chapter 2) Focusing on local systems and contexts, macro theories consider: 'specific phenomena and involve a small number of concepts relating to a restricted range of contexts', such as *sociomateriality* [58 p. 2].

Meat extending: (Chapter 3) Adding data to existing published research without new conclusions [76].

Mechanisms: (Chapter 6) Relevant to realist approaches, mechanisms can be described as: 'underlying entities, processes, or structures which operate in particular contexts to generate outcomes of interest ... [they are] ... usually hidden ... sensitive to variations in context, and ... generate outcomes' [77 p. 368].

Member checking: (Chapter 7) Member checking '... involves the researcher presenting data transcripts or data interpretations to all or some participants for comment. Such sharing is designed to enhance the credibility of data analysis and participant involvement' [49 p. 46]. This is also referred to as respondent or member validation, informant feedback, or dependability checking [49].

Methodology: (Chapter 2) Methodology can be described as: 'theory of method' [28 p. 2].

Micro theory: (Chapter 2) Focusing on individuals, micro theory considers specific phenomena and it is thought to have the narrowest range of interest such as self-determination theory [58].

Middle-range theory: (Chapters 2 and 6) Often related to realist approaches, middle-range theories can be described as: 'formal theories. They often provide a bridge to a wealth of existing research and knowledge about a topic. They are invariably more abstract than programme theories, which seek to explain how and why different outcomes are generated by a specific programme in different contexts' [23 p. 83].

N

Neocolonialism: (Chapter 8) Neocolonialism describes the (typically economic) control of less-developed countries by developed countries [78].

Non-maleficence: (Chapter 3) Avoiding causing harm [18].

Null hypothesis: (Chapter 3) A hypothesis used in inferential statistics that states that any difference between two observable variables is due to chance alone.

O

Objectivism: (Chapters 2 and 5) Objectivism is '... an epistemological notion asserting that meaning exists in objects independently of any consciousness' [66 p.10].

Ontology: (Chapter 2) Ontology considers: 'the nature of reality ... the nature of being' [19 p. 688].

Oppression: (Chapter 8) Unfair treatment or prejudice or undue use of power [45].

Outcomes: (Chapter 6) In the context of realist approaches, outcomes can be described as: '... the anticipated and unanticipated consequences that are brought about by the interaction of different program mechanisms in different contexts' [79 p. 386].

P

Paradigm: (Chapter 9) There are multiple definitions of paradigm; one of the most commonly used in health professions is a basic set of beliefs about ontology, epistemology, methodology, and axiology that guide a researcher's actions [3, 80].

Participant deceit: (Chapter 3) Deception and withholding information from participants [18].

Plagiarism: (Chapter 3) The use of others' ideas without proper credit (thus claiming them as one's own) [81]. See also *self-plagiarism*.

Pluralism: (Chapter 9) An ontological position that multiple theories and perspectives can be true and co-exist, and that multiple methodologies can contribute to these truths [82]. For example, some suggest that: 'different, even conflicting, theories and perspectives can be useful; observation, experience and experiments are all useful ways to gain an understanding of people and the world' [83 p. 18].

Positioning: (Chapter 4) An element of quality that describes how well research is situated within the existing literature [84].

Positivism: (Chapters 2 and 5) Described as a theoretical perspective [66], positivism underpins research from the natural and social sciences that: 'seeks to discover laws of nature, expressing them through descriptions of theory ... [focusing] on explanation and prediction based on the hypothetico-deductive model' [21 p. 691]. Inherent in positivism is belief in the verification (proof) of *a priori* theory, and belief that it is possible to know objective truth [21].

Postcolonialism: (Chapter 8) Such theories: '... are perhaps best conceptualised as a family of theories sharing a social, political, and moral concern about the history and legacy of colonialism – [and] how it continues to shape people's lives, well-being, and life opportunities ... the study of the previous history, politics or culture of an earlier colony that focuses on the human consequences of the exploitation of colonised people and their lands' [85 p. 19]. In the context of health professions education research this may include acknowledgement that colonial ways of knowing continue to shape individuals' access to healthcare and/or healthcare education.

Post-positivism: (Chapters 2 and 5) Post-positivism developed as a critique of *positivism*, and in particular its reliance on the principle of verification [86]. Rather than believing that hypotheses can be proven, post-positivism embraces the falsification (refuting) of hypotheses. Post-positivism concedes that it is impossible to fully comprehend objective truth due to the fallibility of researchers and research methods [86].

Post-structuralism: (Chapter 8) Post-structuralism focuses on: 'identifying meanings that are context specific and that relate to the varying discursive practices operating' [47 p. 667].

Practical theory: (Chapter 2) Practical theory can be described as a loose nexus of ideas in education that might also be called structured reflection. This may relate to: 'craft knowledge, apprenticeship, and ... learning on the job' [87 p. 83].

Predatory journals: (Chapter 11) Predatory journals '... are entities that prioritize self-interest at the expense of scholarship and are characterized by false or misleading information, deviation from best editorial and publication practices, a lack of transparency, and/or the use of aggressive and indiscriminate solicitation practices' [88 p. 211].

Principlism: (Chapter 3) An approach to biomedical ethics that uses a framework of four universal and basic ethical principles: respect for autonomy, non-maleficence, beneficence, and justice [18].

Privilege: (Chapter 8) Privilege can be described as: 'unequal opportunity between groups in respect of access to power and other resources' [89 p. 1348]. For individuals, privilege can reflect a state of being that is carried with them every day without them necessarily realising it such as male or white privilege.

Programme theory: (Chapters 2 and 6) Central to realist approaches, programme theory is: 'the set of assumptions of programme designers (or other actors involved) that explain how and why they expect the intervention to reach its objective(s) and in which conditions' [23 p. 83], or 'why and how the program brought about the changes observed' [90 p. 3].

R

Realist economic evaluation: (Chapter 6) Integrating realist evaluation with economic analyses within a realist framework [91].

Realist evaluation: (Chapter 6) A theory-driven evaluation that evaluates a programme by unpacking how it works (or fails to work), for whom and under what circumstances, and why [92].

Realist interviews: (Chapter 6) A type of interviewing approach that features the teacher–learner (interviewer–interviewee) cycle in the process of gleaning, testing, and consolidating conjectured theories [92, 93].

Realist synthesis: (Chapter 6) An approach for bringing together evidence focused on explanations for how a programme works (or does not work), in what contexts, and why [94].

Reflexivity: (Chapters 2, 7 and 8) A process through which researchers: 'recognise their beliefs and assumptions, acknowledge their relationship to the research topic and participants, and consider how these influence their study' [95 p. 1257].

Relativism: (Chapter 7) Truth is not a pre-existing construct out there in the world to be discovered but is *subjectivist*, influenced by our culture, backgrounds, and past experiences [96].

Reliability: (Chapters 2 and 5) This relates to the extent to which a measure (e.g., scale) is stable, dependable, and consistent under repeated and identical conditions [97].

Reporting guideline: (Chapter 4) A tool designed to help reviewers and researchers ensure that essential information is included in a manuscript so that others can understand the study, replicate it (if applicable), make informed choices about how to use the study's findings, and include the study in a knowledge synthesis. The EQUATOR Network defines a reporting guideline as: 'a checklist, flow diagram, or structured text to guide authors in reporting a specific type of research, developed using explicit methodology' [98].

Reproducibility: (Chapter 5) Reproducibility involves: 'replicability (i.e., the potential for replication) and replication (i.e., multiple instances of the same study)' [86 p. 696].

Research uptake: (Chapter 12) Research uptake involves the extent to which: 'research users have engaged with research' [99 p. 406].

Research use: (Chapter 12) Research use involves the extent to which: 'research users act upon research, discuss it, pass it on to others, adapt it to context, present findings, use it to inform policy, or practice developments' [99 p. 406].

Retroduction: (Chapter 6) Retroduction can be described as the: 'constant shuttling between theory and empirical data, using both inductive and deductive reasoning' [77 p. 374].

Right to withdraw: (Chapter 3) A concept in research ethics where participants have the right to end their participation whenever they choose and despite providing earlier consent [100].

Rigour: (Chapter 4) An element of quality that describes the extent to which the research aligns with established methodological practices and criteria for credibility [101].

S

Salami slicing: (Chapters 3 and 11) This is: '... where papers cover the same population, methods, and question and stresses that splitting up papers by outcomes is not legitimate' [102 p. 1730].

Saturation: (Chapter 7) There are many different types of saturation, with data saturation: 'used in qualitative research as a criterion for discontinuing data collection and/or analysis' [103 p. 1893]. However, Glaser and Strauss introduced the concept of theoretical saturation as part of grounded theory methodology, based on the belief that: 'researchers could identify the point ... at which new data do not add anything new to a developing concept or theory' [49 p. 45]. See *information power* for an alternative approach to determining data sufficiency in qualitative research.

Self-plagiarism: (Chapter 3) Self-plagiarism involves: 'using your own words in more than one document; typically the source document has been published before, hence the plagiarism (negative) label' [81 p. 26]. See also *plagiarism*.

Sense-making: (Chapter 7) Sense-making is a cultural practice through which we play with concepts, language, values, and personal experiences to understand how our world works, who we are in relation to others and elements of the world, and our personal standpoint therein [104].

Social constructionism: (Chapters 2 and 7) This concept focuses on interactions between individuals and how we socially construct meaning through language and action (typically with no claim to cognitive representations) [34]. See also *constructionism*.

Social constructivism: (Chapters 2 and 7) This concept adopts an: 'anti-realist position and states that the process of knowing is affected by other people and is mediated by community and culture' [36 p. 10], with knowledge preceding cognition. See also *constructivism* for a different perspective.

Sociomateriality: (Chapter 2) Sociomateriality involves: 'a focus on materials as dynamic and enmeshed with human activity in everyday practices' [105 p. 47]. Materials can be spaces, technologies, equipment, and so on.

Structuralism: (Chapter 8) 'Any system [for example, social, economic, gender] is made up of a set of oppositional categories embedded in language' [106 p. 33].

Subjectivism: (Chapter 7) Subjectivist research approaches comprise two key assumptions: knowledge is a *social construction* created by communities through *sense-making* activities, who share interpretations, and to understand such constructed knowledge, researchers unpack those meanings by examining a range of non-numerical data [107].

T

Theoretical framework: (Chapters 2 and 10) Some use the terms theoretical framework and *theory* roughly synonymously [108], for example: 'a theoretical framework is a collection of interrelated concepts, like a theory, but not necessarily so well worked-out' [109 p. 92]. Such a theoretical framework is thought to guide the choice of methodology and methods of the study [51].

Theory: (Chapter 2) Although variously described, theory can be seen as: 'an organized, coherent, and systematic articulation of a set of statements related to significant questions ... that are communicated in a meaningful whole. It is a symbolic depiction of aspects of reality that are discovered or invented for describing, explaining, predicting, or prescribing responses, events, situations, conditions or relationships' [110 p. 37].

Transferability: (Chapters 2, 7 and 8) A marker of quality in qualitative research, transferability refers to how applicable study findings are to other groups or contexts such as different countries, or different training stages [64].

Triangulation: (Chapter 7) A marker of quality in qualitative research, triangulation relates to employing multiple sources of data, multiple methods, and/or multiple researchers to find convergence. See an alternative approach of *crystallisation* [49].

Trustworthiness: (Chapters 2, 6, 7, 8 and 9) A marker of quality in qualitative research, trustworthiness is a broad construct relating to issues like internal coherence, credibility, authenticity, and transferability [111].

U

Utilitarianism: (Chapter 3) An ethical theory determining right from wrong by focusing on outcomes. It holds that the most ethical choice is the one that will produce the greatest good for the greatest number of beneficiaries [112].

V

Validity: (Chapters 2 and 5) Validity can mean different things in different contexts but most often in health professions education research relates to assessment validity, i.e., the extent to which something measures what it is supposed to measure [21].

Virtue ethics: (Chapter 3) Virtue ethics mainly deal with the honesty and morality of a person and have been defined as: 'an account of what is involved in making good moral judgments' [113 p. 2], namely, that: 'virtues and vices play a central role in ethics' [113 p. 1].

W

Warranted assertions: (Chapter 9) The beliefs that guide behaviours or lines of action [3]. Used instead of knowledge or evidence, the term warranted assertions conveys the temporal and contextual nature of the products or outcomes of enquiry – particularly to avoid viewing knowledge as fixed and as evidence of causality. Also described as an understanding or solution that seems to 'work' and, as such, can guide future action [114].

Workability: (Chapter 9) The consequences that are likely to follow from behaviours or lines of action taken as part of the enquiry process [3].

REFERENCES

1. Grant C, Osanloo A. Understanding, selecting, and integrating a theoretical framework in dissertation research: creating the blueprint for your "house". *Administrative Issues Journal.* 2014;4(2):12–25.

2. Chirkov V. *Fundamentals of Research on Culture and Psychology: Theory and Methods.* New York and London: Routledge; 2016.

3. Morgan DL. Paradigms lost and pragmatism regained: methodological implications of combining qualitative and quantitative methods. *J Mixed Meth Res.* 2007;1(1):48–76.

4. Lingard B. Thinking about theory in educational research: fieldwork in philosophy. *Educ Phil Theory.* 2015;47(2):173–191.

5. Pigott TD. The role of theory in quantitative data analysis. In Wyse D, Selwyn N, Smith E, et al., eds. *The BERA/SAGE Handbook of Educational Research.* London: SAGE; 2017: 699–710.

6. Vincent S, O'Mahoney J. Critical realism and qualitative research: an introductory overview. In Cassell C, Cunliffe AL, Grandy G, eds. *The SAGE Handbook of Qualitative Business and Management Research Methods.* London: SAGE; 2018: 201–216.

7. Evans C, Stone A. *Open Minds: Academic Freedom and Freedom of Speech in Australia.* Collingwood: Black Inc; 2021.

8. Argyris C. Actionable knowledge: design causality in the service of consequential theory. *J App Behav Sci.* 1996;32(4):390–406.

9. Kelly LM, Cordeiro M. Three principles of pragmatism for research on organizational processes. *Methodological Innovations.* 2020;13(2):1–10.

10. Bradbury H. Quality and "actionability": what action researchers offer from the tradition of pragmatism. In Shani AB, Mohrman SA, Pasmore W, et al., eds. *Handbook of Collaborative Management Research.* Thousand Oaks, Calif.: SAGE; 2008: 583–600.

11. Maggio LA, Meyer HS, Artino AR. Beyond citation rates: a real-time impact analysis of health professions education research using altmetrics. *Acad Med.* 2017;92(10):1449–1455.

12. Warren HR, Raison N, Dasgupta P. The rise of altmetrics. *JAMA.* 2017;317(2):131–132.

13. Mackey E. A best practice approach to anonymization. In Iphofen R, ed. *Handbook of Research Ethics and Scientific Integrity.* Cham: Springer; 2020: 323–343.

14. Gunn A, Mintrom M. Higher education policy change in Europe: academic research funding and the impact agenda. *European Education.* 2016;48(4):241–257.

15. Abdullah D, Abd Aziz M, Mohd Ibrahim A. A "research" into international student-related research: (re)visualizing our stand? *High Educ.* 2014;67:235–253.

16. Lewis-Beck MS, Bryman AE, Futing Liao T. *The SAGE Encyclopedia of Social Science Research Methods.* Thousand Oaks, Calif.: SAGE; 2004.

17. Liamputtong P. *Qualitative Research Methods*, 5th ed. Melbourne: Oxford University Press; 2019.

18. Beauchamp TL, Childress JF. *Principles of Biomedical Ethics*, 5th ed. New York: Oxford University Press; 2001.

19. Varpio L, MacLeod A. Philosophy of Sciences Series: harnessing the multidisciplinary edge effect by exploring paradigms, ontologies, epistemologies, axiologies, and methodologies. *Acad Med.* 2020;95(5):686–689.

20. Varpio L, O'Brien B, Rees CE, et al. The applicability of generalisability and bias to health professions' education research. *Med Educ.* 2020;55(2):167–173.

21. Park YS, Konge L, Artino Jr AR. The positivism paradigm of research. *Acad Med.* 2020;95(5):690–694.

22. Greenhalgh J, Manzano A. Understanding 'context' in realist evaluation and synthesis. *Int J Social Res Method.* 2022;25(5):583–595.

23. Marchal B, Kegels G, Van Belle S. Theory and realist methods. In Emmel N, Greenhalgh J, Manzano A, et al, eds. *Doing Realist Research.* London: SAGE; 2018: 79–89.

24. World Health Organisation. *Code of Conduct for Responsible Research.* Geneva: World Health Organisation; 2017.

25. Sutrop M, Parder M-L, Juurik M. Research ethics codes and guidelines. In Iphofen R, ed. *Handbook of Research Ethics and Scientific Integrity.* Cham: Springer; 2020: 67–89.

26. Banks S, Herrington T, Carter K. Pathways to co-impact: action research and community organising. *Educ Action Res.* 2017;25(4):541–559.

27. Crawford LM. Conceptual and theoretical frameworks in research. In Burkholder GJ, Cox KA, Crawford LM, et al., eds. *Research Design and Methods: An Applied Guide for the Scholar-Practitioner.* Thousand Oaks, Calif.: SAGE; 2020: 35–48.

28. Collins CS, Stockton CM. The central role of theory in qualitative research. *Int J Qual Meth.* 2018;17:1–10.

29. Chugh D, Bazerman MH, Banaji MR. Bounded ethicality as a psychological barrier to recognizing conflicts of interest. In Moore DA, Cain DM, Loewenstein G, et al., eds. *Conflicts of Interest: Challenges and Solutions in Business, Law, Medicine, and Public Policy.* Cambridge: Cambridge University Press; 2005: 74–95.

30. Committee on Publication Ethics (COPE). https://publicationethics.org (accessed 3 December 2022).

31. Waldmann E. Teaching ethics in accounting: a discussion of cross-cultural factors with a focus on Confucian and Western philosophy. *Account Educ.* 2000;9(1):23–35.

32. Iphofen R. Ethical Issues in research methods: introduction. In Iphofen R, ed. *Handbook of Research Ethics and Scientific Integrity.* Cham: Springer; 2020: 371–379.

33. Porter S, O'Halloran P. The use and limitation of realistic evaluation as a tool for evidence-based practice: a critical realist perspective. *Nurs Inq.* 2011;19(1):18–28.

34. Rees CE, Crampton PES, Monrouxe LV. Re-visioning academic medicine through a constructionist lens. *Acad Med.* 2020;95(6):846–850.

35. Burr V. *Social Constructionism.* 3rd ed. London and New York: Routledge; 2015.

36. Amineh RJ, Asl HD. Review of constructivism and social constructivism. *Journal of Social Sciences, Literature and Languages.* 2015;1:9–16.

37. Charmaz K. *Constructing Grounded Theory*, 2nd ed. Thousand Oaks, Calif.: SAGE; 2014.

38. Mckenzie A, Hanley B. *Planning for Consumer and Community Participation in Health and Medical Research: A Practical Guide for Health and Medical Researchers*. Perth: University of Western Australia–Telethon Kids Institute; 2014.

39. Patton MQ. *Qualitative Research and Evaluation Methods: Integrating Theory and Practice*. Thousand Oaks, Calif.: SAGE; 2014.

40. Buccheri RK, Sharifi C. Critical appraisal tools and reporting guidelines for evidence-based practice. *Worldviews Evid Based Nurs*. 2017;14(6):463–472.

41. Critical Appraisal Skills Programme (CASP). Critical skills appraisal programme. https://casp-uk.net/glossary/critical-appraisal (accessed 1 September 2022).

42. Halman M, Baker L, Ng S. Using critical consciousness to inform health professions education. *Perspect Med Educ*. 2017;6(1):12–20.

43. McCartan J, Brimblecombe J, Adams K. Methodological tensions for non-Indigenous people in Indigenous research: a critique of critical discourse analysis in the Australian context. *Soc Sci Hum Open*. 2022;6(1):100282.

44. Charmaz K. The power of constructivist grounded theory for critical inquiry. *Qual Inq*. 2017;23(1):34–45.

45. McLaren P, Kincheloe JL. *Critical Pedagogy: Where are We Now?* New York: Peter Lang; 2007.

46. Cabrera NL. Where is the racial theory in critical race theory? A constructive criticism of the crits. *Rev High Educ*. 2018;42(1):209–233.

47. Given LM. *The SAGE Encyclopedia of Qualitative Research Methods*. London: SAGE; 2008.

48. Paradis E, Nimmon L, Wondimagegn D, et al. Critical theory: broadening our thinking to explore the structural factors at play in health professions education. *Acad Med*. 2020;95(6):842–845.

49. Varpio L, Ajjawi R, Monrouxe LV, et al. Shedding the cobra effect: problematising thematic emergence, triangulation, saturation and member checking. *Med Educ*. 2017;51(1):40–50.

50. Creswell JW. *Research Design: Qualitative, Quantitative, and Mixed Methods Approaches*, 3rd ed. Thousand Oaks, Calif.: SAGE; 2009.

51. Varpio L, Paradis E, Uijtdehaage S, et al. The distinctions between theory, theoretical framework, and conceptual framework. *Acad Med*. 2020;95(7):989–994.

52. Collins English Dictionary. Empiricism. 2022; https://www.collinsdictionary.com/dictionary/english/empiricism (accessed 3 Dec 2022).

53. Butts JB, Rich KL. *Nursing Ethics: Across the Curriculum and into Practice*, 5th ed. Burlington, Mass.: Jones & Bartlett Learning; 2020.

54. Campbell DT, Stanley JC. *Experimental and Quasi-Experimental Designs for Research*. Chicago: Rand McNally; 1963.

55. Cook DA, Beckman TJ. Reflections on experimental research in medical education. *Adv Health Sci Educ*. 2010;15(3):455–464.

56. Blom B, Morén S. Analysis of generative mechanisms. *J Crit Realism*. 2011;10(1):60–79.

57. Pruschak G, Hopp C. And the credit goes to … ghost and honorary authorship among social scientists. *PLoS ONE*. 2022;17(5):e0267312.

58. Reeves S, Albert M, Kuper A, et al. Why use theories in qualitative research? *BMJ*. 2008;337(7670):a949.

59. Friesen F, Baker LR, Ziegler C, et al. Approaching impact meaningfully in medical education research. *Acad Med*. 2019;94(7):955–961.

60. Fleming JI, Wilson SE, Hart SA, et al. Open accessibility in education research: enhancing the credibility, equity, impact, and efficiency of research. *Educ Psychol.* 2021;56(2):110–121.

61. Thomas A, Bussières A. Leveraging knowledge translation and implementation science in the pursuit of evidence informed health professions education. *Adv Health Sci Educ.* 2021;26(3):1157–1171.

62. Malterud K, Siersma VD, Guassora AD. Sample size in qualitative interview studies: guided by information power. *Qual Health Res.* 2016;26(13):1753–1760.

63. US Food and Drug Administration (FDA). Institutional Review Boards (IRBs) and protection of human subjects in clinical trials. 2019. https://www.fda.gov/about-fda/center-drug-evaluation-and-research-cder/institutional-review-boards-irbs-and-protection-human-subjects-clinical-trials#:~:text=Under%20FDA%20regulations%2C%20an%20Institutional,approval%2C%20or%20disapprove%20research (accessed 9 September 2022).

64. Palermo C, Reidlinger DP, Rees CE. Internal coherence matters: lessons for nutrition and dietetics research. *Nutr Diet.* 2021;78(3):252–267.

65. Carter SM, Little M. Justifying knowledge, justifying method, taking action: epistemologies, methodologies, and methods in qualitative research. *Qual Health Res.* 2007;17(10):1316–1328.

66. Crotty M. *The Foundations of Social Research. Meaning and Perspective in the Research Process.* London: SAGE; 2003.

67. Mills AJ, Durepos G, Wiebe E. *Encyclopedia of Case Study Research.* Thousand Oaks, Calif.: SAGE; 2010.

68. Clarivate. Journal citation reports. 2022. http://www.thomsonreuters.com/products_services/science/science_products/a-z/journal_citation_reports (accessed 18 November 2022).

69. SCImago. SCImago journal & country rank. 2022. http://www.scimagojr.com (accessed 15 November 2022).

70. Reed RL, McIntyre E, Jackson-Bowers E, et al. Pathways to research impact in primary healthcare: what do Australian primary healthcare researchers believe works best to facilitate the use of their research findings? *Health Res Policy Syst.* 2017;15(1):1–8.

71. Read R, Cooper A, Edelstein H, et al. Knowledge mobilisation and utilisation. In Levin B, Qi J, Edelstein H, et al., eds. *The Impact of Research in Education: An International Perspective.* Bristol: Bristol University Press; 2013: 23–39.

72. Qi J, Levin B. Introduction and overview. In Levin B, Qi J, Edelstein H, et al., eds. *The Impact of Research in Education: An International Perspective.* Bristol: Bristol University Press; 2013: 1–21.

73. Trimble SW, Grody WW, McKelvey B, et al. The glut of academic publishing: a call for a new culture. *Acad Quest.* 2010;23(3):276–286.

74. Lewis CC, Hurd J. *Lesson Study Step by Step: How Teacher Learning Communities Improve Instruction.* Portsmouth: Heinemann; 2011.

75. Morgan D. Pragmatism as a paradigm for social research. *Qual Inq.* 2014;20:1045–1053.

76. Huth EJ. Guidelines on authorship of medical papers. *Ann Intern Med.* 1986;104(2): 269–274.

77. Astbury B, Leeuw FL. Unpacking black boxes: mechanisms and theory building in evaluation. *Am J Eval.* 2010;31(3):363–381.

78. Tuhiwai Smith L. *Decolonizing Methodologies: Research and Indigenous Peoples.* 3rd ed. London: Bloomsbury Publishing; 2021.

79. Astbury B. Some reflections on Pawson's Science of Evaluation: A Realist Manifesto. *Evaluation*. 2013;19(4):383–401.

80. Denzin NK, Lincoln YS. *The SAGE Handbook of Qualitative Research*, 3rd ed. Thousand Oaks, Calif.: SAGE; 2005.

81. Stewart Jr. CN. *Research Ethics for Scientists: A Companion for Students*. Hoboken, NJ: John Wiley & Sons, Inc; 2011.

82. Johnson B, Gray R. A history of philosophical and theoretical issues for mixed methods research. In Tashakkori A, Teddlie C, eds. *SAGE Handbook of Mixed Methods in Social & Behavioral Research*. 2nd ed. Thousand Oaks, Calif.: SAGE; 2010: 69–94.

83. Johnson RB, Onwuegbuzie AJ. Mixed methods research: a research paradigm whose time has come. *Educ Researcher*. 2004;33(7):14–26.

84. Meyer HS, Durning SJ, Sklar DP, et al. Making the first cut: an analysis of Academic Medicine editors' reasons for not sending manuscripts out for external peer review. *Acad Med*. 2018;93(3):464–470.

85. Browne AJ, Smye VL, Varcoe C. The relevance of postcolonial theoretical perspectives to research in Aboriginal health. *Can J Nurs Res*. 2005;37(4):16–37.

86. Young ME, Ryan A. Postpositivism in health professions education scholarship. *Acad Med*. 2020;95(5):695–699.

87. Thomas G. What's the use of theory? *Harvard Educ Rev*. 1997;67(1):75–104.

88. Grudniewicz A, Moher D, Cobey KD, et al. Predatory journals: no definition, no defence. *Nature*. 2019;576(7786):210–212.

89. Cleland J, Razack S. When I say ... privilege. *Med Educ*. 2021;55(12):1347–1349.

90. Shearn K, Allmark P, Piercy H, et al. Building realist program theory for large complex and messy interventions. *Int J Qual Meth*. 2017;16(1):1–11.

91. Brown S, Dalkin SM, Bate A, et al. Exploring and understanding the scope and value of the Parkinson's nurse in the UK (The USP Project): a realist economic evaluation protocol. *BMJ Open*. 2020;10(10):e037224.

92. Pawson R, Tilley N. *Realistic Evaluation*. London: SAGE; 1997.

93. Manzano A. The craft of interviewing in realist evaluation. *Evaluation*. 2016;22(3):342–360.

94. Rycroft-Malone J, McCormack B, Hutchinson AM, et al. Realist synthesis: illustrating the method for implementation research. *Implementation Sci*. 2012;7:33.

95. Ramani S, Konings KD, Mann K, et al. A guide to reflexivity for qualitative researchers in education. *Acad Med*. 2018;93(8):1257.

96. Berger PL, Luckmann T. *The Social Construction of Reality: A Treatise in the Sociology of Knowledge*. New York: Anchor Books; 1966.

97. Portney LG, Watkins M. *Foundations of Clinical Research: Applications to Evidence-Based Practice*. 4th ed. Philadelphia, Pa.: FA Davis; 2020.

98. The EQUATOR Network. Enhancing the QUAlity and transparency of health research (EQUATOR) network resource center: reporting guidelines for main study types. https://www.equator-network.org (accessed 6 September 2022).

99. Morton BM. Barriers to academic achievement for foster youth: the story behind the statistics. *J Res Child Educ*. 2015;29(4):476–491.

100. Edwards SJL. Research participation and the right to withdraw. *Bioethics*. 2005;19(2):112–130.

101. Gill TG, Gill TR. What is research rigor? Lessons for a transdiscipline. *Inf Sci: The Int J Emerg Transdiscipline*. 2020;23:47–76.

102. Frandsen TF, Eriksen MB, Mortan D, et al. Fragmented publishing: a large-scale study of health science. *Scientometrics.* 2019;119(3):1729–1743.

103. Saunders B, Sim J, Kingstone T, et al. Saturation in qualitative research: exploring its conceptualization and operationalization. *Qual Quant.* 2018;52(4):1893–1907.

104. Schwarz CV, Braaten M, Haverly C, et al. Using sense-making moments to understand how elementary teachers' interactions expand, maintain, or shut down sense-making in science. *Cognition Instruct.* 2021;39(2):113–148.

105. Fenwick T. Sociomateriality in medical practice and learning: attuning to what matters. *Med Educ.* 2014;48(1):44–52.

106. Denzin NK, Lincoln YS. *Collecting and Interpreting Qualitative Materials.* 4th ed. Thousand Oaks, Calif.: SAGE; 2013.

107. Ismaeel M. Philosophical paradigms underlying discourse analysis: methodological implications. In Crossman J, Bordia S, eds. *Handbook of Qualitative Research Methodologies in Workplace Contexts.* Cheltenham: Edward Elgar; 2021: 47–66.

108. Kitchel T, Ball AL. Quantitative theoretical and conceptual framework use in agricultural education research. *J Ag Educ.* 2014;55(1):186–199.

109. Egbert J, Sanden S. Theoretical frameworks: you can't have a how without a why. In Egbert J, Sanden S, eds. *Foundations of Education Research: Understanding Theoretical Components.* 2nd ed. New York and London: Routledge; 2014: 57–72.

110. Meleis AI. *Theoretical Nursing: Development & Progress*, 4th ed. Philadelphia: Lippincott Williams & Wilkins; 2007.

111. Guba E, Lincoln YS. Paradigmatic controversies, contradictions, and emerging confluences. In Denzin NK, Lincoln YS, eds. *The SAGE Handbook of Qualitative Research.* 2nd ed. Thousand Oaks, Calif.: SAGE; 2000: 191–215.

112. Freakley M, Burgh G. *Engaging with Ethics: Ethical Inquiry for Teachers.* Katoomba: Social Science Press; 2000.

113. Van Zyl LL. *Virtue Ethics: A Contemporary Introduction.* New York and London: Routledge; 2019.

114. Hothersall SJ. Epistemology and social work: enhancing the integration of theory, practice and research through philosophical pragmatism. *Eur J Soc Work.* 2019;22(5):860–870.

Index

Note: Page numbers followed by "*f*" refer to figures and "*b*" refer to boxes.
